MENTAL HEALTH RESEARCH
IN ASIA AND THE PACIFIC

Mental Health Research in Asia and the Pacific

EDITED BY
WILLIAM CAUDILL
AND
TSUNG-YI LIN

HONOLULU
EAST-WEST CENTER PRESS

RA
790
A1
C653
1966

The publication of this volume was made possible through grant MH 11900 from the National Institute of Mental Health. The copyright does not apply to Chapters 8 and 29 and to parts of Chapter 9, which were contributed by employees of the United States government.

Contents

EFFECTS OF SOCIAL STRUCTURE AND CULTURE ON HUMAN
BEHAVIOR

Perspectives on Psychological Processes

Introduction

THIS VOLUME contains the papers originally prepared for the Conference on Mental Health Research in Asia and the Pacific held at the East-West Center in Honolulu, March 28–April 1, 1966. We wish here to give something of the background of the conference, discuss the conference itself, and look briefly to the future.

Early in 1964 Dr. Edward W. Weidner, then Vice-Chancellor of the East-West Center, and Dr. Thomas Maretzki, Chairman of the Department of Anthropology at the University of Hawaii, approached the writers concerning the development of a program in the area of the relation between culture and personality to be carried out at the Institute of Advanced Projects of the East-West Center. After an initial exchange of views, the area of study of the program was expanded to include the whole field of mental health. The plan was to invite a small number of scholars from several Asian countries and the United States to be senior specialists in residence for varying periods up to one year during 1965–66 at the Institute of Advanced Projects. The nine scholars who were senior specialists during that year are among the contributors to this volume. They were Dr. Chen-chin Hsu, Dr. Robert I. Levy, Dr. Thomas Maretzki, Dr. Phon Sangsingkeo, Dr. Lee Sechrest, Dr. Alan Stoller, Dr. Shogo Terashima, Dr. Pow Meng Yap, and Dr. S. M. Hafeez Zaidi. In addition, Dr. Yuji Sasaki, also a contributor to this volume, was a postdoctoral fellow at the Institute of Advanced Projects during 1965–66.

In the fall of 1964 it was decided to plan for a one-week conference at the East-West Center on the topic of mental health research in Asia and the Pacific Islands, using the nine senior specialists in residence as the nucleus of the participants in the conference. The writers were asked to be codirectors of the conference and to work with Dr. Maretzki and Dr. George H. Gadbois, Jr., then Associate Director of the Institute of Advanced Projects, in the selection of additional scholars to be invited to the conference as participants and observers.

Our aim was to have a small working conference of about 30 persons equally divided among Asians and Westerners. This design, in itself, made it impossible to have all countries in Asia represented, but we tried to cover as wide a range as we could. Unfortunately, it was not possible for some of those invited to accept because of pressing commitments. We were also sorry to lose the contribution of Dr. Joo Yong Soh of Korea who planned to attend but was unable to do so because of illness. Nevertheless, as can be seen from the institutional affiliations of the authors, Asian scholars were able to attend from the Philippines, Japan, Republic of China (Taiwan), Ceylon, Thailand, Australia, India, Pakistan, and Hong Kong; Western scholars came from the United States, Canada, and Scotland. Roughly half of the participants were Asians and the other half Westerners, as we had hoped.

Our plans called for a focus on research rather than on such topics as treatment or the training of personnel in this first conference. We thought of this first conference as a general stocktaking concerned with methods and findings of research. We hoped thus to provide an opportunity for scholars to exchange views on the best approaches to future research through international collaboration. We did not specify topics or areas to be covered by the scholars in their papers. Instead, we asked each scholar to write what he wanted, suggesting only that he place an emphasis on research which he had carried out in recent years. Happily, almost all the papers were received sufficiently in advance of the conference to permit their prior distribution to participants. The papers were *not* to be read at the conference. Instead, the author was instructed to make a brief, informal summary of his paper and then to open discussion on the paper.

In addition to participants who were specialists on various topics, we invited four "generalists" to listen to and discuss the presentations during the first four days of the conference; then on the fifth day each generalist was assigned the task of summarizing his impressions of the papers and of the discussion from his own particular point of view. As can be seen in the concluding section of this volume, Dr. Wittkower was asked to summarize his thoughts in terms of previous research done in the area of cultural psychiatry in Asia. Dr. Leighton was asked to direct his attention to problems of method and the identification of psychiatric disorders in different cultures. Dr. Wynne was asked to consider the study of the family as a strategic focus for cross-cultural research. Lastly, Dr. Lindemann was asked to focus his remarks around his research on the movement of populations and to make suggestions for future research on problems of social change.

Besides the participants in the conference who prepared papers, we also invited a number of observers who contributed substantially to the discussion. These observers were: Dr. Ari Kiev, of the Department of Psychiatry at Columbia University; Mrs. Margarethe Dalton, of the Asia Foundation; Dr. Joseph C. Finney, of the Department of Psychiatry at the University of Kentucky; and Dr. Richard H. Williams, of the National Institute of Mental Health. We are very appreciative of the contributions made by these observers.

The East-West Center proved to be an ideal place to hold a small working conference. Because it is located in Hawaii, it was a good meeting ground for Asians and Westerners. The facilities provided by the Center were excellent, and the weather was delightful.

In the actual work of the conference, two chairmen—one a Westerner and the other an Asian—shared the burden of monitoring the discussion each day. These cochairmen worked well together, and we are grateful to them for their major role in helping the conference run smoothly. The five pairs of chairmen were: Dr. Erich Lindemann and Dr. Pow Meng Yap, Dr. N. C. Surya and Dr. Lyman Wynne, Dr. Phon Sangsingkeo and Dr. Eric D. Wittkower, Father Jaime Bulatao and Dr. Alexander Leighton, and, on the final day, Dr. Masaaki Kato and Dr. Alan Stoller.

The presentation of the papers at the conference was predominantly by geographical area, except the paper of the keynote speaker on the first day and the papers on the afternoon of the fourth day which were concerned with nosology and research strategy. We felt that the grouping together of papers concerning a particular country would result in discussion giving a cumulative impression of the research on mental health going on in that country. With this idea in mind, we started with the western part of Asia and moved eastward. We began with India, Pakistan, and Ceylon; we then shifted to Burma, Thailand, the Philippines, and Taiwan; turning northward, we discussed papers dealing with mainland China, Okinawa, Korea, and Japan; and, finally, moved westward to the Society Islands and Hawaii.

The discussion among the participants over the five days was very lively, stimulating, and informative, partly because the organization and planning of the conference made it unnecessary to have the papers verbally presented in their entirety. We think other reasons also contributed to the success of the conference. Of primary importance was the small size of the conference. Secondly, as seldom happens in such a conference, the participants were equally divided between Asians and Westerners. Thirdly, and more importantly, by 1966 all of the Asian scholars had at least made an effort to grapple with real research problems (this would not have been true ten years earlier) and hence had pertinent questions of method, analysis, and theory to discuss with their Western counterparts. Finally, the Asian scholars succeeded in speaking meaningfully (if not always fluently) in English, a necessary factor since their Western colleagues, in large part, were unable to speak Asian languages. Thus it was possible for a real dialogue between East and West to take place during the five days of the conference. The gist of the discussion at the conference has been incorporated into the revised versions of the papers published here. This volume presents the findings of the conference, but it cannot convey, in itself, the stimulation of the discussion during the work of the conference.

We have given some thought to the broad issues that seemed to be involved in the dialogue between East and West which took place during the conference. Mental health research draws its theories and techniques mainly from modern psychiatry and social science, both alien to most cultures in Asia. How these new approaches have been accepted, or reacted to, in their actual application is a matter of great interest. How these new approaches have been used in research to further the understanding of the behavioral patterns of people as individuals, in small groups, or in nations in different cultural settings is of equally great interest for theoretical and practical purposes. These two major interests were in mind during the planning of the present conference.

Though we believe in the necessity and merits of a distinct approach for each culture in developing its own mental health program in order that specific needs and resources of local communities can be taken into consideration, special benefits also derive from an international cross-cultural forum. It is through such means that some agreement can be reached with regard to common denominators in human behavior regardless of biological, social, or cultural differences in various national populations; an expansion of horizons also takes place on such occasions through the opportunity to compare one's own familiar approach with the approaches of others using unfamiliar techniques based on different viewpoints. Another obvious benefit deriving from an international forum is the facilitation of communication among workers in the field. There is considerable diversity in the conception of mental health problems in various countries both in the West and the East, and the need for overcoming emotional and cognitive as well as geographic and historical obstacles to communication is great.

Two important considerations, as already indicated, entered into the drawing up of the list of participants for this conference. One consideration had to do with the balance between psychiatrists and social scientists and the other had to do with the balance between Asians and Westerners.

These considerations were met with apparent success, but it should be pointed out that the majority of the Asians invited were psychiatrists and that the majority of the Westerners were social scientists in various disciplines. Moreover, the Western psychiatrists who were invited were doubly trained in psychiatry and in the social sciences. In Asia, however, it is mainly the psychiatrists who are confronted with, and given the task of understanding, human behavior in their daily professional activities; only recently have Asian social scientists started to take an active interest in matters pertaining to mental health. In general, the papers in this volume are focused on specific topics, and coverage of major areas of interest in mental health is uneven. This result is not surprising in view of the latitude permitted the participants in choosing the topics for their papers and in view of the broad purpose of the conference, which was to initiate communication on problems of research in the field of mental health. Yet, as the conference progressed, it became clear that, thanks to the participants' grasp of their subjects and understanding of their cultures, a general picture regarding the trends and range of mental health research in Asia took shape.

We will resist the temptation to include our own comments on particular papers, for this might result in an unfair highlighting of certain papers and a consequent shading of others. In any case, the job of the generalists participating in the conference was to comment on the totality of the papers and the discussion, and they have done their job well in the final section of this volume.

After the conference was over, the participants went home and revised their papers in light of comments made during the discussion. As can be seen in the table of contents of this volume, the chapters are arranged topically although at the conference the papers were discussed predominantly by geographical area. We believe that the topical arrangement which we have adopted here is better suited to the needs of the reader.

The titles of the papers give an indication of their contents within the major divisions of the book, which are addressed, first, to issues in the identification and study of mental illness, and, second, to effects of social structure and culture on human behavior. The four concluding chapters are by the generalists who listened and participated during the first four days and, on the last day, gave constructive criticism on the content of the conference and suggested future directions for training and research.

We believe that this conference represents the first time that a group of Asian psychiatrists and social scientists from a wide range of countries sat down with their Western counterparts to discuss the problems and results of *research* on mental health in Asia and the Pacific islands. Such being the case, this conference should be seen in the perspective of previous and, to a degree, related conferences. If we look back over approximately 15 years, five conferences stand out as helping to lead to the development of mental health research in Asia and the Pacific. The first of these conferences, The Western Pacific Seminar on Mental Health in Childhood, which was sponsored by the World Health Organization, was held in 1953 in Sydney, Australia. The purpose of this seminar was to examine the early development of personality and to consider how knowledge of this subject could be applied to problems concerning the health and education of children. No report was published from this conference, and the main conclusion seemed to be the need for further research. The World Health Organization and the Philippine Family Workshop jointly sponsored a second conference in 1958 in Banguro in the Philippines entitled The First Asian Seminar on Mental Health and Family Life. To some extent, this conference continued the discussion begun in the earlier conference in Sydney, but the discussion was broadened from a focus on childhood to a general concern with family life. Again, there was a wish for additional research and information. Thirdly, the World Health Organization sponsored a seminar held in Manila in 1962 which focused on the epidemiology of mental disorder. The main topic at this conference was how to interest governments and psychiatrists in Asian countries in obtaining factual information about the distribution of mental illness in the populations to serve as a basis for estimating and meeting the need for psychiatric services in each country. Fourthly, the Japanese Society of Psychiatry and Neurology and the American Psychiatric Association held a joint meeting in Tokyo in 1963. This conference was less broad in its geographic coverage but more intensively concerned with research and scientific communication than were the earlier conferences. Finally, there was the annual meeting in 1965 of the World Federation for Mental Health in Bangkok. The theme of this conference was education and mental health, and it emphasized the problems of training mental health workers to meet the psychiatric needs of a changing Asia. These five conferences show a gradually increasing emphasis over the years on problems of research and training. They provided, therefore, a background for our conference, and the experience gained from them helped to make our conference a success. At our conference enough research material was presented to enable us, in a limited and preliminary way, to evaluate methods and results in several countries in Asia.

As for the future, we are happy to report that through the National Institute of Mental Health in collaboration with the East-West Center and the Social Science Research Institute of the University of Hawaii funds have been provided for a five-year program similar to the one which led to the conference reported in this volume. During each year a small group of senior specialists from Asia and the United States will be in residence at the Institute of Advanced Projects at the East-West Center, and there also will be an opportunity to hold several more working conferences of the sort reported here. As a natural development, the subsequent conferences, however, will be more sharply focused. The themes to be emphasized during the first few years of the five-year program include methods in research, problems in the training of personnel for mental health work, and questions of child development.

For the present, the reader can judge the findings of the first conference by the papers presented here. We believe that this volume will be of general professional interest and also will serve a useful purpose in the teaching of mental health research in medical schools and in departments devoted to the several social sciences in universities in Asia and the United States.

William Caudill
Tsung-yi Lin

Bethesda, Maryland
Geneva, Switzerland
March 6, 1968

ISSUES IN THE IDENTIFICATION
AND STUDY OF MENTAL ILLNESS

1. Parameters of Mental Illness and Mental Health:
    A Public Health Approach

ALAN STOLLER, M.R.C.S., F.A.N.Z.C.P., D.P.M.
Mental Health Research Institute
Victoria, Australia

ANY ATTEMPT to measure psychiatric morbidity requires consideration of the ubiquitous character of this phenomenon. Patients with recognized psychiatric disorders, which fit standard nomenclatures, appear at established psychiatric hospitals and clinics; in addition, a large number of persons come to general medical services with hypochondriasis, masked depressions, and psychosomatic and somatopsychic disorders, without any recording of psychiatric disability. Extending into the field of psychosocial problems, one becomes aware of the role of psychiatric morbidity in producing many marital upsets, desertions, and divorces as well as delinquency, crime, suicide and homicide, industrial absenteeism, school and university failures, road accidents, and so on. To look at mental ill-health as a whole or to compare its existence in one country with that in another implies not only that all established psychiatric cases are being recorded and related properly to accurate population statistics but that adequate factual data are being obtained concerning psychosocial problems. We are a long way from such achievements.

It is possible, however, to make useful comparisons between mental hospital statistics of areas with well-developed psychiatric services, for instance, Victoria, Australia; Ontario, Canada; New Zealand; and the United States (Stoller and Krupinski, 1964). Extending such comparisons to total psychiatric morbidity, though, requires a continuing public health effort linked with data sampling through various community and governmental agencies, such as the program in the state of Victoria, which will be described later. It is essential to sample subcommunities in order to build up a picture of the prevalence of psychiatric morbidity in the community as a whole; physical and social as well as psychological characteristics must be evaluated. The Heyfield study, in Victoria, is an example of this type of approach (Krupinski, Stoller, Baikie, O'Day, Polke, and Graves, in press). It is pertinent to note that 53 per cent of the persons in this rural town suffered from some physical disorder, of whom 12.2 per cent had some concurrent psychiatric disability; that 18.6 per cent had a psychiatric disorder, including the aforementioned 12.2 per cent with physical disabilities also; and that only 40.6 per cent could be considered free of any symptom of ill-health. The finding that 18.6 per cent of the townspeople suffered from some psychiatric disorder parallels the findings of general practitioners (Shepherd and Cooper, 1964; Primrose, 1962) and is well below the 30 per cent recorded in the mid-Manhattan study (Srole *et al.*, 1962).

The public health approach has been referred to as a "coarse-grained" approach compared with the "fine-grained" approach by which data are refined for cross-cultural comparisons, especially in regard to the definition of a case. The methodological problems involved in either type of study are enormous. Mishler and Scotch (1965) discussed the difficulties of comparing one of the most characteristic syndromes in psychiatry—schizophrenia—in regard to operative sociocultural factors. In the large number of epidemiological studies they examined, they "attempted to set up criteria for adequacy and relevance . . ." but "found relatively few that met these criteria." Lemkau and Crocetti (1958) laid down the following three essentials for establishing the true incidence of a disease:

> First, the identification of the entity in question should be highly reliable and objective for the investigators, e.g., susceptible of replication. Second, all cases should be known, or the ratio between known or unknown cases clearly established. Third, the population from which the cases are drawn should be clearly defined and carefully enumerated.

These criteria constitute sound public health methodology; ideally, the progressive build-up of as total a picture as possible is desirable. Nevertheless, even with an incomplete recording of incidence and prevalence, patterns emerge which are useful for planning of services and which also indicate social forces operating to produce and maintain disability. The use of large numbers of cases overcomes, to a degree, such problems as diagnosis. In studies of small populations, however, it is essential to agree on a precise definition of a disease, e.g., schizophrenia, though there is the danger that an agreed upon definition may, as Mishler and Scotch (1965) put it, "destroy the phenomenon altogether."

The classical public health approach appears to be as eminently suitable for the study of psychiatric diseases as it has been for physical disorders. This approach has the advantage of being adaptable to the stage of development of psychiatry and to progressive improvements in clinical understanding in a particular country. It is on the basis of *degree of development* that useful comparisons can be made between psychiatric disease in one country and in another. There is every reason to supplement the central collection of data with regular community sampling of determined "groups at risk" and also to undertake, as already mentioned in regard to the Heyfield study, regular total health surveys of sample communities. Lin (1953; personal communication, 1966) has shown the value of this type of incidence and prevalence survey so far as obvious psychiatric disability is concerned and has determined that death rates of schizophrenic cohorts are needed to supplement institutional figures. From the large-scale collection of data, special groups at risk also can be determined for intensive clinical study (Schaechter, 1965). Moreover, it is possible to test clinical hunches through the examination of central records (Stoller *et al.*, 1965) and, in rare instances, to arrive at specific clues to etiology (Stoller and Collmann, 1965b).

The basic philosophy behind the public health approach is bound up with the definition of mental health, which should bear a clear relation to concepts of physical health. The so-called mental health of a community represents the degree of mental health which is possessed by the individuals who make up the community. In essence, a mentally healthy person is one who can come to terms with himself and with others reasonably well and who can exercise his creative potential to a satisfactory degree. Indefinable in absolute quantitative terms, mental health is, as stated by Stoller (1965), an:

> optimal state for each individual, dependent on a number of
> variables, including such factors as age, sex, economic status,
> social setting and cultural surroundings. . . . Mental illness,
> conversely, implies a deviance in behavior, which is foreign
> to that expected of a person of a certain age, a certain
> sex, in a certain social setting and with a particular cultural
> background.

Mental illness can be recognized in any society (Ross, 1965) as persisting behavior which is unnecessary or inappropriate in regard to environmental changes; which is ego-alien, felt beyond the person's control, and possibly forced upon him by external agencies; which is repetitive, with needs for satisfaction unmet; which expresses incompatible strivings; which contributes to discomfort by a reduction of efficiency, contentment, or relations with others; and which is disproportionately intense in reaction to an evoking stimulus. Such a picture demonstrates emotional maladjustment, even if hospital treatment is not indicated. As Ross put it: "Whether his social group condones or condemns is quite beside the point. The Shaman who has delusions when he wishes not to have them and fulfils the foregoing criteria is psychotic, irrespective of his cultural setting." How society reacts to the illness, however, has significance for the provision of health services and for public health planning in general.

It was a reasonable aim of the public health approach initially to locate and treat cases of rickets. Recognition of the special socioeconomic characteristics resulting in poor nutrition and lack of sunlight which lead to the disorder, however, made it not only imperative to counter these lacks with vitamin D but also drew attention to the poor housing conditions and the overall lack of physical growth in the social class affected by the disease. The introduction, then, of diet supplements in elementary schools helped overcome the defect, and the physical health of young people rose to a new optimum. Similarly, the treatment of established mental disorders in adults should reduce the number of people who potentially may communicate psychopathology to children; the treatment of psychopathology in children should lessen the number of abnormal adults; while the creation of mentally healthy persons, through family and school education, should lessen both the former. Whether this hypothesis is actually so must be determined by sampling and follow-up of representative population cohorts, a procedure which implies long-term longitudinal studies. Improvement in mental health as a whole, as in physical health as a whole, finally will depend not only on the reduction and prevention of mental illness but also on the improvement of the biogenetic, social, and cultural factors which are important in the production of mental abnormality. Before proceeding with a description of the public health approach developed in Victoria, some present-day concepts of the relations of society and culture to mental illness will be considered.

Society, Culture, and Mental Illness

Social psychiatry, according to Ruesch (1965), focuses upon the "structure of the community, the significance of the group for the individual, and the mechanics of communication." Among its functions is the description of social organizations and values, as seen by anthropologists, which seem significant to people participating in "psychiatric transactions." The epidemiological and ecological points of view are more strictly medical and reflect "attempts to relate the overall social and environmental conditions to the occurrence of disorders of behavior." The latter frame of reference involves the observer more clearly than does the former in assessing the individual as sick and in determining the relation of his sickness to his social setting; it is the main theme of this chapter.

Social psychiatry involves union with the social sciences. Since the scientific method involves a breakdown into smaller and smaller units whereby the original pattern gets lost, Ruesch postulated that a new investigative approach, based on group functioning, is necessary. Anthropologists provide insights regarding the significance of "preferences and values," such as ethnic values and social status.

Certain groups—e.g., geriatric, delinquent, or criminal—may manifest abnormality to a greater extent than their numbers in a population warrant, as determined by statistical analysis of factors such as age, sex, and social, occupational, and educational status. Sociologists help identify types of social order—e.g., agricultural, urban, primitive, technological—and aspects of social and cultural change—such as geographic mobility, social mobility, ethnic acculturation, and economic change—which may be associated with special stress to the individual.

No really practical definition of stress has yet been evolved. Cattell (Medical News Report, 1964), after measurement and factor-analysis of more than "400 experimentally measured alleged manifestations of anxiety over a ten-year period, has defined a single anxiety dimension . . . which can be measured with equal validity by an objective test battery, the objective-analytic (OA) battery, . . ." or by a questionnaire of 20 overt items "which anyone can see involve anxiety . . ." and 20 covert items "which would be hard to fake because they do not apparently involve anxiety, though they correlate equally with the anxiety factor and separate patients equally." In terms of biological stress patterns, such as 17-ketosteroid excretion, however, anxiety correlates only partially. Furthermore, there is a clear distinction between anxiety and neurosis, even though many normal persons are anxious temporarily and some neurotics develop defenses of denial or indifference. Similar distinctions will limit any neurophysiological measurement. The extent to which biological and psychological stress patterns are manifest in people subjected to sociocultural change, their persistence, and the relation of such reactions to those of a control group have yet to be determined. Efforts are being made to determine indexes of sociocultural change, both normal (Allen and Bentz, 1965) and pathological (Gordon and Gordon, 1964); the former authors have estimated such aspects of change as variation in cost of living, population growth, industrial-urban development, and educational provision; the latter have used such indexes as statistics on suicide, infanticide, divorce, desertion, and attendance at psychiatric outpatient clinics. Other indexes may be suggested; they need to apply to the community in general as well as to special groups within the community, if meaningful comparisons are to be made between their existence in one country and in another. Indeed, it still has to be shown how these phenomena meaningfully reflect psychopathology arising from social change. One very necessary proviso is that data be collected regularly and accurately on a long-term basis from a sizable population at risk.

Further concerns of social psychiatry are the functioning of small groups in the community, whether supportive or deviant—in special situations such as industrial groups, military camps, and new housing areas; in unusual situations such as disasters, war, famine, or unemployment; and in optimal social milieux in institutions under various social therapies ("therapeutic communities").

Ruesch (1965) referred to the epidemiology and ecology of mental disease, "formerly the province of public health," as a central concern of social psychiatry. It may be argued conversely that social psychiatrists are essential keystones of present-day public health practice. Shepherd and Cooper (1964) have supported the latter viewpoint and the overlap between psychiatry and general medicine:

> Epidemiological methods are fundamental to the aims of
> social medicine, which stands or falls by the ecological
> approach to illness—and especially to non-infectious chronic
> illness where mental diseases take their natural place among
> Ryle's (Ryle, 1948) diseases of prevalence, which also have
> their epidemiologies and must eventually be considered
> to be in greater or lesser degree preventable.

Finally, a quotation from Ginsberg (1956) is relevant: "Though the individual consists largely of his social relations, there is a core of individuality in each person which is uniquely his own and which is in the last resort unshareable and uncommunicable."

Turning to cultural influences on psychiatry, Ruesch (1965) considered cultural psychiatry a branch of social psychiatry. Wittkower and Rin (1965) challenged this position, although they did not express any considerable opposition to it. They stressed that cultural psychiatry is at present predominantly a research technique of value to a practicing psychiatrist (or survey interviewer) in that it requires him to take into account the culture of his patient in relation to his own, to take cultural considerations into account in planning health services, and, as they stated, "it is *hoped* that additional knowledge of sociocultural variables noxious to mental health will assist in the prevention, or at least reduction, of mental illness." There is a need to focus on "behavior that would be regarded as abnormal by trained observers irrespective of the culture in which it is observed."

In regard to methodology, Wittkower and Rin referred to the determination of qualitative and quantitative differences and attempts to explain these in terms of sociocultural variables; they stressed the need for a team approach by psychiatrists, anthropologists, social workers, or psychologists to transcultural studies. The tools of research include clinical observations, field surveys, hospital and governmental records, psychological tests, and questionnaires. The difficulties in the cultural approach concern "variability of nomenclature, of locale of observations, of methodology and of cooperation." There is still a need for "systematic, well-designed comparable field studies," and they consider that all the psychological tests used "are to some extent culture bound and cannot be used in a standard fashion cross-culturally." This was certainly the case in regard to the use of Western tests in an attempt to evaluate child development in Thailand (Stoller, 1959).

[I agree with the observation that primitive people tend to act out their unresolvable anxiety through gross hysterical manifestations or through aggressive panics. It must be remembered how the gross conversion hysterias of World War I gave place to the more common anxiety and psychosomatic states of World War II. Evidence is now accumulating that no society is free of psychosis or, indeed, of neurosis. Both in Thailand (Stoller, 1959) and Indonesia (Stoller, 1963), the frequency of neurotic and psychosomatic disorders has been recorded, not only by trained psychiatrists but also by local general practitioners. It is as hard to visualize a culture completely devoid of persons genetically predisposed to a poor tolerance to anxiety as it is to visualize no persons, in either Thailand or Indonesia, in chronic anxiety states resulting from involvement in interpersonal problems.

The problems of comparing epidemiological findings cross-culturally have already been mentioned (Mishler and Scotch, 1965). The WHO Study Group on Schizophrenia (1959) stressed the different cultural themes in the expressions of schizophrenics which have implications for diagnosis:

> The themes, the ways of behavior and expressing oneself,
> the use of language, the accepted modes of thought, and the
> symbolic interpretation of the world and of our personal
> existence differ greatly and they infallibly colour those
> psychological phenomena upon which the diagnosis of
> schizophrenia turns.

The changing pattern I have observed in the frequency and then the virtual disappearance of catatonic schizophrenia in Western countries, however, makes it hard for me to accept the supposition that the frequency of catatonic schizophrenia in India reflects, to a degree, the "postures adopted by certain types of *sanyasi* or *yogi*" (WHO, 1959). On the other hand, the patterns of delusions of influence have changed with the advance of modern science from electricity, through X-rays, to the atomic bomb. It does not appear difficult to recognize well-established "process" schizophrenics in any culture, and these groups should be the initial subjects for cross-comparison, in my view. The broadening of the definition of schizophrenia raises virtually insuperable problems in regard to its assessment in a single community, let alone in comparisons of its existence in one community with that in another. The frequency of paranoid reactions in refugee migrants from Eastern Europe has been noted in many areas of the world, including Australia, and is undoubtedly a reflection of uprooting, persecution, loss of loved ones, and difficulties associated with resettlement.

Depressive states, formerly thought to be rare, now are being recorded even in primitive communities. The previous lack of recognition was related to the tendency of a society to look on the phenomenon as a matter of spirit possession or even to accept it as an unfortunate change of personality. This was certainly the case in Thailand, where an experienced female psychiatrist often was able to perceive depressive changes in middle-aged women whose families thought such changes were just one of the "natural phenomena" they had to come to terms with (Stoller, 1959).

In developing countries acute confusional excitements also have been noted, but whether they represent toxic or exhaustive states has not yet been settled. Follow-up of the culture-bound disorders also has been inadequate to determine the extent to which they represent recognizable psychiatric syndromes. Over a period of three months in Indonesia, I did not meet with one case of *amok*, and widespread questioning of psychiatrists failed to elicit any recent knowledge of a case, though they mentioned acute states of excitement of hysterical, depressive, and schizophrenic origin. Nevertheless, Yap, in Chapter 3, looks on culture-bound disorders as "reactive psychoses" and has proposed a nosological grouping for them.

There has been a trend by many investigators toward assuming that certain cultures produce personalities especially vulnerable to mental disorders. This area has been examined by Leighton and Hughes (1961), who concluded that supportive evidence is insufficient, especially since culture-bound psychological tests have been used and adequate quantitative estimates of mental illness have not been made in the communities studied.

From the foregoing, it must by now be obvious that we are far from having developed a suitable model for comparing mental illness in communities of differing social development and with varying cultural values. In a "coarse-grained" way, it is possible to compare developing communities of comparable social development but only through the concerted action of a multi-professional group, which will also make sure, as did Lin (1953), that the population at risk is defined properly. Meanwhile, as I have already indicated, it is possible to find a base line of comparable data for developed countries, where population statistics are adequate and where a high proportion of the more disturbing cases are hospitalized. It is still necessary for each community, both developing and developed, to operate a central public health agency which will continue to collect and process whatever data is available, supplementing this wherever possible by special epidemiological studies. Even if the rates for psychoses in developed countries were being recorded adequately, there still would be the problems of incipient psychoses and unrecorded psychoneuroses, personality disorders, and psychosocial problems.

Mental Health Services in Victoria

Prior to 1950, the Mental Health Department of Victoria operated to a large degree through its mental hospitals, which were grossly understaffed and overcrowded. Admissions were relatively few, patient stay was long, and discharges were correspondingly few (Stoller, 1955).

Since 1950 the department has expanded considerably, now being responsible for more than 80 units throughout the state of Victoria, either directly or through subsidy. These include over 30 outpatient units, some 35 day training centers for mentally retarded children, and a wide range of facilities, extending from a personal emergency advisory service center through social clubs, hostels, sheltered workshops, outpatient centers, early treatment units, continued treatment hospitals, and long-term rehabilitation hospitals. The developments of the first decade of this comprehensive program are described in *Asylum to Community* (Dax, 1961).

The state government provides all mental health services without cost. A pattern of regionalization has developed with the aim of giving all residents access to facilities, and usage is indeed high as was demonstrated in the Heyfield survey (Krupinski, Stoller, Baikie, O'Day, Polke, and Graves, in press). Each region is aiming to develop a continuum of services, from the advisory service to the long-term facility, for all types of mental illness and mental retardation. Melbourne itself, which comprises two million people (two-thirds of the total population of the state of Victoria), is split into four regions, and the rest of the state into seven regions, with populations of around 150,000. There are special facilities in the Melbourne area for research, special diagnosis, surgical and neurosurgical treatment, university teaching, and child and adult forensic problems; the majority of sheltered industry is in Melbourne also. This bare description hardly does justice to the widespread availability of psychiatric advice and care.

A public relations program has brought a wide group of voluntary organizations into practical contact with mental health facilities—in fact, it has been said that one in four adults have been involved in some way through these community groups in furthering mental hygiene in the state. This fact has had a widespread effect on community attitudes. In 1955 a supplementary mental health education program aimed at professional and semiprofessional groups was added. Although its long-term objective is based on the belief that the *informed* opinion of this generation becomes the *general* opinion of the next, this special program has affected public attitudes toward mental illness even in the decade it has been operating.

The Mental Health Department has 11,000 beds compared with about 300 in general and private hospitals and some 200 in the veterans' program. There are some 30–40 psychiatrists in private practice, but the limited availability of private beds and the cost of mental illness bring many of their patients, especially the severely ill, to state facilities in due course. Outside the metropolitan area, private psychiatry is limited; regional outpatient services, therefore, handle a wide spectrum of cases, making possible statistical comparison with the general intake into the department.

Since 1950 standards in hospitals and clinics have been upgraded markedly. Admissions have increased almost fourfold, and discharges have risen correspondingly. Despite a rapid increase in population, the number of beds has remained relatively stationary, a factor which seems to suggest diminishing incidence, though, in fact, as the result of the increase in population there is some resistance to admissions of severe psychogeriatric patients and mentally retarded persons of poor prognosis. Hospitals have been opened largely on the basis of the progressive therapeutic formula—classification, segregation, treatment, occupation, freedom, socialization, rehabilitation, resettlement in the community—and, with the provision of hostels and sheltered industry, it has been possible to resettle in the community many adult persons of apparently poor prognosis. The situation, however, is being watched to determine how far it merely represents a displacement of family responsibility. The degree to which it is advisable for the "open door" to become the "revolving door" has not yet been determined.

The high proportion of persons with mental health problems receiving care through a wide range of state facilities has significance for the epidemiological program.

Epidemiological Program in Victoria

In 1955 the Mental Health Authority of Victoria established the Mental Health Research Institute, one of its main aims being to map the nature and distribution of patterns of mental illness and mental retardation in the state of Victoria.

At that time two epidemiological studies already were under way: (1) a mapping of the geographic incidence of all schizophrenic admissions to the main early treatment center, which was responsible for almost 90 per cent of all admissions; and (2) a community prevalence study of Huntington's Chorea. The former study suffered from the fact that the expanded admission policy had not yet been instituted fully; consequently, a smaller proportion of more severe schizophrenics had been admitted than would now be encountered. Nonetheless, the findings showed the same type of concentration of cases in inner Melbourne areas as did a study by Faris and Dunham (1939) in Chicago. The study of Huntington's Chorea has continued to the present; central recording of cases has enabled correct diagnosis of many new cases and subsequent useful counseling. The collection of these cases also has facilitated a study of the natural history of the disease (Brothers, 1964).

The first task undertaken after the opening of the Mental Health Research Institute was a survey of juvenile delinquency (Barry, Stoller, and Barrett, 1956). This study has provided a useful base line for subsequent departmental activities in relation to child forensic problems. The rate of delinquency, as evidenced by records of children's courts, declined considerably over 50 years, with peaks during the two world wars and a low incidence in the depression years (early thirties) attributed to the father's being home. This interpretation was supported by a study of "breaking and entering" cases, where 70 per cent of the boys had lost their fathers early through death, divorce, or desertion. It was found that delinquency was predominantly a male phenomenon (10:1). Analysis of police records on 1000 consecutive offenders showed that two-thirds of the crimes were committed before the age of 25. A high proportion of recidivist juvenile offenders commenced their antisocial history with truancy around the age of 9 and their first offenses around the age of 11, a finding which put the responsibility for detection and prevention firmly with the Education Department. Most juvenile crimes were committed after school or work hours, on week ends, or during holidays. Psychiatric diagnoses were not attempted in this study, but referrals to the children's courts' clinic are treated within the context of the general pattern of delinquency found, which was confirmed in a further study five years later. The fact that the special courts' clinic of the Mental Health Department and children's remand homes work closely together makes possible further epidemiological analysis of problems; a study in depth has just been arranged to sample the population coming into the main remand center. Referrals to the courts' clinic, of course, are recorded regularly through the main statistical system.

The next venture was into the field of mental deficiency. As a first step, it was decided to investigate the syndrome of mongolism, the most easily recognizable condition. An attempt was made to determine whether mongolism occurred regularly in relation to the prevailing population, maternal ages, and so on, in other words, whether it was genetic, or whether variations in time and place of occurrence might suggest an environmental influence. Environmental influence has been established (Stoller and Collmann, 1965a, 1965b); there are regular peaks of incidence; the latest peak was forecast; and a close statistical relation has been demonstrated between the epidemiology of infectious hepatitis and mongolism. As a possible indicator of virus-chromosome interaction without observable gross chromosomal change, it also has been noted that the epidemiology of hydrocephaly shows concordant peaks with mongolism (Stoller and Collmann, 1965c). Meanwhile, the epidemiological characteristics of hydrocephaly, anencephaly, and spina bifida also have been determined for the state of Victoria. As by-products of these studies, it has been possible to produce up-to-date life tables and survival rates for mongolism (Collmann and Stoller, 1963a, 1963b) and to estimate prevalence in western communities. Another side line has been the establishment of the first figures on blood-group distributions in the normal Australian maternal population. In line with the etiological hypothesis which has emerged for mongolism, an experiment has been devised to try to demonstrate a biological virus-chromosome link in mothers and their mongoloid infants.

Meanwhile, the original aim of mapping the prevalence of mental deficiency in Victoria has continued, and, in line with the policy of beginning with readily recognizable states, a study of the prevalence of moderately and severely retarded persons now has been completed (Krupinski, Stoller, Macmillan, and Polke, in press). The fact that Victoria's prevalence rate is lower than that found in comparable studies of the United Kingdom is attributed to the screening of immigrant children for mental retardation, the high proportion of hospital deliveries (almost 100 per cent), and the relative absence of poor socioeconomic groups. It is interesting that the ratio of mongoloid children to the total number mentally retarded is comparable to that found in other studies.

The mapping of mental deficiency in Victoria has been supplemented by other departmental interests and activities. The total population of the largest mental deficiency institution in Victoria (800 beds) has been examined in depth (Pitt and Roboz, 1965), and some modification of Heber's classification has been suggested. The origin of almost 60 per cent of the cases still remains unknown. Epidemiological studies also have been carried out on the occurrence of all congenital anomalies in a year's admissions to the Royal Women's Hospital, Melbourne (Pitt, 1962a, 1962b), and on the effects of rubella in the first trimester of pregnancy throughout Australia, with follow-up to the ages of four to eight years (Pitt and Keir, 1965a, 1965b; Keir, 1965). Other current epidemiological studies relate to the incidence and prevalence of phenylketonuria (Pitt and Wilmot, 1965) which is now being extended by the application of the Guthrie test; children with a double handicap of hearing and sight (Pitt, 1965); tuberose sclerosis; toxoplasmosis; lead intoxication; and chromosomal and dermatoglyphic anomalies. All data can be tested against known hospitalized prevalence (including those on waiting lists), and studies are being extended to all 35 day-training centers throughout the state. Data are collected centrally on a regular basis and are supplemented by data from the Heyfield community study. Now, there is a growing need to extend the mapping of adult mental deficiency beyond hospital patients in order to determine community need for sheltered industry (Stoller, 1965).

At this point, it is appropriate to mention the Statistical-Epidemiological Unit of the Mental Health Research Institute, which has become a focus for the development of epidemiological studies in Victoria. As already indicated, there is a central recording of data. An individual card is prepared for each person admitted as an inpatient or outpatient. All subsequent changes of status, discharges, readmissions, and so on, are noted. It is intended to build up a picture by these means of the natural history of persons with various psychiatric conditions, especially in a state where such a high proportion of psychiatric morbidity is covered. The program has commenced with a historical review of records of all departmental facilities on admissions, discharges, and deaths from 1882–1959 analyzed in terms of incidence, prevalence, and outcome, based on differences in sex, age, diagnosis, marital status, and educational and occupational backgrounds (Krupinski and Stoller, 1962a, 1962b, 1962c). In mid-1961, a statistical system was introduced covering the entire Mental Health Department, and a base line census of all resident patients was carried out to coincide with the national census (Krupinski and Stoller, 1962b). Bulletins are issued annually analyzing all new admissions. After the July, 1966, census, it will be possible to analyze morbidity and hospitalization trends over a 5-year period and to compare the statistics with those on cohorts established from the historical study (5 per cent samples of admissions during 5-year periods centered around census years from 1921 on, with the first cohorts followed up for over 40 years). Shifts in diagnostic emphasis have been taken into account in evaluating the historical data, and reasonable concordance in departmental diagnosis currently is being effected by the use of a diagnostic manual and by regular discussions between consultants; additionally, the large numbers of cases involved (7500–8000 first admissions annually) and the treatment of diagnostic entities in broad groupings tend to overcome personal variations in diagnosis. Populations involved in department researches now are being related as far as possible to the total statistical data so that they will be representative of the whole and also related to equivalent population incidences.

Space does not allow consideration in detail of the various other areas of epidemiological research opened up in Victoria. Progressively more data are being accumulated on disorders among immigrants, adult forensic problems, suicides, homicides, alcoholics, marital conflicts, and so on. These studies are increasingly more effective because of the progressive spread of psychiatric services throughout the community. The forensic program, for instance, gains by being linked to prison services and, through another clinic, to probation services and also to a center of services for alcoholics and other asocial and antisocial individuals. The forensic and alcoholism pictures are being mapped not only through these sources but additionally through the general patient intake to the Department (800 new cases of alcoholism per annum) and even through a psychiatric service to the Salvation Army, where research on their vagrant population is now being done. These two problems also are being assessed in relation to research sponsored by the Marriage Guidance Council of Victoria (Krupinski, Polke, and Stoller, 1965a). The size and nature of the psychogeriatric problem also are emerging slowly.

Special studies of specific psychosocial problems are being instituted periodically. Studies of mental disorders in immigrants, for instance, have determined five groups which run a greater risk than is warranted by their proportions in the population. Young United Kingdom migrants run a greater risk of becoming alcoholics and breaking their marriages than do others. Southern European middle-aged females apparently tend to assimilate poorly, remain relatively isolated from the community, progressively lose contact with their own family members, and therefore are prone to breakdowns. Eastern Europeans, who suffered the worst war experiences, as expected, run a greater risk than is usual, as do migrants of professional status whose qualifications are not recognized. Finally, a picture is beginning to emerge of a higher than normal incidence of personality disorders in adolescent and young adult second-generation migrants (Krupinski and Stoller, 1965).

In regard to completed suicide (Krupinski, Polke, and Stoller, 1965b), the following groups are special risks: cases of attempted suicide diagnosed as having personality disorders or alcoholism; middle-aged depressives; and males over 65 who have suffered bereavement or are isolated in the community. In regard to murder, influences frequently are alcoholism and depressive states and occasionally schizophrenia.

In mapping pictures such as those above, it becomes necessary to compare their validity with community prevalence studies. The first such comparison has been completed in Heyfield, a rural town of approximately 2000 inhabitants, 128 miles from Melbourne. Its social characteristics were determined, a census was taken, and questionnaires on 98 per cent of its inhabitants were completed by fifth-year medical students. In addition to socioeconomic data, physical and psychological disturbances were recorded. A preliminary analysis has been carried out, and full correlations between the various items of data are being programmed for computer analysis. Enough has emerged to show that there is a higher rate of psychiatric morbidity in the community than comes to the attention of the general practitioner, let alone to a psychiatric service. Among interesting trends which have emerged are: an increase in alcohol intake by adult males is paralleled by pill-taking by females; there is a decrease in the number of excessive drinkers from ages 55–60, paralleling the general picture of the age distribution of alcoholics; alcoholic parents produce more psychiatric problems in children than do psychotic parents; only 35.9 per cent of those with psychiatric diagnoses had actually sought help compared with 75 per cent of those with physical disorders; and psychiatric sufferers had far less tendency to consult unlicensed practitioners than had those who were physically ill (Krupinski, Stoller, Baikie, O'Day, Polke, and Graves, in press).

To sum up, the Mental Health Research Institute, through its Statistical-Epidemiological Unit and its stimulation of research throughout the Department, gradually is building a mosaic of patterns of mental ill-health and retardation from an increasing number of investigations. There is, and will continue to be, a constant feedback to illuminate hypotheses, and, as far as possible, initial researches will sample larger groups at risk than they have in the past.

Concluding Remarks

As I stated over ten years ago (Stoller, 1957), mental health programs have to be geared to the state of development of a society:

> As financial resources and numbers of specialist personnel are limited, mental health priorities have to be determined. This can only be done through a central administrative and investigatory organisation, proceeding on public health lines and attached to a central government. Mental health workers in such a central body must be part of a total health department and trained in broad epidemiological aspects of public health, thinking in such terms, just as they expect others to think in terms of human relations and the individual personality. Psychiatric, sociological, anthropological, epidemiological, administrative and educational viewpoints should all be represented. The mental health body must be

prepared to give an advisory service to other government departments and mobilise community agencies to help them. It could give help in the framing of those laws which have important sociological implications. It should also be responsible for the dissemination of educative mental health materials and could disperse research resources to best advantage. Mental health would thus be a unitary consideration, located within a general health programme and pervading those aspects of government concerned with disturbances in human relationships.

My thesis is that countries of similar stages of social development can find certain standards for comparison. Models, however, will need to be produced to attain scientific accuracy. Models will not be satisfactory if they do not include progressive development from a basic recording of illnesses to the assessment of psychosocial disorders, contributions from all social sciences, and close collaboration with clinical and preventive medicine. Lambo (1965), in his concluding remarks in "Psychiatry in the Tropics" stated:

> Massive preventive programmes against nutritional deficiencies, and infections and other endemic diseases, would reduce psychiatric morbidity in the tropics by well over 40 % . . . . Better understanding and appreciation of community and social factors, more refined studies of urban ecology, and better medical and social services are all equally necessary. . . . Important as psychopathological reactions may be, the physical basis demands much further research, since nutritional and general psychopathological problems underlie many of the psychiatric conditions. There must be close collaboration between psychiatry, clinical and preventive medicine, and the social sciences.

These factors are essential to a mental health program for any country at any stage of development. While it is fundamentally necessary to approach ill-health as a whole and initially establish the frequency and interrelation of both physical and mental health in a community, lack of attention to social circumstances and cultural factors will prohibit the proper development of curative services, obscure important clues to etiology, and reduce opportunities for prevention. Independently of the prevention of detectable ill-health, one also needs to be looking hopefully for the social and cultural approaches which will foster resilient personalities, optimally adaptable to the demands which will be the lot of the forthcoming generation.

REFERENCES

Allen, F. R., and W. K. Bentz. 1965. Toward the measurement of socio-cultural change. Social Forces 43:522–35.

Barry, J. V., A. Stoller, and D. Barrett. 1956. Report of Juvenile Delinquency Advisory Committee. Melbourne, Victoria Government Printer.

Brothers, C. R. 1964. Huntington's Chorea in Victoria and Tasmania. Journal of the Neurological Sciences 1:405–20.

Collmann, R. D., and A. Stoller. 1963a. A life table for mongols in Victoria, Australia. Journal of Mental Deficiency Research 7:53–59.

—————. 1963b. Data on mongolism in Victoria, Australia; prevalence and life expectation. Journal of Mental Deficiency Research 7:60–68.

Dax, E. C. 1961. Asylum to community. Melbourne, Cheshire.

Faris, R. E. L., and H. W. Dunham. 1939. Mental disorders in urban areas. Chicago, University of Chicago Press.

Ginsberg, M. 1956. On the diversity of morals. London, Heinemann.

Gordon, R. E., and K. K. Gordon. 1964. Psychiatric challenges of the 1960's. International Journal of Social Psychiatry 10:223–31.

Keir, E. H. 1965. Results of rubella in pregnancy. II. Hearing defects. Medical Journal of Australia 2:691–98.

Krupinski, J., P. Polke, and A. Stoller. 1965a. An analysis of activity of an Australian marriage guidance council. Journal of Marriage and the Family 27:502–508.

—————. 1965b. Psychiatric disturbances in attempted and completed suicides in Victoria during 1963. Medical Journal of Australia 2:773–78.

Krupinski, J., and A. Stoller. 1962a. Survey of institutionalized mental patients in Victoria, Australia, 1882 to 1959. I. Admissions to and residents in mental hospitals. Medical Journal of Australia 1:269–76.

—————. 1962b. Survey of institutionalized mental patients in Victoria, Australia, 1882 to 1959. II. Analysis in terms of diagnosis. Medical Journal of Australia 1:314–21.

—————. 1962c. Survey of institutionalized mental patients in Victoria, Australia, 1882 to 1959. III. Duration of stay and outcome. Medical Journal of Australia 1:359–67.

—————. 1962d. A statistical system introduced for the evaluation of the epidemiology of psychiatric disorders in Victoria, Australia. Health Bulletin 3:127–28.

—————. 1965. Incidence of mental disorders in Victoria, Australia, according to country of birth. Medical Journal of Australia 2:265–69.

Krupinski, J., A. Stoller, A. Baikie, D. O'Day, P. Polke, and G. Graves. In press. Heyfield community health survey: preliminary analysis.

Krupinski, J., A. Stoller, C. Macmillan, and P. Polke. In press. Epidemiology of mental deficiency in Victoria: severely and moderately retarded persons below the age of 17 years.

Lambo, T. A. 1965. Psychiatry in the tropics. Lancet 2:1119–21.

Leighton, A. H., and J. H. Hughes. 1961. Cultures as causative of mental disorder. *In* Causes of mental disorders: a review of epidemiological knowledge. New York, Milbank Memorial Fund.

Lemkau, P. Y., and G. M. Crocetti. 1958. Vital statistics of schizophrenia. *In* Schizophrenia: a review of the syndrome. L. Bellak, ed. New York, Logos Press.

Lin, T. 1953. A study of the incidence of mental disorder in Chinese and other cultures. Psychiatry 16:313–36.

Medical News Report. 1964. Anxiety. Journal of the American Medical Association 188(3): 49–53.

Mishler, E. G., and N. A. Scotch. 1965. Sociocultural factors in the epidemiology of schizophrenia. International Journal of Psychiatry 1:258–305.

Pitt, D. 1962a. Congenital malformations: a review I. Medical Journal of Australia 49:82–87.

————. 1962b. Congenital malformations: a review II. Medical Journal of Australia 49:121–24.

————. 1965. Children with a double handicap of hearing and sight. Medical Journal of Australia 2:829–31.

Pitt, D., and E. H. Keir. 1965a. Results of rubella in pregnancy. Part I. Medical Journal of Australia 2:647–51.

————. 1965b. Results of rubella in pregnancy. Part III. Medical Journal of Australia 2:737–41.

Pitt, D., and P. Roboz. 1965. A survey of 782 cases of mental deficiency. Journal of Mental Deficiency Research 9:4–23.

Pitt, D., and A. E. Wilmot. 1965. Phenylketonuria in Victoria. Medical Journal of Australia 1:33–39.

Primrose, E. J. R. 1962. Psychological illness: a community study. London, Tavistock Publications.

Ross, B. 1965. Mental health in Papua and New Guinea. Medical Journal of Australia 1:478–80.

Ruesch, J. 1965. Social psychiatry: an overview. Archives of General Psychiatry 12:501–509.

Ryle, J. A. 1948. Changing disciplines. London, Oxford University Press.

Schaechter, F. 1965. Previous history of mental illness in female migrant patients admitted to the psychiatric hospital, Royal Park. Medical Journal of Australia 2:277–79.

Shepherd, M., and B. Cooper. 1964. Epidemiology and mental disorder: a review. Journal of Neurology, Neurosurgery and Psychiatry 27:277–90.

Srole, L., T. S. Langner, S. T. Michael, M. T. Opler, and T. A. C. Rennie. 1962. Mental health in the metropolis: the midtown Manhattan study. New York, McGraw-Hill.

Stoller, A. 1955. Mental health facilities and needs of Australia. Canberra, Commonwealth Printer.

————. 1957. An Australian looks at the under-developed world. *In* Mental health and world community. Fraser Brockington, ed. London, World Federation for Mental Health.

————. 1959. Assignment report on mental health situation in Thailand. WHO Project: Thailand 17. Mimeographed document No. 7.

————. 1963. Assignment report on mental health situation in Indonesia. WHO Project: Indonesia. Mimeographed.

————. 1965. Industrial opportunities for mentally retarded persons. *In* Industrialization and mental health: Proceedings of the 17th Annual Meeting of the World Federation for Mental Health. Geneva, World Federation for Mental Health.

————. In press. Man's humanity to man. *In* Proceedings of the 18th Annual Meeting of the World Federation for Mental Health, Bangkok.

Stoller, A., and R. D. Collmann. 1965a. Virus aetiology for Down's syndrome (mongolism). Nature 208:903–904.

————. 1965b. Incidence of infective hepatitis followed by Down's syndrome nine months later. Lancet 2:1221–23.

————. 1965c. Patterns of occurrence of births in Victoria, Australia, producing Down's syndrome (mongolism) and congenital anomalies of the central nervous system: a 21-year prospective and retrospective survey. Medical Journal of Australia 1:1–4.

Stoller, A., and J. Krupinski. 1964. Admissions, discharges and deaths, 1962. Statistical Bulletin No. 3, Mental Health Authority, Victoria. Melbourne, Victoria Government Printer.

Stoller, A., J. Krupinski, A. J. Christophers, and G. K. Blanks. 1965. Organophosphorus insecticides and major mental illness: an epidemiological investigation. Lancet 1:1387–88.

WHO. 1959. [Report of] Study Group on Schizophrenia, Geneva, September 9–14, 1957. American Journal of Psychiatry 115:865–72.

Wittkower, E. D., and H. Rin. 1965. Transcultural psychiatry. Archives of General Psychiatry 13:387–94.

2. Some Issues in Intercultural Research on Psychopathology

LESLIE PHILLIPS, Ph.D.
Institute of Human Sciences
Boston College
Boston, Massachusetts

JURIS DRAGUNS, Ph.D.
Department of Psychology
Pennsylvania State University
University Park, Pennsylvania

TWO CONCEPTUALLY independent and contrasting commitments have guided investigation in the intercultural study of psychopathology. One is directed at the delineation of a fixed set of mental disorders whose clearcut manifestations presumably are obscured by the distorting influence of cultural diversity. This objective traditionally has been pursued in psychiatric cross-cultural research. The alternative position, which originates in cultural anthropology, views cross-cultural differences in the expression of psychiatric disorders as clues to the divergent attitudes, values, and aspirations which demarcate one society from another. We are aware, of course, that not all psychiatrists engaged in cross-cultural research are associated with the psychiatric tradition. Similarly, it would be incorrect to suggest that all cultural anthropologists concerned with deviant and disturbed behavior espouse the contrasting conceptual position. Nevertheless, even at the risk of oversimplification, it is not inappropriate to suggest that a primary goal of transcultural psychiatry is the search for constancy, and of cross-cultural anthropology, diversity. In this chapter the intent is to explore the consequence of these divergent goals on the research strategies which characterize cross-cultural research on mental disorders and to propose a reformulation of issues which eventually may permit integration of these two approaches in the search for both constancies (or culture-free universals) and divergences (or culture-bound particulars) in deviant or maladaptive behavior.

The psychiatric tradition in the cross-cultural study of psychopathology goes back to Kraepelin (1904; *see also* Benoit, 1964b; Lauter, 1965). It is based on the presumed substantive and immutable character of the various mental disorders. Depression, schizophrenia, and sociopathic behavior are regarded as entities that may at times be camouflaged but which, in principle, are detectable, once stripped of their culture-bound covering. The belief in the substantive nature of psychiatric disturbance has sparked three varieties of psychiatric intercultural research. The first, initiated by Kraepelin (1904), involves the comparative study of incidence rates of the major nosological categories in several countries and continents. This type of research has been pursued vigorously in the recent past. The results have been reviewed by Wittkower and Rin (1965) in a sophisticated and balanced account of both the achievements and the limitations of the diagnostic approach to transcultural psychopathology. They observed that the major variants of psychopathology, schizophrenia in particular, are world-wide in their distribution, although prevalence rates vary in accordance with several dimensions along which cultures can be classified. In their own words: "Schizophrenia is known to occur all over the world. The framework of the schizophrenic process is the same wherever it is found; in fact, it has been emphasized by most authors that the similarities in the clinical picture are more striking than the dissimilarities . . ." (Wittkower and Rin, 1965, p. 391).

Many authors (Aronson, 1965; Benoit, 1946b; Enright and Jaeckle, 1963; Wittkower and Fried, 1959; WHO, 1959) have agreed, however, that only limited significance can be attached to such findings. Empirical as well as conceptual difficulties abound in classifying individuals according to diagnostic categories which have been imported from an alien Western culture. The value of cross-cultural comparisons conducted along diagnostic lines is perhaps greatest when the results are not regarded as tallies of some presumably substantive disease entity but as clues to cultural sensitivities and blind spots of the psychiatric observers and of the societies which they represent. Examples of such an interpretation of cross-cultural diagnostic research have been provided by Aronson (1965). They are compatible with the position espoused by us that diagnosis is an inferential, second-order judgment rather than a designation for a process that has an aura of substantive reality.

A second variety of psychiatric cross-cultural study has been devoted to a description and case enumeration of unique symptom states such as *latah, koro,* and *amok,* which are thought to be equivalents of the Western forms of psychiatric disorder, hysteria, mania, and schizophrenia. Yap (1951) and Linton (1956), in informative reviews, underscored the remarkable inventiveness of human beings in devising highly original if self-defeating solutions to their conflicts and predicaments. More recent but limited accounts of culture-bound psychiatric states have been contributed by Ponce (1965) and Rubel (1964). Carothers (1948) also has expressed the belief that the unusual symptomatology of African psychiatric patients corresponds to the Western disorders of depression and schizophrenia, although stripped of their secondary and uniquely Western elaborations. The clinical description of the exotic variants of psychopathology is a worthwhile undertaking in its own right, yet, for the most part, it has been carried on with the intent of fitting manifestations into one of the rubrics of traditional Kraepelinian nosology.

A third group of psychiatric investigators start with the acceptance of conventional diagnostic designations but proceed to a comparison of patients in several cultures according to their actual symptom manifestations. Examples include the intercultural investigations of depression and schizophrenia co-ordinated by Murphy, Wittkower, and their associates (Murphy, et al., 1963; Murphy, Wittkower, and Chance, 1964), the comparisons of depressive symptomatology in Japan and Germany undertaken by Kimura (1965), and the comparative research on Japanese and American schizophrenics reported by Schooler and Caudill (1964). In all these studies symptom differences are considered in the context of some one diagnostic category, without questioning the substantive reality of that form of mental disorder.

In contrast to the three varieties of psychiatrically oriented investigations just described, those carried out within an anthropological tradition have emphasized cultural diversity in symptom expression. These studies have been guided by the assumption that the various forms of deviant reaction in some way reflect the styles of life which dominate various cultural settings. The review by Kennedy (1961) and reports by Hallowell (1959) and Spiro (1959) exemplify this approach. More recent investigation in Japan of the possible links between culture and psychopathology also reflect this orientation (Caudill, 1962; Doi, 1962). These studies are important sources of information on the relation between antecedent cultural conditions of socialization and impulse control and the consequent variables of self-defeating, deviant behavior patterns.

Viewed collectively, the anthropological investigations of psychiatric disorder constitute a fascinating mosaic of specific links between social characteristics and psychopathological manifestations. The limits of this approach readily become apparent, however, as one attempts to use the wealth of anthropological data on psychopathology to map interculturally valid functional relations between society and maladaptation. The *modus operandi* of anthropological investigators provides few avenues for transcending cultural uniqueness. Undeniably, anthropological studies form an important and substantial source of data for the student of transcultural psychopathology. The information, however, needs to be supplemented and integrated with findings and methods originating in other approaches to the cross-cultural study of psychiatric disorder.

To restate, we have identified and described, perhaps in a somewhat exaggerated form, the differences between the two traditions of transcultural research in psychopathology. The two approaches differ in both methods and goals, in tactics as well as in strategy. Typically, the psychiatrist proceeds from the disorder to the culture; the anthropologist goes from the culture to the disorder. Social milieu, while recognized as influential by both groups of scientists, is accorded a subsidiary role in psychiatric writings; its role is paramount in anthropological formulations. Psychiatrists rely heavily upon statistical compilations; anthropologists excel in providing qualitative information. Yet both these groups of investigators work with the same "raw data," the disordered and deviant versions of human behavior in their panoramic diversity.

We are committed strongly to the proposition that these two divergent conceptual orientations in the field of intercultural research in psychopathology are mutually complementary rather than antagonistic. Specifically, it is proposed that certain universal principles which guide human behavior must be articulated in order to understand the nature of psychopathology. Further, the relative frequencies of the various disorders within any one society presumably reflect the dominant attitudes, values, and aspirations of that society.

In brief, two major issues confront the field of cross-cultural psychiatry: (1) what are the universals in human behavior which are relevant to an understanding of psychopathology, and how can they be measured; and (2) what is the nature of the relation between cultural forms, attitudes, and values, on the one hand, and corresponding dominant forms of pathology? In stating the issues in this fashion, our position overlaps those of at least three recent theoretical formulations: Caudill's (1962) differentiation of "universals" and "diversity" as the basic concerns of psychoanalysis and anthropology, respectively; Benoit's (1964a) contrast between the "centripetal" and "centrifugal" objectives of intercultural psychiatric research; and Zubin and Kietzman's (1966) distinction between the culture-dependent and culture-free aspects of psychiatric disorder.

Our own framework easily accommodates some of the salient aspects of both the psychiatric and the anthropological positions. With the psychiatrists, we share concern with the world-wide constants of psychopathological expression. Yet we do not believe that the traditional diagnostic scheme provides a useful base for the search for these universals. Rather it is our conviction that an understanding of universal aspects of psychopathology must be derived rationally, e.g., from modern personality theory, and demonstrated empirically, e.g., through the techniques of factor analysis. At the same time we, in agreement with the anthropologists, try to place the observable aspects of psychopathology in their unique social context. Unlike at least some of the proponents of the anthropological approach (e.g., Benoit, 1964a), however, we do not despair of the possibility of studying the relation between the culture and its pathology in a systematic, quantified, and interculturally comparable fashion. Our position represents a blend of the psychiatric and anthropological orientations to the cross-cultural investigation of mental disorder. We will illustrate our approach by referring to the basic formulations and the preliminary findings of certain of our studies in psychopathology at Worcester State Hospital.

This research is based on the following set of propositions:

1) Psychiatric disorder is not to be conceived of as an alien and pathological process imposed on the individual personality independent of a person's life circumstances. On the contrary, pathology *is* the person attempting to cope, albeit inappropriately and ineffectively, with life circumstances beyond his adaptive resources. This proposed continuity in life pattern between adaptive and pathological phases is implied by the observed relation between ecology and disorder (e.g., Faris and Dunham, 1939), social class and disorder (e.g., Hollingshead and Redlich, 1958; Myers and Roberts, 1959), social competence and disorder (e.g., Phillips and Zigler, 1964; Zigler and Phillips, 1960), and ethnic origin and disorder (e.g., Enright and Jaeckle, 1963; Opler and Singer, 1956; Piedmont, 1965; Rin and Lin, 1962; Roussin and Fredette, 1963; Sanua, 1961).

2) A key personality characteristic associated with susceptibility to disorder is the individual's adaptive potential which can be measured both by psychological development (Lane, 1955) and by achieved level of social competence. Between them, these measures have been related to the form (Zigler and Phillips, 1962) and outcome (Phillips, 1953; Zigler and Phillips, 1961) of disorder.

3) The form of the disorder can be conceptualized as reflecting the individual's life style (Phillips, Broverman, and Zigler, 1966). For this purpose, symptom manifestation can be classified according to two dimensions which we have named role orientation and sphere dominance. "Role orientation" refers to the relative dominance of pathological symptoms indicative of a "turning against the self" (e.g., guilt feelings, suicidal attempt), a "turning against others" (e.g., threatened assault, destructive outbursts), or "avoidance of others" (e.g., suspiciousness, withdrawal). It is proposed that the individual's dominant role orientation indicates his capacity to accept responsibility for both his own life and destiny and the welfare of others who are dependent upon him. Those who feel that they have not met their obligations and that they are responsible for their failures in life turn against themselves in their symptom manifestation; those who are relatively immature or who feel that others are to blame for the vicissitudes of their existence either destructively turn against others or avoid others who threaten them.

Acceptance of personal responsibility, or, to phrase it differently, seeing the locus of control as within oneself rather than as dependent on the whim of others (or on an impersonal fate), is considered an index of psychological or personal maturity. It was hypothesized, therefore, that dominance of symptoms indicative of "turning against the self" would be associated with a high level of premorbid social competence, indicating personal maturity in the adaptive or normal phase of social interaction. Similarly, it was expected that symptoms of both "turning against others" and "avoidance of others" would be associated with a low level of premorbid social competence. This hypothesis has been confirmed in North American patients. Its intercultural generality is suggested by its replication in both Argentine (Draguns *et al.*, 1964, 1966) and Japanese (Draguns *et al.*, in press) samples.

"Sphere dominance" refers to the tendency for a patient's symptoms to be concentrated in one of the four possible spheres of organismic expression, viz., action, thought, affect, or somatic processes. We have observed that "thought over action" symptom dominance is associated with high levels of achieved premorbid social competence (Phillips and Zigler, 1961). Further, we have found that an emphasis on ideational symptomatology occurs primarily in those engaged in ideational occupations, and action symptoms, in those whose work is predominantly manual in nature, independent of the required level of skill. These observations again indicate the continuity in "preferred" or dominant life style from the adaptive to the deviant phases of the life pattern.

Although some of the studies just outlined transcend the boundaries of our own culture, we do not consider them truly cross-cultural. Rather they are attempts to test the universality of a set of psychological and behavioral relations. Our work also has extended into testing the way in which cultural differences in life style express themselves in pathological states. In such investigations it is important to control for variables known to influence the symptoms expressive of life style even within the confines of a single culture. These include all variables which define the individual's social role, viz., his sex, age, and social class (measured in terms of educational achievement and occupational skill); his level of social competence; and the diagnosis of his pathological state. This last variable was added in spite of our doubts about the validity of diagnostic criteria in cross-cultural work. Lacking access to complete psychiatric population pools, we attempted to compensate by controlling the diagnostic composition of our samples in order to guard against the fortuitous overrepresentation within our samples of a particular type of pathology that might bias the comparison of symptom manifestation.

In studies in which we have controlled patient samples on all these variables, we have obtained striking cultural differences in symptom expression. We have found that Argentine patients are relatively more passive and dependent than are North American patients, while North Americans are comparatively more tense, active, and destructive (Draguns *et al.*, 1964, 1966). In terms of the symptom dimensions described above, these differences are expressed in a prevalence of the role orientation of "turning away from others" in Argentina and that of "turning against others" in the United States as well as in an overrepresentation of somatization in the former country and of affective symptoms in the latter. These findings, we have been fascinated to discover, support a high degree of correspondence between the typical symptom manifestations of Argentine patients and an attitude of passive response to stress which allegedly is characteristic of at least some Latin American cultures (Diaz Guerrero, 1964).

We have observed, too, striking differences between symptom expressions of Japanese and United States male psychiatric patients, again when the above complex of variables is controlled carefully (Draguns *et al.*, in press). These contrasts appear, for the most part, as a relatively diffuse response to stress (e.g., impulsivity, emotional lability) among the Japanese and more goal-directed, although equally maladaptive behavior (e.g., suicidal ideas, perversions) among the Americans.

The results that we have obtained so far bear on both intercultural universals and on culture-bound particulars. To accommodate the former, we have developed an explicitly conceptual rationale which is outlined above. But what theoretical sense can be made out of the culture-bound differences observed in symptom manifestations? At this point, quite frankly, we pose the question without providing an answer. Ideally, we would like to fit our findings in with empirically established knowledge of cultural and personality characteristics in Argentina, Japan, and the United States, for conceptually we propose that psychopathology is not a behavioral aberration *sui generis* but is related in some manner to the cultural characteristics of the milieu in which it appears. That is, we propose a correspondence, or perhaps complementarity, between the typical behavior patterns of the normal and the deviant members of a society. The task of the intercultural investigator is to articulate the correspondence. Yet, this task rarely has, if ever, been attempted. Rather, we are impressed by the fact that intercultural studies of psychopathology, on the one hand, and of normal personality and behavior, on the other, have been carried on in airtight isolation.

In particular, three kinds of theoretical and empirical literature seem to have been exploited only rarely and incompletely in cross-cultural psychopathological research. First, an imposing body of writings can be described as general culture and personality literature. Such material, which is relevant to both cultural themes and behavioral patterns, is particularly abundant on Japanese society (e.g., Benedict, 1946; Gorer, 1943; LaBarre, 1945). Second, one of us (Phillips, 1963) has proposed relating statistical information on educational and technological achievements within each country to the prevalence of various forms of psychopathology. At first glance, the task of relating such indexes as the number of telephones or automobiles or books published in a country to its dominant modes of aberrant behavior may appear farfetched. Yet these two types of data conceivably may represent the technological and psychological facets of the same cultural characteristic. Finally, and most pertinently, a number of empirical studies have analyzed national character (Duijker and Frijda, 1960; Inkeles and Levinson, 1954) or a country's "basic sociocultural premise" (Diaz Guerrero, 1964). We note also the monumental investigation of the normal Japanese by Muramatsu (1962) and a considerable body of work conducted on specific theoretical issues by Caudill and Scarr (1962), Stoetzel (1955), and others. In addition, pilot comparative studies of normal samples of Argentines and North Americans are available (Havighurst *et al.*, 1963).

Practical and methodological problems abound in any attempt to apply the results of these studies to the interpretation of findings obtained in cross-cultural psychiatric work. Consequently, none of these three bodies of literature can substitute for the simultaneous empirical study of both normal and abnormal individuals drawn from two or more culturally and geographically distinct locales. Specifically, we propose that intercultural psychopathological research should proceed according to the following tri-partite scheme: (1) a comparison of normal individuals drawn from diverse cultures; (2) a comparison of psychiatrically recognized abnormal persons from the same settings, matched with their normal counterparts and with each other; and (3) a comparison of the differences between normal and abnormal individuals which cut across cultural lines. Of course, major practical problems of sampling as well as availability of normal subjects who would match the demographic characteristics of the patient samples would ensue, if such studies are undertaken. Even if these problems are overcome, the investigator will be faced with serious methodological issues, such as the choice of techniques and measures applicable to both normal and pathological individuals as well as to those of culturally divergent societies.

How are these difficulties to be resolved? At this point, we can offer only the most tentative lead toward their solution. We have noted in our studies on psychopathology the pervasive explanatory and predictive power of social competence as both a concept and a measure. We have proposed elsewhere (Phillips and Morrissey, MS) that the construct of competence development may serve as a co-ordinating principle for a variety of social action programs in the fields of mental retardation, delinquency, mental disorder, poverty, and even in developmental programs in technologically less advanced societies. We ask, therefore, whether the study of social competence and its nature and origins in personality development and culture may not serve as a vehicle for the study of both normal and pathological individuals in different cultures. To this end, we have devised a set of psychological and interview procedures, to be administered in group form, which permit the exploration of social competence variables in relation to attitudes, values, early family experiences, the sense of anomie or alienation, and so on. We have used these measures in the study of American normal adults of different social classes. We believe it feasible to extend these studies to other societies as well.

We then could attempt to use empirical data in answering such general conceptual questions as these: Do the maladaptive responses found within a given society represent a contrast to or an exaggeration of its modal behavior patterns? Schooler and Caudill's (1964) results, which highlight the prevalence of aggressive manifestations of the Japanese, would at first glance, favor a contrast interpretation. On the other hand, our own data from Argentina (Draguns *et al.*, 1964, 1966) suggest that psychopathological individuals express an exaggeration of the prevailing cultural behavior pattern. Be that as it may, we are committed strongly to the proposition that a necessary next step in intercultural research is the systematic study of deviant behavior in contrast to behavior expected by society.

In conclusion, the fact that investigators from both psychiatry and anthropology as well as other disciplines are contributors to this book provides convincing evidence that the divisions in transcultural research increasingly will be overcome—divisions that separate the psychiatric and anthropological approaches to the cross-cultural study of psychopathology and those that stand between the cross-cultural studies of psychopathology and the investigations of culture and normal personality relations. To these ends, we have advanced certain theoretical and methodological proposals derived from the field at large and from our own emerging program of transcultural research. Investigations in this complex field of endeavor can and must explore both what is universal and what is unique in culture and personality interactions and what is common and discrepant in normal and deviant behavior. The study of such complex issues requires the joint efforts of all the clinical and social science disciplines.

ACKNOWLEDGMENT

The preparation of this paper was facilitated by the Dementia Praecox Research Project, Worcester State Hospital, and by a research grant (M-6369) from the National Institute of Mental Health, United States Public Health Service.

REFERENCES

Aronson, J. 1965. Schizophrenia in transcultural perspective. Transcultural Psychiatric Research 2:12–13 (abstract). Paper presented at the First International Congress of Social Psychiatry, London, 1964.

Benedict, R. 1946. The chrysanthemum and the sword. Boston, Houghton Mifflin.

Benoit, G. 1964a. Qu'est-ce que la psychiatrie transculturelle? L'Information Psychiatrique 40:529–38.

――――――. 1964b. Legitimité et racines de la psychiatrie transculturelle. L'Information Psychiatrique 40:539–54.

Carothers, J. C. 1948. A study of mental derangement in Africans and an attempt to explain its peculiarities, more especially in relation to the African attitude to life. Psychiatry 11:47–86.

Caudill, W. 1962. Anthropology and psychoanalysis. *In* Anthropology and human behavior. T. Gladwin and W. C. Sturtevant, eds. Washington, Anthropological Society of Washington.

Caudill W., and H. A. Scarr. 1962. Japanese value orientations and culture change. Ethnology 1:53–91.

Diaz Guerrero, R. 1964. La dicotamía activo-pasiva en la investigación transcultural. *In* Proceedings of the Ninth Interamerican Congress of Psychology. M. B. Jones, ed. Miami, Interamerican Society of Psychology.

Doi, L. T. 1962. "*Amae*"—a key concept for understanding Japanese personality structure. *In* Japanese culture: its development and characteristics. R. J. Smith and R. K. Beardsley, eds. Chicago, Aldine Publishing Company.

Draguns, J. G., M. Knobel, T. A. de Fundia, I. K. Broverman, and L. Phillips. 1964. Social competence, psychiatric symptomatology and culture. *In* Proceedings of the Ninth Interamerican Congress of Psychology. M. B. Jones, ed. Miami, Interamerican Society of Psychology.

————. 1966. Sintomatología psiquiátrica y cultura: investigación intercultural. Acta Psiquiátrica y Psicologica de la América Latina 12:77–83.

Draguns, J. G., L. Phillips, I. K. Broverman, and S. Nishimae. In press. Psychiatric symptoms in relation to social competence and culture: a study of Japanese psychiatric patients. *In* Proceedings of the Tenth Interamerican Congress of Psychology. C. F. Hereford, ed. Austin, University of Texas Press.

Duijker, H. D. J., and N. H. Frijda. 1960. National character and national stereotypes. Amsterdam, North Holland Publishing Company.

Enright, J. B., and W. B. Jaeckle. 1963. Psychiatric symptoms and diagnosis in two subcultures. International Journal of Social Psychiatry 9:12–17.

Faris, R. E. L., and H. W. Dunham. 1939. Mental disorder in urban areas. Chicago, University of Chicago Press.

Gorer, G. 1943. Themes in Japanese culture. Transactions of the New York Academy of Sciences (Series 2) 5:106–24.

Hallowell, A. I. 1959. Psychic stresses and culture patterns. *In* Culture and mental health. M. K. Opler, ed. New York, Macmillan.

Havighurst, R. J., M. E. DuBois, M. Czikszentmyhalyi, and R. Doll. 1963. Las actitudes personales y sociales de adolescentes de Buenos Aires y de Chicago. Washington, Panamerican Union.

Hollingshead, A. B., and F. C. Redlich. 1958. Social class and mental illness. New York, Wiley.

Inkeles, A., and D. J. Levinson. 1954. National character: the study of modal personality and sociocultural systems. *In* Handbook of social psychology. Vol. 2: Special fields and applications. G. Lindzey, ed. Cambridge, Massachusetts, Addison-Wesley.

Kennedy, D. A. 1961. Key issues in the crosscultural study of mental disorders. *In* Studying personality crossculturally. B. Kaplan, ed. Evanston, Row, Peterson.

Kimura, B. 1965. Vergleichende Untersuchungen über depressive Erkrankungen in Japan und in Deutschland. Fortschritte der Neurologie, Psychiatrie und ihrer Grenzgebiete 33:202–15.

Kraepelin, E. 1904. Vergleichende Psychiatrie. Zentralblatt für Nervenheilkunde 15:433–37.

LaBarre, W. 1945. Some observations on character structure in the Orient: the Japanese. Psychiatry 8:319–42.

Lane, J. E. 1955. Social effectiveness and developmental level. Journal of Personality 23:274–84.

Lauter, H. 1965. Kraepelins Bedeutung für die Kulturpsychiatrie. Transcultural Psychiatric Research 2:9–12 (abstract).

Linton, R. 1956. Culture and mental disorders. Springfield, Thomas.

Muramatsu, T. ed. 1962. Nihonjin: Bunka to pasonariti no jisshō-teki kenkyū. (Reviewed by T. Sofue in Transcultural Psychiatric Research 1:100–102, 1964.)

Murphy, H. B. M., E. D. Wittkower, and N. A. Chance. 1964. Crosscultural inquiry into the symptomatology of depression. Transcultural Psychiatric Research 1:5–18.

Murphy, H. B. M., E. D. Wittkower, J. Fried, and H. Ellenberger. 1963. A cross-cultural survey of schizophrenic symptomatology. International Journal of Social Psychiatry 9:237–49.

Myers, J. K., and B. H. Roberts. 1959. Family and class dynamics in mental illness. New York, Wiley.

Opler, M. K., and J. L. Singer. 1956. Ethnic differences in behavior and psychopathology: Italian and Irish. International Journal of Social Psychiatry 2:11–23.

Phillips, L. 1953. Case history data and prognosis in schizophrenia. Journal of Nervous and Mental Disorder 6:515–25.

————. 1963. Social maturation and psychopathology. Paper presented at the Eighth Interamerican Congress of Psychology, Mar del Plata, Argentina.

————. In press. The severe disorders. *In* Abnormal Psychology. P. London and D. Rosenhan, eds.

————. In press. The competence criterion for mental health programs. Journal of Community Mental Health.

Phillips, L., I. K. Broverman, and E. Zigler. 1966. Social competence and psychiatric diagnosis. Journal of Abnormal Psychology 71:209–14.

Phillips, L., and J. Morrissey. MS. Social competence as a unifying principle in social action programs.

Phillips, L., E. Zigler. 1961. Social competence: the action-thought parameter and vicariousness in normal and pathological behaviors. Journal of Abnormal and Social Psychology 63:137–46.

————. 1964. Role orientation, the action-thought dimension and outcome in psychiatric disorder. Journal of Abnormal and Social Psychology 68:381–89.

Piedmont, E. B. 1965. Ethnicity as a dimension in mental health research. Community Mental Health Journal 1:91–99.

Ponce, O. V. 1965. Historia de la psiquiatría peruana. Transcultural Psychiatric Research 2:41–43 (review).

Rin, H., and T. Lin. 1962. Mental illness among Formosan aborigines as compared with the Chinese in Taiwan. Journal of Mental Science 108:134–46.

Roussin, M., and M. Fredette. 1963. La dépression chez les Canadiens-francais. Paper presented at the 17th International Congress of Psychology, Washington.

Rubel, A. J. 1964. The epidemiology of a folk illness: susto in Hispanic America. Ethnology 3:268–83.

Sanua, V. 1961. Sociocultural factors in families of schizophrenics. Psychiatry 24:246–65.

Schooler, C., and W. Caudill. 1964. Symptomatology in Japanese and American schizophrenics. Ethnology 3:172–77.

Spiro, M. E. 1959. Cultural heritage, personal tensions, and mental illness in a South Sea culture. *In* Culture and mental health. M. K. Opler, ed. New York, Macmillan.

Stoetzel, J. 1955. Without the chrysanthemum and the sword. New York, Columbia University Press.

Wittkower, E. D., and J. Fried. 1959. Some problems of transcultural psychiatry. *In* Culture and mental health. M. K. Opler, ed. New York, Macmillan.

Wittkower, E. D., and H. Rin. 1965. Transcultural psychiatry. Archives of General Psychiatry 13:387–94.

WHO. 1959. [Report of] Study Group on Schizophrenia, Geneva, September 9–14, 1957. American Journal of Psychiatry 115:865–72.

Yap, P. M. 1951. Mental illness peculiar to certain cultures: a survey of comparative psychiatry. Journal of Mental Science 97:313–27.

Zigler, E., and L. Phillips. 1960. Social effectiveness and symptomatic behaviors. Journal of Abnormal and Social Psychology 61:231–38.

――――――. 1961. Social competence and outcome in psychiatric disorder. Journal of Abnormal and Social Psychology 63:264–71.

――――――. 1962. Social competence and the process-reactive distinction in psychopathology. Journal of Abnormal and Social Psychology 65:215–22.

Zubin, J., and M. L. Kietzman. 1966. A crosscultural approach to classification in schizophrenia and other mental disorders. *In* Psychopathology of schizophrenia. P. H. Hoch and J. Zubin, eds. New York, Grune and Stratton.

3. The Culture-bound Reactive Syndromes

POW MENG YAP, M.D.
Hong Kong Psychiatric Center
Hong Kong

INQUIRY into the problems of comparative psychiatry and systematic examination of *latah,* the possession syndrome, *koro,* and the hypereridic state [1] indicate that the so-called exotic psychoses can be classified properly under the rubric of the "psychogenic psychoses" as described by Faergeman (1963) and others before him. In 1962 I suggested that the term "atypical, culture-bound psychogenic psychosis" be adopted to embrace these conditions. For general purposes I would retain the adjective "atypical" because each of these psychoses is relatively unfamiliar even in its own cultural milieu, but I would now substitute "reactive" for "psychogenic," in spite of its more narrow connotation, and "syndrome" for the more controversial "psychosis."

The Need for Nosology and Standard Nomenclature

The need for a generally accepted nomenclature and classification of mental illness is nowhere more urgent than in transcultural psychiatry (Yap, 1962). Rigidity in basic nomenclature has its value, but if classification of mental illness is to fulfill its function we must temper inflexibility by the demand for assimilating new observations. On the one hand, common disease concepts are needed for purposes of communication; on the other, a need exists to integrate new knowledge into old or, conversely, to allow application of accumulated knowledge to fresh clinical problems. It is possible for excessive insistence on the simple communicative function of nosological systems to blind us to unusual phenomena, hampering further investigation of them. The interpretative function of nosological classification needs emphasis, although it varies according to the nature of the axis employed for differentiating one disorder from another. The more etiologically fundamental the axis, the narrower is the possible range for its use when studying puzzling new conditions. The more symptomatically conceived the disease category, the less valuable it is in helping to define and trace the causes of unfamiliar illnesses, for measurements of variables in a broad and necessarily heterogeneous group will not appear to be significant, although they are significant for a smaller homogeneous one. For example, the frequency of positive urine tests in phenylketonuric amentia is not statistically significant when a random sample of children is examined rather than a narrowly defined clinical group of retarded children.

Most present-day classifications rely on a mixture of symptomatic and etiological differentiating axes, and, unfortunately, there is no agreement on any one overall scheme (Stengel, 1959; Meyer, 1961a, 1961b). The nosology of the culture-bound reactive psychoses, however, is simplified by the fact that the category of reactive or psychogenic psychosis already is recognized in the majority of classification systems employed in continental Europe, the Soviet Union, and Japan (Yap, 1962). In the United States a curious situation exists. According to the investigations of Hollender and Hirsch (1964), five out of six professors of psychiatry use the term "hysterical psychosis," although it is not accorded official recognition. On the other hand, the predominantly psychodynamic orientation of the American Psychiatric Association Classification is given special weight in the mention of "gross stress reaction," "transient situational personality reaction," and "psychoneurotic depressive reaction"; the latter is stated to be synonymous with "reactive depression," and the diagnostic criteria prescribed differ little from those of the classical German psychiatry. No attention is given to the fact that stress of less than catastrophic degree can lead to disturbances of consciousness. In Great Britain the term "pseudo-psychotic hysteria" has to suffice for the reactive psychoses, although the term is unwieldy and ascribes to "psychosis" a meaning that is not always clear. The World Health Organization Classification does not have a place for the reactive psychoses, and Odegaard (1959) has pointed out that it overlooks the vast number of functional psychoses outside schizophrenia and manic-depressive insanity.

While it is not necessary to create anew the concept of reactive psychosis, it is desirable to clarify its connotation and to define precisely, if we can, the key words "psychogenic," "reactive," and "psychosis." "Psychogenesis" means the process whereby mental experience brings about an abnormal reaction in a predisposed subject. The predisposition may be conceived in wholly or partly somatic terms, as by Jaspers (1962) in discussing psychologically incomprehensible extraconscious mechanisms or by Schneider (1959) in referring to a "psychic ground," partly physical and partly psychological but not identical with the Freudian unconscious. It may be framed purely in psychological terms as by psychoanalysts who insist on the continued effects of infantile experiences, though mediated by the psychophysical constitution. The subjective values and imaginative power and attitudes of the patient are always relevant, since these determine for him whether or not a special experience is traumatic. More technically, Faergeman (1963) has defined "psychic trauma" as the excessively anxious reaction of the individual, having been sensitized by infantile frustrations, to a catathymic [2] event. He also has pointed out that it is possible for an overwhelming experience—such as a catastrophic accident for an adult or an initial loss of a mothering figure for an infant—to be traumatic in itself without the need for catathymic preparation.

The term "reactive" (which is not to be confused with "exogenous") means that an abnormal reaction has been produced by an external traumatic shock of great severity in a mechanical manner or has been brought into open expression in a predisposed subject by an external, experiential stress. Since most cases of psychogenic psychosis are of the latter type, the term "reactive," when applied to them, must be understood in that sense. In practice, it is not possible to relate the response to the stress without further taking into account the direct effect of sociocultural factors in patterning affective and behavioral responses to pernicious stimuli.

It is hardly possible to give an accurate definition of the word "psychosis" that will be acceptable to all schools of thought. The simplest way in which it can be used is to denote a severe degree of abnormal psychic functioning manifested in behavior. If further specification is required, severity should be measured according to the following dimensions: loss of insight; loss of contact with reality as indicated by delusions, hallucinations, or significant impairment of the ability to understand and use language; loss of control over instinctual life; and drastic change in the whole personality and impairment of adaptive powers. Such usage does not relate the term to a specific etiological theory, as preferred by Schneider (1959) in reserving the word for conditions with a real or assumed organic basis.

Justification for the Class of "Reactive Psychosis"

There is little difficulty in accepting the existence of states of ego-disorganization following acute stress, perhaps accompanied by the eruption of unconscious thoughts and feelings, with or without an element of wish-fulfillment. Bond pointed out that the hysterical psychosis is the same as Freud's *übervaltingungspsychose*, in which the ego is overwhelmed (cf. Hollender and Hirsch, 1964). It is my task to show that a formal diagnostic category comprising these states is of value for several reasons.

A standard objection to the concept of reactive psychosis is that it fails to do justice to the multifactorial nature of mental disease. The objection can be resolved into the assertion that experiential factors are much less important in causing mental disorder than are somatic factors. The basic reason for such an attitude is the difficulty in identifying causally significant, traumatic psychological factors. It is trite to point to the rarity of cases fulfilling Jaspers' (1962) criteria for reactivity—criteria such as a meaningful relation between the precipitating cause and the content of illness and a parallel time relation between the two. It also is arbitrary to attribute acute brain syndromes to physical lesions. The fundamental difficulty in discussing psychogenesis lies in applying the idea of causality to mental phenomena, when the subject-predicate grammar of the Aryan type of language constrains us to think of mind as a *substance,* but one without position and spatial extension (Northrop, 1963).

The multifactorial approach is appropriate to the complexity of the problem, but it should not be allowed to disguise what is really reductionism. It would be self-deceiving to accept only a primary neurophysiological lesion, relegating all other factors to vague epiphenomena, and not bothering to enumerate, much less demonstrate, them or to test hypotheses implicating them. When confronted with a patient, serious scientists are responsible for evaluating significant etiological factors and assigning them some order of importance: which factors are necessary but not sufficient, and which factors perhaps are sufficient by themselves? To regard a case as reactive does not exclude appreciation of constitutional factors, which are after all partly the result of earlier psychic experience, but emphasizes the outstanding importance of experiential factors, which may sometimes, if severe, be sufficient in themselves to bring about illness.

The restriction of the term "disease" to mean only the structural alterations caused by physical lesions is unacceptable. Not only are organic disorders like asthma, tetany, migraine, and essential hypertension defined in terms of functional symptoms, but so also are the functional psychoses— manic-depressive insanity and schizophrenia—and the psychoneuroses. If one is persuaded by Slater (1965) to deny hysteria the status of a disease because it is a purely psychological disorder without genuine physical symptoms, the same reasoning must be extended to the functional psychoses and the other psychoneuroses. Roth (1963) has pointed out the illogic of attempts to separate medical and behavioral parts of medicine because all functional psychiatric syndromes, when defined in terms of symptoms and signs, include a minority of cases associated with organic disease in a causally significant way, e.g., schizophrenia in rare cases with amphetamine intoxication, and depression in the aged sometimes with physical disease.

I agree with Roth that in some respects the contrast drawn by Jaspers and Schneider between normal development and pathological process has been overemphasized, inasmuch as there exist borderline conditions labeled pseudo-neurotic schizophrenia, schizophreniform psychosis, and, of course, the psychogenic psychoses, which have not been duly taken into account. Little is to be gained by debating the distinction between quantitative and qualitative abnormality, but it often is forgotten that the extremes of apparently normal psychological functioning do demand clinical attention. It is possible to speculate that in these cases specific and partly independent neurophysiological mechanisms are brought into play by stress, but these need not be the sole criteria of abnormality, although generally it should be easier to identify these somatic mechanisms than the psychological ones that may be involved.

Rudolph Virchow,[3] the founder of cellular pathology, strove to formulate physiological definitions of disease and held that pathology was only physiology in the wrong context. "Disease" can be defined broadly as a state of imbalance or disharmony between the various parts of an organized system, but "parts" can mean different entities at different levels of organization. It is basic to psychiatry that social and psychological phenomena be included in its purview. Most cases of disease, whether mental or physical, represent a disturbance of social adaptation, i.e., of the social functioning of the patient. It is this disturbance which brings the subject to a recognized professional for help. Where a biological lesion or focus of dysfunction is detected, the patient is treated legitimately by the medical healer. Where there is no social disharmony, even the presence of a definite though benign biochemical or structural anomaly is not regarded as abnormal in the sense of requiring medical attention, e.g., pentosuria and flat-foot in certain persons. For dysfunction at the psychological level, e.g., disturbances of particular performances, of psychological "part-functions" (Lewis, 1953), the critical case is one in which social disharmony is evident without any somatic abnormality. The difficulty in using such a criterion for abnormality is not that the view of normal function is subjective and takes the form of a value judgment, for one should be able to discover the norm by statistical survey. Rather, the difficulty lies in the vagueness of the concepts of psychological functions, e.g., volition, and in the obstacles to isolating and measuring them. It must be recognized that reactions which are regarded merely as extreme variations of normal mental life involve bizarre and psychologically incomprehensible symptoms, such as depersonalization-derealization, hallucinations, automatic obedience, and echo-reactions, that are dysfunctional at their own level, quite apart from reflex and psychophysiological changes, perhaps with structural changes ensuing, that can be extreme in states of terror.

It will be helpful, finally, to invest bare doctrine with some substance to see how the concept of reactive psychosis has been employed in clinical research. Two recent studies show the clinical characteristics of the condition, characteristics that can be regarded as *typical* and perhaps found universally, even in countries where atypical culture-bound forms also exist. Astrup, Fossum, and Holmboe (1962) and Faergeman (1963) have shown in follow-up studies that reactive psychoses do not end in schizophrenic deterioration, nor are they schizophrenic in the Bleulerian sense. Astrup,

Fossum, and Holmboe drew attention to the following characteristics of their 206 cases: the patients had sensitive, hysterical, or neurotic personalities; the illness was precipitated by mental trauma, sex conflict, childbirth, or physical illness; the onset was acute; the patients often were unintelligent and came from low social classes; and genetically the patients were related to recovered rather than deteriorated schizophrenic or manic-depressive patients. Faergeman in his study of 79 cases found that most were women between the ages of 29 and 40; three-quarters had a familial predisposition, including "psychopathy, psychogenic reactions, neuroses and the like." Many had abnormal premorbid personalities, either psychopathic or neurotic, but low intelligence was not common.

The Position of the "Exotic Syndromes"

Arieti and Meth (1959), Ellenberger (1965), and Kiev (1965) have given accounts of the "exotic syndromes." Arieti and Meth suggested that they are unclassifiable. On the contrary, it is my belief that systematic analysis places the "exotic syndromes" within the psychogenic psychoses grouping, although patients may not always be disturbed enough in the sense discussed earlier to merit being called "psychotic." These syndromes are culture-bound in that certain systems of implicit values, social structure, and obviously shared beliefs produce unusual forms of psychopathology that are confined to special areas. Social and cultural factors bring about special forms of mental illness, although these are only atypical variations of generally distributed psychogenic disorders. It is necessary to avoid over-generalizing about the relation between culture and mental disorder from the material available. In theory, there are almost a dozen ways in which this relation can be spelled out (Murphy and Leighton, 1965). Van der Kroef (1958) has made an elaborate attempt to explain *latah* and *amok* in terms of the Indonesian ethos, relying heavily on Jung, and Wallace (1961) has propounded an ecological theory of mental disorders which he calls "bio-cultural," with special reference to Eskimo *piblokto*. It does not appear that any one schema, however, can do justice to all the facts. For the whole group of culture-bound reactive syndromes, diverse links are traceable between illness and its sociocultural background, although the subject is not considered systematically in this chapter.

It is mistaken to suppose that all these syndromes are rare. Psycho-genic death from extreme terror in its complete form (so-called than-atomania) may be rare and of scientific interest only as an example of the utmost limits of psychophysiological derangement, but *amok, latah,* "malignant anxiety," and to a less extent *koro* are not uncommon. Indeed, the psychiatrist in his ordinary practice is faced with the inescapable prob-lem of diagnosing and classifying such cases for which he has no guide, since these disorders are treated in textbooks only as remote medical curio-sities. Certainly, they are at the very least of the same order of frequency as cases of sexual deviation. Schmidt (1964) stated that in Sarawak *amok* is only one of many "short-lived explosive psychoses" and that *latah* is still common. Sangsingkeo (personal communication) has found *latah* common in Thailand. Both Maguigad (1964) and Zaguirre (1957) reported that *amok* is frequent in the Philippines; in fact, the latter recorded that it has become more common since World War II. As for the undifferentiated syndrome of panic that Lambo (1962) has called "malignant anxiety," all workers in Africa agree on its frequency. Lambo was able within a period of six years to gather 98 cases of persons so afflicted charged with offenses involving capital punishment.

Many cases of the "exotic syndromes" may not come to the attention of the clinician because they are not severe, or, as best exemplified in the very wide-spread possession syndrome, the reactions may be exploited socially so that doubt arises over their medical abnormality. Possession may be valued in various religious contexts and in spiritualistic mediumship. *Amok*-like behavior has in the Philippines found expression in ritually supported *jurmentado,* and it appears that Philippine law enforcement agencies tend to be lenient toward homicidal violence. The reactions, however, may become quite uncontrolled on the part of the subject so that he commits serious antisocial acts. Medico-legal issues arise, and psychiatric expertise, if only in differential diagnosis, is called for. For this reason, Lambo has stressed the forensic importance of malignant anxiety in Africa, and an early paper by Lloyd-Still (1940) gave case histories illustrating the forensic significance of *latah* in Burma. In Burma according to Hazel Weidman (personal communication), *amok*-like behavior can arise out of the startle reaction. The criminological aspects of *amok*, which need hardly be elaborated, have been dealt with by Zaguirre (1957). The reality of psychogenic death in Africa sometimes becomes a practical issue in death inquiries (Lambo, 1962).

The successful exploitation of some minor or moderate examples of a number of these reactions by both the patients themselves and society should not obscure the fact that the fully developed forms exhibit abstruse and psychiatrically technical phenomena, e.g., depersonalization, dissociation, hypereridism, echo-reactions, command automatism, and psychophysiological changes. The fact that illness is capitalized upon by society is not an argument *per se* against its abnormality; similar exploitation of physical diseases occurs, for instance, exhibiting midgets, giants, and Siamese twins in circuses, using deformed children for beggary, or training the blind for mediumship (as happens in certain parts of northern Japan).

It should not be overlooked that characteristically developed forms of these reactions are regarded by their own societies as abnormal, although, as far as possession is concerned, the abnormal may not always be clearly distinguished from the preternormal and numinous, so that the social response is ambiguous. Devereux (1963) has suggested that in folk cultures patients who consider themselves unfit in one way or another seek to define themselves in terms of some socially supported model of insane behavior in order to obtain certain satisfactions associated with the sick role and to avoid being treated as criminals. Such a formulation is overgeneralized, ignores the fact that cultural patterning of abnormal behavior must take place on the basis of individual psychological or psychiatric dysfunction, overestimates the degree of self-control in the patient, and also exaggerates the freedom of choice open to him in expressing his disabilities. Moreover, Devereux wrongly sees all mental illness as merely psychogenic, as does Szasz (1961). The insight of the ethnologist needs to be balanced by the perception of the clinician interested in the structural analysis of mental disease.

There are typical and atypical forms of the reactive psychoses everywhere, the atypical forms appearing in puzzling ways because of specific cultural forms and social structure. Atypical culture-bound variations of psychogenic reactions in European and American countries include homosexual-panic; depression, which Hutterites call *anfectung* and regard as surrender to Satanic design; mass excitement, sometimes accompanied by fainting of female adolescents at the sight of popular male idols; and perhaps also school-phobia and anorexia nervosa. These reactions have not been dignified as basic syndromes in themselves, partly because they are not common to all cultures and partly because the conceptual apparatus of psychiatry has not been applied to their fundamental analysis. The same cannot be said of the "exotic syndromes" in general. Table 1 attempts to draw parallels between these and related conditions that are typical and generally distributed, the aim being to expound the basic psychopathological nature of the "exotic syndromes." Certain conditions, e.g., the *piblokto* [4] of the Arctic, the *banga* of the Congo, and the *misala* of Malawi, are not included because they are only vague generic terms for mental illness or denote only ordinary, unspecialized hysterical reactions. Such terms should not be allowed to creep into the psychiatric literature. One of the purposes of this paper is to prevent their proliferation.

Psychopathologically, it is possible to distribute the less familiar atypical reactive syndromes into the four groups indicated. In the unlikely event that new conditions are discovered, they also probably could be accommodated in these groupings. The culture-bound fear reactions occupy a prominent place, a factor which cannot be surprising, for fear, even more than rage, has the power to impair ego functioning and ultimately bring about a level of mental functioning that is nondiscriminative, impulsive, and thus rudimentary. At this level, cultural forces can build up distinct and unique patterns of abnormal behavior. Kretschmer (1934) called mental functioning on this plane "hypobulic-hyponoic" or "primitive" in contrast to individual personality reactions of a less regressive kind; he also stressed the ease with which hysterical reactions grew out of them. Furthermore, it is not surprising that the specialized primary fear reactions (as opposed to the culturally inculcated phobias) are found in simple folk societies, for

Table 1: Atypical and Typical Syndromes of Reactive Psychoses

Atypical "Exotic Syndrome"	Typical Prototype
Primary Fear Reactions	
Malignant anxiety	Undifferentiated states of acute anxiety and panic with varying degrees of ego-disorganization
Latah reaction, including *mali-mali, mir-yachit, imu, bah-tschi, young-dah-hte;* "jumping"	States of hypersuggestibility with echo-reactions following psychogenic shock, commonly with other predisposing causes, e.g., toxic-exhaustive; "startle neurosis"
Susto, including *espanto*	Traumatic anxiety-depressive states with psychophysiological changes
Psychogenic "magical" death or "thanatomania"	Severe psychophysiological disorganization with surgical shock from terror in catastrophic situations
Hypereridic Rage Reaction	
Amok (including *negi-negi?*)	Acute psychopathic reaction issuing from states of morbid hostility in predisposed personalities
Specific, Culturally Imposed Nosophobia	
Koro	Depersonalization states associated with severe anxiety, arising from unrealistic fears, e.g., "venereophobia"
Trance Dissociation	
Possession syndrome, including *windigo* psychosis, *hsieh-ping*	Possession states, with varying degrees of social sanctioning, often poorly delimited and beyond patient's control

being technically backward such peoples have inadequate mastery over their environment and live in a psychological world hostile beyond the comprehension of metropolitan man.

Classification of Reactive Psychoses by Syndrome

A formal ordering of the reactive psychoses within an acceptable and relevant nosological scheme is needed for clinical, didactic, forensic, and administrative purposes. A widely used classification is that of Schneider (1959), which has been adopted by Stromgren and Faergeman. It subdivides the generic grouping of psychogenic (reactive) psychosis into paranoid and emotional syndromes, and disorders of consciousness. The suggestion is tentatively offered that the culture-bound syndromes can be fitted usefully into the classification shown in Table 2. *Latah, amok,* and the possession state involve disturbances of consciousness, as does severe malignant anxiety. *Koro* and *susto* belong rather more to the emotional syndrome, although an intense reaction may be accompanied by clouding in the case of *koro*, and perhaps also in *susto*. Possession, *koro,* and *susto* implicate delusional beliefs, but only in a special sense, since the social consensus in the patients' subcultures buttresses these beliefs. Psychogenic death is prefaced by such unusual behavior and involves such extreme psychosomatic reactions that at present it also can be considered psychotic.

As any other classification, Table 2 is unduly neat and precise. It is based on clinical symptoms, but it cannot take into account minor variants and mixed pictures in differentiating one form from another. As a classification it is, in our present state of knowledge, zealously comprehensive,

Table 2: Tentative Classification of Atypical Culture-bound Reactive Syndromes

1. Paranoid syndrome	
2. Emotional syndrome	2.1 Depersonalization state: *koro*
	2.2 Fear-induced depressive state: *susto*
3. Syndrome of disordered consciousness	3.1 Impaired consciousness: *latah* reaction
	3.2 Turbid states: malignant anxiety, *amok, negi-negi*
	3.3 Dissociated consciousness: certain types of possession syndrome, *hsieh-ping, windigo* psychosis

Note: It may be possible with further information to add to the three main headings a meaningful fourth: Extreme and irreversible psychophysiological disorganization from terror: psychogenic death.

but it is offered mainly to provoke thinking and discussion. The various syndromes require further elaboration.

Koro. This is a culture-conditioned acute depersonalization syndrome, with localized depersonalization confined to the penis, occurring in the context of a panic state with fears of impending death (Yap, 1965a; Rin, 1965; Gwee, 1963). It is encountered in Hong Kong and Southeast Asia where the belief in a mortal *koro* illness with penile shrinking intensifies ordinary guilt and anxiety over real or fancied sexual excess, especially auto-erotic activity, and also determines specifically the unique presenting symptom in a psychologically comprehensible way. Cultural forms therefore can be pathogenic as well as pathoplastic. Immaturity of personality, an anxious temperament, and cold are contributing factors; sudden fright can precipitate an attack.

It occurs in all degrees of severity, leading rarely to clouding of consciousness with extreme panic. It is never welcome and always feared; consequently *koro* is never exploited for social ends. The institution of polygamy in one form or another, with its demands for adequate male sexual performance, may be a precondition for its occurrence in any society, as is the tradition of ancestor veneration with its emphasis on maintaining the family line.

Comparable abnormally intense fear reactions induced by socially-supported beliefs have been described among the Saulteaux, who learn to be unrealistically frightened of certain snakes and caterpillars (Hallowell, 1934). These specifically imposed and pathological fears have to be distinguished from abnormal primary fear reactions.

Susto, Including Espanto. This illness, which occurs in the people of the Andean highlands, is usually brought on by fright, e.g., from a fall, a thunderclap, or meeting a ferocious animal. It affects mainly children and adolescents, but no age group is immune. The symptoms are insomnia, asthenia, apathy, loss of appetite and weight, depression, and anxiety with its physiological accompaniments. It is treated by indigenous ritualistic psychotherapy (Sal y Rosas, personal communication; Leon, 1965; Rubel, 1964).

The illness is ascribed to contact with supernatural agencies, e.g., witches' saliva, "black-magic," the "evil eye," supernatural punishment, and "bad air" from dangerous places such as caverns and cemeteries. The result is thought to be loss of the soul. The original inhabitants of the New World and dwellers in the sub-Arctic regions of the Old World attributed trance states to soul loss. These trances have to be distinguished from the less common ritual soul projection of shamans, used as a technique of clairvoyance. Linton (1956) suggested that trance states put down to soul loss are comparable to trance states ascribed to possession by an alien soul or spirit, with opposite explanations being used in the two instances. From the clinical viewpoint, however, the former show no automatism or glossolalia, nor does dissociation of consciousness occur as it does in the equally psychogenic possession syndromes of the Old World. *Susto,* although it is precipitated by fright as is *latah,* presents a dissimilar picture. The crucial part that cultural conditioning plays in determining responses to fear is plain.

Latah. I have used this one term to cover a number of different terms which describe the same reaction in widely separated countries (North Africa, Southeast Asia, Siberia, Hokkaido, North America) in order to emphasize the psychodynamics of the reaction (Yap, 1952). *Latah* is identical with the "jumping" of Maine, to which Stevens (1965) has devoted a recent paper. Thorne (1944), without being aware of *latah* or "jumping," described in white American draftees what he called "startle neurosis," in which a sudden stimulus such as a slap or putting the finger in the gluteal fold ("goosing") produces acute distress with trembling, jumping, or whirling around. This reaction could be provoked repeatedly in the same subject to the point of exhaustion.

Latah is based on a variant of Kretschmer's "primitive reactions," and exhibits hypersuggestibility, automatic obedience, coprolalia, and echolalia. It is very much like the traumatic neuroses described by Kardiner (1959) in that it sometimes becomes progressively more severe, with permanent psychic changes attributable to a reduction of the adaptive powers of the ego, leading to social incapacity. The part that organic factors play in determining such a course is not clear. The *latah* subject is unable to cope with sudden stress, or shock, which may in itself be quite ordinary, and reacts to it with severe ego-disorganization and anxiety. Many cases develop after an acute traumatic experience, although the experience may in some be traumatic only because of idiosyncratic fears, e.g., of certain worms and animals. The reaction may be precipitated even by mention of the feared objects, or—of great psychopathological interest—by tickling.

As a rule, *latah* patients are nervous and yielding; Aberle (1952) attempted to interpret this fact in terms of ambivalence toward submission, arising from "an unconscious connection between submission and a dreaded and desired passive sexual experience akin to being attacked." It is true that most patients are females and moreover females of low social class. Cross-culturally, an explanation in terms of class may be apposite, though it would not exclude psychodynamic formulations. Carluccio, Sours, and Kolb (1964) have sought to explain echo-reactions as mocking behavior, as well as on the basis of identification with the aggressor. I have interpreted *latah* in terms of gestalt field concepts and pointed out that echo-reactions are the simplest responses a psychologically disorganized subject can exhibit when placed in a demanding situation, since the figural stability and dominance of the impaired ego is overcome by the valences that bind it to the behavioral field (Yap, 1952). In technologically backward societies, the sense of hazard is so diffuse and pervasive that it is not practicable to develop a definite psychological set toward distinguishable dangerous objects in the environment; consequently powers of mastery are ill-developed and the ego weak. The *latah* reaction provides a clear example of impairment of consciousness produced by purely psychological factors and is thus important for general psychopathology.

Latah, like other (including somatic) diseases, is not regarded as abnormal unless it is of a certain degree; infrequently, severe cases involve homicidal complications, requiring expert diagnosis (Lloyd-Still, 1940).

Malignant Anxiety. This is the name given by Lambo (1962) to a common African syndrome of chronic anxiety without latent or manifest psychosis of separate etiology. It runs a progressive and socially crippling course but does not end in schizophrenic or organic deterioration. It is marked by tension and hostility, which in men (who more often show it) may lead to homicide, and in women to suicide. The patients often have markedly sensitive, moody, restless, and egotistic personalities and are usually preoccupied by fear of bewitchment. The bouts of intense anxiety with confused excitement not followed by amnesia cannot be explained on the basis of cerebral dysrythmia or hypoglycaemia. Lambo examined 29 patients and mentioned the occurrence of three major epidemics of this disorder. French workers in Africa also have described it and remarked on its frequency (Yap, 1962).

Malignant anxiety can be regarded as a clinically undifferentiated form of the hypereridic state, in which hostility accumulates in the patient without conversion into depression or psychoneurotic symptoms and may ultimately issue in destructive behavior either against himself or others, or, since ego-disorganization occurs, against both at the same time. The direction which aggression takes depends on a number of personality and environmental factors; when a culture prescribes a certain mode of aggressiveness against others following frustration, malignant anxiety can give the appearance of *amok*.

Amok. I have defined *amok* as a strictly psychogenic reaction based on hypereridism (Yap, 1958b). It therefore is to be placed alongside the acute psychopathic reactions described in constitutionally predisposed or intellectually subnormal persons under stress, familiar to psychiatrists everywhere; and should not be confused with apparently similar behavior caused by schizophrenia, epilepsy, or acute brain lesions resulting from toxic, exhaustive, or infective causes.

The only systematic clinical study of this reaction familiar to me is by Zaguirre, Professor of Neuro-Psychiatry at the University of the East in Manila (1957), whose little-known paper deals with military cases examined and observed in hospital. Most of his cases—17 out of a series of 25—were purely psychogenic. He did not adopt the category of reactive psychosis; instead he diagnosed dissociation reaction in 6, hysterical fugue in 1, immaturity reaction (aggressive type) in 5, obsessive-compulsive reaction in 2, psychopathic personality in 2, and low intelligence (moron grade) in 1. Apart from obsessive-compulsive reaction, it would be legitimate to put all the above diagnoses aside in favor of reactive psychosis of the *amok* type; it is questionable whether Zaguirre would have given prominence to obsessional symptoms in the 2 patients had the term reactive psychosis been a diagnostic division available in the basically American scheme he used.

Amok is associated with dazing or clouding of the sensorium and subsequent amnesia, preceded by frustration. Too much weight should not be given to the element of learning involved in this reaction. The argument that all psychoneurotic behavior is due to maladaptive learning is no longer novel, and does not affect clinical diagnosis. *Amok* is definitely maladaptive and deviant and requires medical attention, as Zaguirre's material so well illustrates. No doubt many attacks are aborted because prompt measures are taken; the patients are kept in custody after their initial violence has been curbed but are not charged (Sechrest, personal communication). The report that the incidence in Java fell after *amok* runners were captured alive and jailed need mean no more, even if true, than that social measures can change the pattern and therefore the incidence of psychogenic reactions. It is not an argument against the abnormality of *amok*. Because of certain cultural forms, people in areas where *amok* occurs tend to develop a low frustration tolerance to interpersonal stress, reacting to such stress with blind rage. Such rage, however, is regarded as abnormal in its own milieu, and only a small minority exhibit this extreme reaction. It is mainly because of the significant cultural influence in the patterning of this reaction that the ordinary label of "acute psychopathic reaction" is not appropriate to it.

A psychogenic *amok*-like reaction occurring in Puerto Rico has been described by Rothenberg (1964) under the name of "Puerto-Rican syndrome" or *mal de pelea*. It is desirable to analyze such conditions going under their native designations in relation to the better-known *amok*. Rothenberg pointed out that in the local language the word "nervous" also means "angry."

Negi-Negi. This condition in the New Guinea Highlands has been reported upon recently by Langness (1965). He quoted the field and clinical observations of Sinclair (1957), who used the term "acute hysterical psychotic state." A similar condition in Papua under the name of *lulu* affects only males and takes the form of aggressive behavior which may be homicidal. Usually it is associated with the death of a relative, but the essentially involved frustration and hostile tension arising from it suggests a relation to *amok*. It is accompanied by fears of the departed and, as might be expected, is thought to be caused by spirit possession. More information is needed about this disorder. Although glossolalia is absent, perhaps it lies closer to the trance possession states than to *amok*.

Trance (Possession) States. It is useful to follow the example of Bourguignon and Haas (1965) and Bourguignon and Pettay (1964, 1965) and make a distinction between trance states and states of possession. I mean by trance any state of dissociated consciousness, psychologically in-duced and reversible, which is not associated with primary schizophrenic symptoms. From a certain point of view, dissociated consciousness also may be said to be narrowed or restricted. Automatism may appear in thematic speech and semipurposive behavior out of keeping with the subject's normal personality. Trance may be viewed in different cultures or sub-cultures as a mystical state, a disease per se, soul loss, or possession either by a feared or a benign spirit. Possession by benign spirits and, to a lesser extent, possession by evil spirits may not be considered within the field of medicine, but even when it occurs in a religious context the trance behavior may become so extravagant and uncontrolled that the subject is taken to a psychiatrist. It is true that in folk societies the medical and priestly func-tions of the shaman are not clearly separated, reflecting the uncertainty with which such reactions are regarded by the group. In terms of the modern psychiatrist's professional orientation, however, most instances of possession must be defined as abnormal. I have analyzed a series of patients who were brought to the psychiatric clinic because of spontaneous possession or possession with behavior so excessive that relatives and neighbors could not reconcile it with accepted spiritualistic cults or professional mediumship (Yap, 1960). As a rule, in such patients there is some degree of clouding and incoherence, but often it is possible to discern a thematic content in the symptoms, understandable in the light of the patients' real difficulties.

Because of differing social attitudes toward trance and because of the need for diagnosis differentiating trance, especially trance possession, from other illnesses, a clearcut definition of possession is necessary. I have offered the following basic definition (Yap, 1960), which utilizes a funda-mental concept of G. H. Mead and H. S. Sullivan, to identify the condition even in little-known and disparate cultures:

> It is a condition where problem-solving processes result in an
> unusual dramatization of the "me" part of the Self, that
> aspect being constituted by previous partial identification with
> another personality, believed to be of transcendental nature,
> whose relationship to the subject is not tested in reality
> but is elaborated in fantasy. The nature of the possessing
> personality can be psychologically understood in the light of
> the subject's own personality needs; his life situation; the
> personality characteristics either historical or symbolical of the
> possessing agent; and the subject's cultural background, which
> determines the normality or otherwise of such a condition.

Windigo. This psychosis, called *witigo, witiko,* and so on, is another example of a culturally patterned possession syndrome, occurring among the Indians of northeast Canada. The most systematic account of it is that by Teicher (1960), but Parker (1960) has offered the most pain-staking discussion of its relation to sociocultural and psychological factors. *Windigo* always is regarded as undesirable, deviant behavior which can culminate in homicide through cannibalism. The patient shows prodromal depression and anxiety before becoming possessed by the *windigo,* a giant monster with a skeleton and heart of ice feeding on human beings. The intrusion of this spirit sometimes cannot be resisted; subjects in the prodromal stage even may ask to be killed themselves. A *windigo* patient is treated first by shamanistic techniques, but once he becomes cannibalistic he is put to death. Experience with and fears of winter famine make the thematic content of this disorder comprehensible, but they cannot explain the clinical form it takes.

A further example of the possession syndrome goes under the name of *hsieh-ping* in Taiwan; it has no remarkable features (C. C. Hsu, personal communication) and appears to be similar to syndromes I have studied in Hong Kong. The introduction of this term into the literature was fortuitous and is a reminder that we must be on guard against a meaningless terminological explosion in comparative psychiatry.

Psychogenic "Magical" Death. The existence of this condition, —bearing also the deceptive name of "thanatomania"—must remain scrupulously *sub judice,* yet it is of outstanding importance for psychosomatic medicine. Cannon (1942) urged observers to give serious attention to it and even outlined simple clinical examinations for use in the field to test his hypothesis of the cause of death. Cannon's hypothesis is that grossly excessive sympathetic activity causes vasoconstriction in the visceral blood vessels and consequent damage through anoxemia to the capillary endothelium, leading to loss of blood plasma and blood volume, ultimately resulting in a fatal fall in blood pressure. He compared this process to the death of a decorticated cat from sympathetic overexcitement when the sympathetic system was intact. He also drew attention to deaths of men suffering from surgical shock, who are caught in a vicious circle of progressive hypotension, and pointed out that the relevance of psychological factors in this condition have long been recognized. Cannon's "emergency reaction" has its modern parallel in the "alarm reaction" of Selye; but facts accumulated in the study of the latter have yet to be applied to the subject here. Richter (1957), based on evidence from a study of sudden deaths provoked in laboratory rats, has suggested that excessive parasympathetic stimulation may be involved, but whatever the mechanism of death it is probable that an uncontrolled and unbalanced autonomic response based on terror is implicated (*see also* Barnett, 1964). Whether a cataleptic reaction similar to "decerebrate rigidity" arising from vascular, physiological decortication of the brain also takes place is a matter for speculation. Examples of stuporous conditions with shock occurring in war, accident, and disaster have been reported by many writers. In such cases, loss of fluid intake could have aggravated shock fatally. It is reported that patients succumbing to "voodoo death" are so convinced that they are about to die that they no longer eat or drink, but death comes too rapidly to be due to dehydration. In rural Hawaii, belief in the potency of Kahuna sorcery is still so strong that a case was reported recently of a child allowed to die of illness without the parents' attempting to seek medical treatment (Johnson, 1964).

Psychogenic death has been described in Polynesia, Australia ("boning"), and Africa. Lambo (1962) mentioned that African patients with malignant anxiety from fear of bewitchment may die unless indigenous psychotherapy is instituted. Cannon quoted reports of such patients, including several by medical men in the field; some of these reports stated that breaking of the spell by the same or another witch doctor led to sudden recovery. These examples seem to exclude the possibility of poisoning; in any case, a knowledge of powerful but subtle poisons or of their antidotes is not likely in most of the tribes where psychogenic death has been reported. This subject also has been surveyed by Ellenberger (1951). Needed now are alertness to the problem on the part of ethnologists and medical field workers, proper facilities for observation, and additional concrete findings which can stand up to criticism. It is relevant to draw attention to the *British Medical Journal* of November and December, 1965, wherein a number of clinicians in Britain gave admittedly anecdotal accounts of cases in which psychogenic factors appeared to be decisive in the deaths of patients seen in their ordinary practice. Psychogenic death, however, is more probable among primitives who can be plunged into unrestrained terror as a result of the absolute conviction that they are being killed by magical means than it is among others; even among them, it is likely that the psychophysiological reactions can appear in varying degrees of severity short of death. If this relativistic point of view is adopted, the condition becomes one of great interest to the student of medical psychology.

Further Research

The principal aim of this chapter is to show that it is possible to place the "exotic syndromes" in the context of present-day clinical psychiatry. Once this idea is accepted, the way is open to the use of various tested clinical research techniques to explore the nature of these syndromes, much as the reactive psychoses have been studied in psychiatrically developed countries. Undoubtedly modifications in tool and method will have to be made. It is important that first steps be taken in an effective direction. Detailed and systematic nosographic effort, as we have seen, is still required; [5] attempts should be made to distinguish essential from accessory symptoms, to tease out possible associations with other psychiatric and somatic illnesses, and to trace the natural history of each disorder in its elementary psychogenic form. From such studies, a consistent definition of each disorder in terms of modal symptomatology, and eventually, psychopathology, can be arrived at and provide a firm basis for further clinical research.

Much can be expected from the expert application of epidemiological techniques in this area, although it always will be necessary to find or to produce collateral demographic and socioeconomic control data in order to evaluate the significance of variations in incidence among different groups. Where social and cultural variables are difficult to interpret, they can be illuminated by life-history studies, which enrich and stimulate epidemiological research.

The skills and insight of the anthropologist are needed to help identify role and value conflicts and to analyze the belief systems at their basis. Personality formation as it is related to early training still merits attention, although interest in later life experiences should be given more careful scrutiny. It is necessary to find out why certain specific ego-defenses are employed rather than others more commonly encountered in ordinary clinical practice. Another approach would be to inquire how cultures specially organize biologically founded emotional responses, particularly the fear and rage responses, into unusual patterns that can become deviant even within their own cultures. Interesting data may be accumulated to enlarge understanding of ego development and, of crucial importance, ego strength.

Sophisticated inquiries of this kind can be expected to add a new dimension to classical controversies associated with such names as Bonhoeffer, Kleist, and Stertz over (1) the determination of clinical symptomatology by trauma; (2) whether there is a specific link between reaction and trauma; and (3) the extent to which fundamental human reaction forms as well as individual constitutional and personality predispositions determine responses to trauma. It seems, for example, that culture can induce highly nonadaptive, abnormal reactions to ordinary trauma which otherwise occur only after massive calamity. It appears also that symptoms normally associated with the acute brain syndrome can be produced by psychogenic, nonphysical factors, given the requisite cultural background. Indeed, it might be queried whether examples exist of specific psychological stress or trauma directly bringing about singularly abnormal behavior. Quite apart from practical gains, the identification of the "exotic syndromes" as atypical culture-bound variants of reactive psychosis thus raises a number of interesting questions for research, questions that touch on some of the basic problems of psychiatry.

NOTES

1.   The term "hypereridism" was introduced by Lindemann (1950) to denote a state of undifferentiated, morbid hostility. As general background for this chapter see Yap (1951, 1952, 1958a, 1958b, 1960, 1962, 1965a, 1965b).

2.   H. W. Maier uses "catathymic" to refer to an affect-laden complex in the Unconscious influencing conscious mental activity and behavior.

3.   Virchow's fame as the founder of cellular pathology has masked the fact that his general theoretical position was not narrowly atomistic and mechanistic. In 1848 he founded a new journal, *Die medizinische Reform*, in the first number of which he prominently stated: "Medicine is

a social science." His concept of the nature of disease logically led him
to the idea of social medicine (*see* Ackerknecht, 1953).

4.   Wallace (1961) has collected existing reports on *piblokto* and hazarded
the guess that it is only a manifestation of tetany. I believe it is hysteria
exhibiting a wide range of symptoms, including fits, because the disorder
is found everywhere, even among people not suffering from lack of
calcium. It is true that hysterical hyperventilation can produce alkalosis
and localized tetanic spasm.

5.   In the case of *amok*, *latah*, and *koro*, however, nosographic work almost
has reached the point of diminishing returns. Some 330 papers on these
subjects, mostly descriptive, have been listed by Professor Alfred G.
Smith of Emory University.

REFERENCES

Aberle, D. F. 1952. "Arctic hysteria" and latah in Mongolia. Transactions of the
New York Academy of Sciences (Series 2) 14:291–97.
Ackerknecht, E. H. 1953. Rudolf Virchow. Madison, University of Wisconsin Press.
Arieti, S., and J. M. Meth. 1959. Rare, unclassifiable, collective, exotic syndromes.
In American handbook of psychiatry. Vol. 1. S. Arieti, ed. New York,
Basic Books.
Astrup, C., A. Fossum, and R. Holmboe. 1962. Prognosis in functional psychoses.
Springfield, Thomas.
Barnett, S. A. 1964. Psychogenic death from stress in mammals. Viewpoints in
Biology 3:203–18.
Bourguignon, E., and A. Haas. 1965. Transcultural research and culture-bound
psychiatry. Paper presented at Meeting of the Western Division of the
American Psychiatric Association, Hawaii.
Bourguignon, E., and L. Pettay. 1964. Spirit possession and cross-cultural research.
In Proceedings of the 1964 Annual Spring Meeting of the American
Ethnological Society. J. Helm, ed. New York, American Ethnological
Society.
————. 1965. The self, the behavioral environment and the theory of spirit
possession. *In* Context and meaning in cultural anthropology. M. E.
Spiro, ed. Glencoe, Free Press.
Cannon, W. B. 1942. Voodoo death. American Anthropologist 44:169–81.
Carluccio, C., J. A. Sours, and L. G. Kolb. 1964. Psychodynamics of echo-reactions.
Archives of General Psychiatry 10:623–29.
Devereux, G. 1963. Primitive psychiatric diagnosis. *In* Man's image in anthro-
pology and medicine. I. Galdston, ed. New York, International Uni-
versities Press.
Ellenberger, H. F. 1951. Der Tod aus Psychischen Ursachen bei Naturvölken
("voodoo death"). Psyche 5:333–44.
————. 1965. Ethnopsychiatrie. *In* Encyclopédie médico-chirurgicale: psychi-
atrie. Paris, 18 Rue Seguier VIe.
Faergeman, P. 1963. Psychogenic psychoses. London, Butterworth.
Gwee, A. L. 1963. Koro—a cultural disease. Singapore Medical Journal 4:119–22.
Hallowell, A. I. 1934. Culture and mental disorder. Journal of Abnormal and
Social Psychology 29:1–9.

Hollender, M. H., and S. J. Hirsch. 1964. Hysterical psychosis. American Journal of Psychiatry 120:1066–74.

Jaspers, K. 1962. General psychopathology. (Translated into English by M. W. Hamilton and J. Hoenig.) Manchester, University Press.

Johnson, H. M. 1964. The Kahuna Hawaiian sorcerer. Archives of Dermatology 90:530–35.

Kardiner, A. 1959. Traumatic neurosis of war. *In* American handbook of psychiatry. Vol. 1. S. Arieti, ed. New York, Basic Books.

Kiev, A. 1965. The study of folk psychiatry. International Journal of Psychiatry 1:524–50.

Kretschmer, E. 1934. Textbook of medical psychology. (Translated into English by E. B. Strauss.) London, Chatto and Windus.

Lambo, T. A. 1962. Malignant anxiety. Journal of Mental Science 108:256–64.

Langness, L. L. 1965. Hysterical psychosis in the New Guinea Highlands. Psychiatry 28:258–77.

Leon, C. A. 1965. El "espanto": sus implicaciones psiquiatricas. Transcultural Psychiatric Research 2:45–48 (abstract). (Lecture to Second Latin-American Congress of Psychiatry, Mexico.)

Lewis, A. 1953. Health as a social concept. British Journal of Sociology 4:119–24.

Lindemann, E. 1950. An epidemiologic analysis of suicide. *In* Epidemiology of mental disorder. New York, Millbank Memorial Fund.

Linton, R. 1956. Culture and mental disorders. Springfield, Thomas.

Lloyd-Still, R. M. 1940. Remarks on the aetiology and symptoms of young-dah-hte with a report on four cases and its medico-legal significance. Indian Medical Gazette 75:88–93.

Maguigad, L. C. 1964. Psychiatry in the Philippines. American Journal of Psychiatry 121:21–25.

Meyer, J. E. 1961a. Problems of nosology and nomenclature. *In* Field studies in the mental disorders. J. Zubin, ed. New York, Grune and Stratton.

————. 1961b. An internationally acceptable diagnostic scheme suitable for comparative psychiatric studies. *In* Comparative epidemiology of the mental disorders. P. Hoch and J. Zubin, eds. New York, Grune and Stratton.

Murphy, J. M., and A. Leighton. 1965. Approaches to cross-cultural psychiatry. Ithaca, Cornell University Press.

Northrop, F. S. C. 1963. The neurophysiological meaning of culture. *In* Man's image in medicine and anthropology. I. Galdston, ed. New York, International Universities Press.

Odegaard, O. 1959. Psychiatric terminology. *In* Report of the Second International Congress for Psychiatry. Zurich, Orell Füssli.

Parker, S. 1960. The wiitiko psychosis in the context of Ojibwa personality and culture. American Anthropologist 62:603–23.

Richter, C. P. 1957. On the phenomenon of sudden death in animals and man. Psychosomatic Medicine 19:191–98.

Rin, H. 1965. A study of the aetiology of koro in respect of the Chinese concept of illness. International Journal of Social Psychiatry 11:7–13.

Roth, M. 1963. Neurosis, psychosis and the concept of disease in psychiatry. Acta Psychiatrica Scandinavica 39:128–45.

Rothenberg, A. 1964. Puerto Rico and aggression. American Journal of Psychiatry 120:962–70.

Rubel, A. 1964. The epidemiology of a folk-illness. Ethnology 3:268–83.

Schmidt, K. E. 1964. Folk psychiatry in Sarawak. *In* Magic, faith and healing. A. Kiev, ed. Glencoe, Free Press.

Schneider, K. 1959. Clinical psychopathology. (Translated into English by M. W. Hamilton.) New York, Grune and Stratton.

Sinclair, A. 1957. Field and clinical survey report of the mental health of the indigenes of the territory of Papua and New Guinea. Port Moresby, Government Printer.

Slater, E. 1965. Diagnosis of hysteria. British Medical Journal 1:1395–99.

Stengel, E. 1959. Classification of mental disorders. Bulletin of the World Health Organization 21:601–63.

Stevens, H. 1965. Jumping Frenchmen of Maine. Archives of Neurology 12:311–14.

Szasz, T. S. 1961. The myth of mental illness. New York, Hoeber-Harper.

Teicher, M. I. 1960. Windigo psychosis. *In* Proceedings of the 1960 Annual Spring Meeting of the American Ethnological Society. V. F. Ray, ed. New York, American Ethnological Society.

Thorne, F. C. 1944. Startle neurosis. American Journal of Psychiatry 101:105–109.

Van der Kroef, J. M. 1958. Indonesian social evolution: some psychological considerations. Amsterdam, Van der Peet.

Wallace, A. F. C. 1961. Mental illness, biology and culture. *In* Psychological anthropology. F. L. K. Hsu, ed. Homewood, Dorsey Press.

Yap, P. M. 1951. Mental diseases peculiar to certain cultures. Journal of Mental Science 97:313–27.

————. 1952. The latah reaction. Journal of Mental Science 98:515–64.

————. 1958a. Hypereridism and attempted suicide in Chinese. Journal of Nervous and Mental Disease 127:34–41.

————. 1958b. Suicide in Hong Kong, with special reference to attempted suicide. London, Oxford University Press.

————. 1960. The possession syndrome: a comparison of Hong Kong and French findings. Journal of Mental Science 106:114–37.

————. 1962. Words and things in comparative psychiatry, with special reference to the exotic psychoses. Acta Psychiatrica Scandinavica 38:163–69.

————. 1965a. *Koro*—a culture-bound depersonalization syndrome. British Journal of Psychiatry 111:43–50.

————. 1965b. Phenomenology of affective disorder in Chinese and other cultures. *In* Transcultural psychiatry. A. V. S. de Reuck and R. Porter, eds. London, Ciba Foundation.

Zaguirre, J. C. 1957. "Amuck." Journal of the Philippine Federation of Private Medical Practitioners 6:1138–49.

4.   Mental Health Surveys in Ceylon

M. G. JAYASUNDERA, Ph.D.
Mulleriyawa Hospital
Angoda, Ceylon

EARLY IN 1959 a Ceylon association affiliated with the World Federation for Mental Health met with representatives of government departments and interested groups and individuals to discuss Ceylon's contribution toward the World Mental Health Year in 1960. Two activities were decided upon at this gathering: (1) to disseminate propaganda widely in order to promote a better popular understanding of mental health problems; and (2) to undertake a prevalence survey to provide information for operational purposes. These two projects were undertaken by separate committees working with a co-ordinating committee having overall responsibility.

Knowing that surveys of mental illness in populations of Germany, Japan, and Taiwan had been costly in money or time or both, the Ceylon research committee hoped to obtain a close enough approximation to the true rate by utilizing the 3,400 village headmen in the country. These headmen often had been used for various types of censuses, had full lists of householders in their areas for food rationing purposes (since World War II), and, above all, their use would overcome the difficult problem of finding adequate funds. If approaches were made through the heads of government departments, the village headmen would not require additional payments for making a simple census of people known or suspected to be mentally ill.

The department heads sent out forms to the village headmen calling for such simple information as the name, age, and sex of all persons in each village during May, 1959, who met the following definition of mental disorder: *by mental disorder is meant any disorder of the mind, either congenital or acquired; all doubtful cases should also be included.* (Patients in government mental hospitals were to be excluded, since these figures were available from hospital records.)

Despite the expectation that the wide-open definition and stress upon inclusion of doubtful cases would result in overreporting, underenumeration was general. The obviously low and unlikely rate of 0.1 per cent was returned for all mental disorders in the villages. At this stage, Prof. G. Morris Carstairs visited Ceylon, and he and I visited a few village headmen. They appeared to have ignored the definition given them to follow. Their own individual concepts of mental disorder varied considerably, but it was obvious that in general they viewed the mentally disordered as "crazy" and probably dangerous people.

In 1960 as an outgrowth of the two committees already mentioned, the Ceylon Mental Health Association (C.M.H.A.) was established. Its research committee, having gained experience from the first survey attempt, decided to do house-to-house prevalence surveys of typical villages in different provinces to cover major representative groups of the population. Before planning any new mental health services, the first task was to gain some fairly reliable estimate of the number of persons needing psychiatric services and, as far as possible, their geographic location.

Before describing the method and procedure of the surveys, it may be useful to convey some idea of the setting and background of the research. The island of Ceylon is 25,332 square miles in size, and its population in 1960 was 10 million persons (recent figures approach 12 million). Although there are nine provinces, the island can be divided geographically into four zones. The southwest, which produces coconut, rubber, and rice, is well populated; the central hills, the tea-producing area, has a large immigrant Indian population; the flat dry zone is sparsely populated; and along the northeast coast the inhabitants are chiefly Ceylon Tamils and Moors. Ceylon's population is multiracial, with widely divergent traditions and practices. The Sinhalese form approximately 70 per cent of the population, the Indian Tamils 12 per cent, the Ceylon Tamils 11 per cent, and the Moors 7 per cent. In religion, approximately 64 per cent are Buddhists; 20 per cent Hindus, 9 per cent Christians, and 7 per cent Muslims. The Sinhalese and Tamils speak their own languages, and about 8 per cent of the population, including the Ceylon Burghers who are of European origin, speak English. Another three or four dialects, modifications of Sinhalese and Tamil, are used in particular geographical areas.

Investigating mental illness in such a heterogeneous culture presents many problems. Nevertheless, the research committee of C.M.H.A. planned to determine the prevalence rates in each of six or seven well-differentiated socioeconomic groups by single-day case-finding surveys. To date, four surveys using similar procedures have been conducted in order in the following areas:

1) *Aluthgama-Bandaragama* (September, 1960). The area surveyed consisted of two hamlets, about 19 miles east of Colombo, containing a combined population of 2,506 persons living in 440 households. Almost all were Sinhalese Buddhists engaged in agriculture.

2) *Seeduwa* (November, 1961). This village, about 20 miles north of Colombo on the western seaboard, had a population of 2,212 living in 394 households. Again the population was almost entirely Sinhalese, but the majority were Methodists or Roman Catholics, predominantly the latter. Employment was varied because some industrial concerns and the Katumayake Airport serving Colombo are situated within a few miles of the village. A considerable number of villagers, however, worked daily in Colombo business firms and government offices. Weaving and poultry raising were profitable spare-time employments.

3) *Vadukoddai* (May, 1962). The area surveyed consisted of two adjoining hamlets on the Jaffna Peninsula, 200 miles north of Colombo. The population numbered 1,519 and was almost entirely Ceylon Tamil, and Hindu.

4) *Uda Peradeniya-Urawela* (September, 1964). These two adjoining villages are in central Kandyan Province, 70 miles from Colombo but close to Kandy, the second largest city in Ceylon. The combined population of the two villages was 2,497 persons at the time of the survey who lived in 400 households. Almost all were Sinhalese, and Buddhists. Although some villagers still cultivated their paddy fields, many worked instead as unskilled laborers on the campus of the nearby University of Ceylon.

An interview schedule was designed to be completed for each household by the interviewers, who were medical students with some clinical experience. Because of the general reluctance of the population to admit mental illness owing to the attached stigma, it was thought that a direct inquiry into mental illness would defeat the main purpose of the survey. It was decided therefore to design the inquiry as a general health survey, putting the interviewee at ease by first obtaining general socioeconomic data, gradually probing into physical illness, epilepsy, and finally, mental illness. After the first survey, the interview schedule had to be revised and minor alterations made to overcome some difficulties in coding the initial results.

It was reasonable to expect that psychotic illness would be identified easily but that psychoneurotic illness could be missed easily. To avoid this happening as far as possible, detailed instructions were both printed in the schedule and included in the briefing sessions, mainly to introduce the interviewers to the common beliefs of the average person about mental illness and its manifestations. The interviewers were briefed to note every suspicious case. It was hoped that a wide enough net thus would be spread at the primary case-finding stage to assure that a subsequent visit by a psychiatrist to all cases of possible mental illness would establish reliable identification.

Once the area for each survey was delimited, at least two months were spent on essential preliminary work. The survey organizers visited the village together with the public health inspector of the area, an official who knew the area and was familiar with its residents. The purpose and method of the survey and any likely difficulties were discussed with him and a plan of action decided upon. Help in organizing the survey was solicited from all influential people in the area, such as community leaders, the village headmen, religious leaders, heads of schools and school teachers, and *ayurvedic* [1] physicians. The public health inspector mapped out the houses in the area, grouped them into sections based on a suitable working headquarters, such as a community center, school, or the health unit office, and allocated houses to each interviewer, the number varying according to difficulties such as access and distance. In the first two surveys, each interviewer visited about 10 houses, while in the third and fourth the number was 15. The public health inspector also prepared household lists, fixed numbers on all houses, and selected suitable guides to help the interviewers, at least one guide per interviewer. The guides generally were school children who knew the houses in their own areas intimately. The guide also was able to obtain help from an organizer at each center, whenever an interviewer had difficulty scoring a questionnaire.

Through the good offices of the Dean of the Faculty of Medicine and the President of the Medical Students' Union of the University of Ceylon, third- and fourth-year medical student volunteers with clinical experience who were accustomed to history taking were selected to conduct the interviews. About 60 medical students took part in each of the first two surveys, 30 students in the third, and 40 in the fourth. They underwent intensive training by means of formal lectures and discussions, with emphasis on elementary psychiatric symptomatology, interview techniques, and specific problems of interpretation that might arise. The medical students who took part in the actual interviewing were familiar with the language of the area, e.g., in Aluthgama-Bandaragama all spoke Sinhalese and in the Vadukoddai survey Tamil. On the day of the survey the interviewers were handed the household lists for the houses allocated to them. In all four surveys the number of households allocated to each interviewer permitted him ample time to complete his work. The assistance and advice of psychiatrists who were in charge of the separate sections were always available to the interviewers. These persons conducted a sample check on the interviewers' work to ensure accuracy.

The completed interview schedules were scrutinized carefully, and a team of psychiatrists returned about a month later to interview all persons even suspected to be mentally ill and to diagnose actual illness. The shortness of the interval between survey and diagnosis ruled out to a great extent the possibility of complete remissions.

The voluntary medical student interviewers differed for each survey, except that a few interviewers in the second survey also had taken part in the first. The organizers and screening psychiatrists were nearly the same for the first two surveys. Few organizers participated in the third and fourth surveys, however, because some of the original workers were away, and, of the few remaining, some had become apathetic. Undoubtedly, the results must have been influenced considerably by the flagging enthusiasm.

It is interesting to note in Table 1 the variations in the prevalence rates of mental illness among the areas surveyed. The highest rate of 1.0 per cent was recorded in the first survey, 0.5 per cent in the next, 0.6 per cent in the third, and 0.4 per cent in the last. Many factors could be responsible for the high rate of 1.0 per cent in the first survey. The fact that the people of Aluthgama-Bandaragama were used to various types of house-to-house surveys resulted in a ready response. Voluntary organizers and interviewers were at the highest level of enthusiasm and interest during the first survey, as evidenced by the participation of 60 medical student volunteers (more than the required number, allowing for stand-by helpers) compared with 50, 45, and 40, respectively, in each of the other surveys. A total of 116 cases of possible mental illness (including suspected) were found in the first survey compared with 60, 30, and 43, respectively, in the other three surveys.

The second area, Seeduwa, differed from the others in that it had the highest proportions of Christians, persons in high income groups, and persons regularly employed, as shown in Table 2. The reduction of the mental illness prevalence rate to 0.5 per cent in the second survey from 1.0 per cent in the first survey in Aluthgama-Bandaragama is somewhat understandable because of the affluence in the Seeduwa area.

Although the procedure in the four surveys was generally the same, the third and fourth surveys differed from the first two in some important aspects that may have influenced the results considerably. For instance, there was some difficulty in organizing the last two surveys because of the distance from the capital city, the headquarters of the C.M.H.A. The survey in Vadukoddai required overnight train travel and the weather was very bad on the day of the survey, facts which must have influenced the results considerably. Further, the ethnic-religious group in Vadukoddai, the Tamil-Hindu, is extremely conservative and has strong, deeply rooted beliefs and customs, which are known to affect adversely information gathering on such matters as stigma-ridden mental disease. As shown in Table 1, 66 per cent (six of the nine cases) of those considered mentally ill had resorted to indigenous remedies, possibly because Western psychiatric treatment was available only in Colombo, 200 miles away. Most cases were identified on the day of the interview by only two psychiatrists; a few left-over cases were screened by a psychiatrist a month later. All these factors are likely to have caused the prevalence rate to be lower than the true figure, although the range of difference is comparatively small.

In the fourth survey, that of Uda Peradeniya-Urawela, only 10 cases were found of the 43 screened. Screening was again done on the

Table 1 : Number of Personnel Used, and Number and Characteristics of Cases Identified, in Four Surveys

Item	Survey 1: Aluthgama-Bandaragama	Survey 2: Seeduwa	Survey 3: Vadukoddai	Survey 4: Uda Peradeniya-Urawela
Personnel				
Interviewers (medical students)	60	50	45	40
Screening psychiatrists	6	6	3	4
Cases				
Total screened	116	60	30	43
Identified as mental illness				
Male	10	8	4	5
Female	15	3	5	5
Total	25	11	9	10
Prevalence rate (per 100 population) of total identified cases	1.0	0.5	0.6	0.4
Diagnosis				
Schizophrenia	13	5	2	8
Affective illness	3	2	6	0
Organic psychosis	5	3	1	0
Neurotic illness	4	1	0	2
Total	25	11	9	10
Types of Treatment (in percentage)				
Western psychiatric	16	27	12	40
Ayurvedic	24	9	66	5
Other	8	9	—	5
None	52	55	22	50
Total	100	100	100	100

day of the interview by four psychiatrists. As in the third survey, distance of the area from Colombo caused considerable difficulty in organization. The enthusiasm of the organizers had reached its lowest ebb and the Secretary of the C.M.H.A. had to organize the survey more or less by himself.

Considering the procedures adopted and the overall results obtained from the four surveys, the first two surveys appear to be more reliable than the latter two. The prevalence rate in the first survey of 1.0 per cent (or 10.0 per 1,000 population) approaches the figure of 10.8 per 1,000 population produced in a survey conducted in Taiwan by psychiatrists screening total households in selected areas (Lin, 1953). As was necessary, cost per survey was extremely low, less than £50, because most of the work was done by volunteers or regular government employees.

To complete the original plan of surveying representative population groups, additional surveys are planned of a Muslim group, an Estate Tamil-Hindu group, and a combined Muslim-Tamil group living together in the eastern province of Ceylon. Two of these are expected to be completed in 1966.

The survey results can be criticized for not revealing the true prevalence rates, because each member of the population group was not screened. It is claimed, however, that such surveys suffice, at least for operational purposes, because they use the locality's criteria of mental illness in combination with a general health inquiry by properly briefed, medically trained interviewers reporting all probable cases, which subsequently are screened by psychiatrists. This claim is supported by the fact that the results obtained in the first survey, when participation was most effective, approach closely the figures Lin (1953) obtained by psychiatric screening of total households. Further, it is necessary to recognize that the community criteria of mental illness are of great importance in organizing mental health services catering to the community's needs.

In addition to the prevalence rates of mental illness, other important information was derived from the surveys. Only a comparatively small proportion of the mentally ill seek Western psychiatric treatment, and, probably of even more significance, around 50 per cent of the mentally ill were under no treatment at all, as indicated in Table 1.

Brief mention has been made of government mental hospitals and of indigenous treatment of mental illness, and more should be said about both. Most existing government mental health services are concentrated around the capital city of Colombo, which has a population of about one million. A large mental hospital (1,800 beds) at Angoda, 7 miles from Colombo, now is so overcrowded that it reminds one of the custodial care era. Nine miles from Colombo is the open-ward Mulleriyawa Hospital (850 beds), and at Pelawatte in the rubber growing southwestern district is a 300-bed mental hospital. Daily outpatient mental health clinics are conducted at the General Hospital in Colombo and recently in all the

Table 2: Percentage Distribution of Characteristics of the Populations in the Four Areas Surveyed

Characteristic	Survey 1: Aluthgama-Bandaragama	Survey 2: Seeduwa	Survey 3: Vadukoddai	Survey 4: Uda Peradeniya-Urawela
Total Population of Area	2,506	2,212	1,519	2,497
Ethnic Group				
Sinhalese	100.0	98.9	—	90.8
Tamil	—	0.8	100.0	6.7
Moor	—	—	—	2.0
Others	—	0.3	—	0.5
Total	100.0	100.0	100.0	100.0
Religion				
Buddhist	99.5	10.6	—	87.3
Hindu	—	0.2	99.3	4.8
Christian	—	24.5	0.7	1.5
Catholic	0.5	64.7	—	2.3
Muslim	—	—	—	2.0
Others	—	—	—	2.1
Total	100.0	100.0	100.0	100.0
Occupation of Head of Household				
Self-employed	6.5	7.1	4.8	7.3
Professional	—	—	—	3.0
White collar worker	6.8	18.9	15.4	4.3
Skilled worker	5.7	21.7	9.0	20.3
Unskilled worker	65.0	29.2	49.0	56.6
Pensioner	5.4	9.9	10.3	—
Unemployed	10.6	13.2	11.5	8.5
Total	100.0	100.0	100.0	100.0
Income per Month of Head of Household				
Less than 100 rupees (£8)	56.0	38.0	45.0	42.0
101-200 rupees (£9- 16)	29.0	27.0	26.0	30.0
Over 200 rupees (> £16)	10.0	17.0	10.0	8.0
Unspecified	5.0	18.0	19.0	20.0
Total	100.0	100.0	100.0	100.0

mental hospitals. Such clinics now are held thrice weekly at two other general hospitals about 30 and 60 miles, respectively, from Colombo.

At present there are 17 psychiatrists in Ceylon, all trained in the United Kingdom except 2 who were trained in Canada. Although it is proposed to spread the mental health services throughout the country by appointing psychiatrists to the major provincial general hospitals, up to now all psychiatrists have operated from Angoda Mental Hospital.

Indigenous *ayurvedic* medicine is practiced widely throughout the country, and a few practitioners cater especially to the mentally ill. A few centers provide inpatient treatment. At Vadukoddai an indigenous medical practitioner from another village had a treatment center where, on the day of the survey, two nonvillagers were noticed—a recovering maniacal patient (kept chained) and a psychotic female being cared for by her husband. A large and popular treatment center is run by a physician Buddhist priest at and around a temple at Neelammahara, about 12 miles from Colombo. Treatment there consists mainly of unpleasant unctions of oils, bitter decoctions of herbs, and somewhat painful means of restraint. Spontaneous remissions of fresh cases must constitute a good proportion of the accredited cures effected; patients reach this place very early in their illnesses. It is more or less the rule that every patient within range of this center who seeks Western psychiatric care has been under treatment there first. Many other remedies, such as "charming" by a *Kattadiya* ("charmer") or more elaborate "devil dancing" and other exorcising methods, are all exhausted before a patient ultimately sees a Western-trained psychiatrist. It is seldom that a patient is seen by the latter within one or two years of the onset of the first attack, although it appears that this period is becoming shorter. An investigation is in progress to determine the type of remedies resorted to, their frequency at each episode of a mental illness, and the time consumed by each of them, using a random sample of admissions to the Angoda Mental Hospital, which has about 6,000 admissions a year.

Granting that a considerable proportion of mental illness remits spontaneously, yet it is widely accepted that modern Western treatment helps the majority of patients to achieve earlier social recovery than does *ayurvedic* treatment. An attempt should be made to provide Western mental health treatment facilities for as many patients as need them, at the same time adopting known preventive measures. By working through the already well-organized Ceylon Public Health Services, results might be achieved relatively rapidly.

I shall conclude this chapter by outlining briefly certain ways in which such a program could be implemented, based on past experience with community health services.

The Ceylon public health system has a long history and a uniquely successful record by comparison with most developing countries of Southeast Asia. Over 35 years ago a health unit system was instituted; in these units medical and paramedical personnel carry out planned intensive health programs among 50,000 to 80,000 people in defined geographic areas, usually a small urban area and some surrounding rural areas. The importance of these health units, now numbering about 30, for an extended program of mental health work lies in the fact that their efforts are directed toward community co-operation in various projects involving traditional beliefs and attitudes.

In each health unit, a medical officer of health is in charge. He may have one or more assistant medical officers. Other important members of the unit are a public health inspector, a public health nurse, and a public health midwife. The duties of these staff members are largely those suggested by their titles, with the addition of an extensive school health program involving all members of the unit except the midwife.

Initially almost all activities of the health units met with considerable public opposition. In part, this opposition resulted from a lack of proper health education and prejudice carried over from past approaches to certain problems. Perhaps the chief difficulties arose, however, because the new measures involved a break with traditions, habits, and cultural or group beliefs of the population. In addition, the village quack healer, the soothsayer, and the untrained village midwife were vehemently concerned with maintaining the status quo to protect their own means of livelihood.

The sanitary inspector was indirectly responsible for much of the opposition. In earlier days his visit to a village elicited complaints about some sanitary provision on the premises of a man who knew no better or who lacked the wherewithal to provide required facilities. Such a man was often taken to court, fined or otherwise punished, and returned home none the wiser in matters of health education but full of fear and dislike for the sanitary inspector as a sort of policeman. The health unit approach of tact, persuasion, and health education to improve and provide environmental sanitation changed this situation. The usefulness of the sanitary inspector to the mental health programs was shown by the assistance he was able to provide in the village surveys already completed. His work load in sanitation is so heavy, however, that the sanitary inspector can do little more than lend his co-operation to furthering mental health programs.

Other major resistance to Western health work in the community centered about maternity and child welfare. The untrained village midwife, who was firmly established in every village, having successfully brought forth almost all that survived (the dead not being considered her responsibility), could not be dislodged easily. The villager could not understand why she was not good enough, having had such "success." Any maternal or infant deaths were put down to acts of God or the devil. At first the villagers could not believe that the young, usually unmarried, trained midwife could practice midwifery having had no experience herself in bearing children. Some of the earliest trained midwives even worked in fear of physical harm. They began, however, to pay domiciliary visits to each pregnant woman, giving valuable advice. With much persuasion, they brought her to prenatal clinics and gradually obtained her confidence. The authorities began to judge the midwives' work by the number of mothers brought to prenatal clinics, the deliveries conducted by them, and the amount of domiciliary work. Their tact and powers of persuasion were taxed to the limits. In spite of all prenatal care, often the untrained village midwife and the trained midwife both attended at the confinement of many an early subject, and the competition grew keen and acute at times. The breakthrough came gradually, with the aid of some legal provisions dealing with the untrained midwife.

The public health nurse supervised the midwife's field and clinical work. The earlier public health nurses were mostly married women with families, who took up field work in many cases because married women were not allowed to work in the ordinary hospitals as nurses or sisters. The public health nurse helped the young midwife to establish herself as a useful field officer in the maternity care service.

Maternity homes got established in certain areas where the public health personnel could provide institutional services complete with medical attention by the medical officer of health, often where a hospital was out of easy reach. Child welfare centers and clinics got established gradually to look after infants, though not a few early patrons came mainly to obtain a supply of dried milk which these centers often provided.

The main load of a mental health program operated through public health personnel must necessarily fall on the midwife and the public health nurse. The midwife has almost the same basic education as the public health nurse—a year's training in all. It is easily possible to include basic mental health training in the midwife's training program and to combine her with a public health nurse as an effective team for mental health work. They could do valuable work in mental health education during times when those they are caring for are most receptive, and greatly help in effecting preventive measures against known factors detrimental to the mental health of mothers and children and the family in general. They also could detect early causes of psychiatric disturbances.

The same approach used in establishing maternity homes and child welfare centers by public health authorities could be applied to instituting mental health programs to provide local outpatient and domiciliary care as well as short-term inpatient care in local hospitals in towns or in rural and cottage hospitals in the villages. Within the cultural context of an extended family system in Ceylon, with a strong stigma attached to mental illness and an attitude of reluctance to institutionalize their sick, a community care system should be welcome. The hospitals could house patients while relatives cared for them, if necessary. The rural and cottage hospitals easily could apportion a quota of beds for mental care provided by local physicians under the guidance of psychiatrists who could pay regular visits to such treatment centers scattered over a wide area.

Moreover, the oganized school health team of medical officer and health nurse with the public health inspector and midwives of the area where the village school is located could form an important mental health organization, aided by the co-operation of the schoolteachers in detecting, treating, and general settlement of emotionally disturbed children and defectives. In establishing school health work, few difficulties were encountered as long as the teachers co-operated as they usually did. A few deaths of children occurring after treatment with the early toxic drugs and some severe reactions to immunization created some prejudice and resistance, but these are almost completely forgotten now, and increased health consciousness has been achieved by health education and propaganda. The village school now forms the center of many a health drive and ready co-operation of all concerned is the rule. If the present health unit examinations at three levels of each student's career could include mental health aspects, it would be a natural, comparatively easy step toward identifying the mental health problems of many children which now are known only to teachers.

NOTE

1.   *Ayurvedic* medicine is an indigenous system of medicine widely practiced in Ceylon. It is derived from old Eastern systems of medicine largely utilizing herbs, oils, brews, and distillations. Diagnosis is based primarily on assessment of various features of the pulse. In treating mental disease, some practitioners still use stocks and other forms of restraint of varying levels, while various herbs and oils are applied to the head for long periods; drastic purgatives and decoctions also are used. For centuries this system of medicine has been passed from master to pupil at a personal level, mainly through the Buddhist clergy in Ceylon. Even today, most mental diseases are treated in a few *ayurvedic* centers operated by Buddhist priests.

      The government of Ceylon has given increasing recognition to this system of medicine recently and has set up a medical college to train additional practitioners. Efforts to establish the system on an acceptable scientific basis include the recent founding of a research center.

REFERENCE

Lin, T. 1953. A study of incidence of mental disorders in Chinese and other cultures. Psychiatry 16:313–36.

5. Mental Disorders in Taiwan, Fifteen Years Later:
    A Preliminary Report

TSUNG-YI LIN, M.D.

Mental Health Unit
World Health Organization
Geneva, Switzerland

HSIEN RIN, M.D.

Department of Neurology and Psychiatry
National Taiwan University Hospital
Taipei, Taiwan

ENG-KING YEH, M.D.

Department of Psychiatry
Medical College
National Taiwan University
Taipei, Taiwan

CHEN-CHIN HSU, M.D.

Taipei Children's Mental Health Center
National Taiwan University Hospital
Taipei, Taiwan

HUNG-MING CHU, M.D.

Department of Psychiatry
Medical College
National Taiwan University
Taipei, Taiwan

THIS CHAPTER presents some of the major findings of two successive epidemiological studies carried out at an interval of 15 years in three communities in Taiwan (Formosa)—Baksa, a rural area; Simpo, a small town; and Amping, a section of the city of Tainan. The emphasis in this chapter is on prevalence rates of various types of mental disorders among the Taiwanese inhabitants in relation to sociodemographic data collected simultaneously with the psychiatric investigation of all the inhabitants of the three communities. Taiwanese, as used here, refers to Chinese who were resident in Taiwan before the end of World War II and their descendants, as distinct from the mainland Chinese who came to Taiwan after the war and their descendants. At the time of the first study, the inhabitants of the three communities were practically all Taiwanese. The findings on the mainland Chinese who were included in the second study will be reported separately.

The first study was carried out between 1946 and 1948 to obtain objective data on psychiatric conditions which could be utilized as the basis for planning a mental health program as well as for further scientific investigation on mental disorders in Taiwan (Lin, 1953). The application of the findings of this study to actual planning of the mental health program has been reported elsewhere (Lin, 1961), and the survey has provided a continuing basis for research in Taiwan, e.g., a comparative study of mental disorders of Chinese and Formosan aborigines (Rin and Lin, 1962) and an epidemiological study of psychophysiological reaction (Rin, Chu, and Lin, 1966).

The combination of several favorable circumstances made it possible to attempt a continuing epidemiological study of mental disorders in Taiwan. Of primary importance has been the stability of the research team. The investigators who participated in the first survey have stayed with the Department of Psychiatry, National Taiwan University, and maintained an interest in the same field of psychiatric research. The Department of Psychiatry, the only psychiatric center in the country at the time, was entrusted with planning the mental health program and therefore has developed a special interest in the epidemiological approach; this interest invariably has had an impact on the research orientation of the staff as well as on the content of teaching programs for medical students. In fact, a number of students who collaborated in the first study as field investigators joined the staff of the Department and played a leading role in the second study.

The stability of the research team extends to the research technique. The case-finding technique used in the 1946–48 study also was used in a study of mental disorders among aborigines (1949–53), through which experience was gained in applying the same technique to a population group with different sociocultural backgrounds. During this study and also during ensuing years in which data were analyzed, it was felt that the diagnostic criteria used were maintained practically unchanged. Not only the continuity of the principal investigator and his team but also the fact that the Department of Psychiatry is the only training center for psychiatrists in Taiwan made it more feasible to apply an identical research technique using similar diagnostic criteria to different population groups or to the same population groups at different times or both.

As stated in the report on the 1946–48 study (Lin, 1953), the cordial co-operation obtained from the communities, i.e., the officials, elders, teachers, doctors, and almost all the inhabitants, was a decisive factor in carrying out a successful survey. This excellent contact with the key leaders of the communities was maintained after the completion of the first survey, partly through established personal relations and partly through frequent professional contacts in follow-up studies of psychiatric cases discovered during the first survey or referrals of new cases for treatment.

A final factor of critical importance to a continuing study of mental disorders in Taiwan has been the availability of basic information about the population in relation to social change. One might think of Taiwan as an island of social upheaval in view of the influx of Chinese mainlanders, military tension, and rapid industrialization and urbanization, conditions which might vitiate any attempt at objective demographic investigation as a basis for a psychiatric epidemiological study. Carefully collected census data on all Taiwan inhabitants, frequently revised, sometimes once every two years, has made it possible, however, to obtain fairly reliable demographic information on the communities. The original records on the people that were filed for each household were made available to the investigators, thanks to the co-operation of the officials of the respective communities.

Methodology

The techniques used in the first study were duplicated in the second study, to the best knowledge and effort of the research team, in obtaining both the demographic data and psychiatric findings on inhabitants of the three communities.

The first stage of the investigation lasted for about four to six months in each community. Visits were made to all the leaders of the community: the administrative chief (the mayor, the district chief, or the village chief); officials of the administrative offices, particularly those dealing with census, welfare, and health; members of the town council; elders; doctors; nurses; principals and teachers of the schools; and police. These visits were intended, firstly, to explain the purpose of the proposed field investigation and to obtain their understanding and support, and, secondly, to acquire firsthand, intimate knowledge about the community in general, particularly the major changes that had taken place during the 15 years since the last study. Precoded schedules were used for copying demographic information from the original census records. These schedules were designed to contain information about each family and data on its individual members: name, date of birth, sex, family relationship including sibling order, education, occupation, health, duration of residence, housing, and religion. In addition to psychiatric information volunteered during contacts with the leaders of the community, efforts were made to obtain the names of possible psychiatric cases by asking a set of standard questions to a number of selected informants, such as doctors, teachers, police, and elders of the community, who possessed intimate knowledge regarding the professional, business, and personal affairs of the inhabitants. The set of questions referred to gross signs of abnormal behavior, attempted suicide, poor work record, poor school record, poor health record, police record, and addiction. The family record sheets copied from the census records were most useful for this purpose, since they enabled the informants to consider each member of a family systematically.

The second stage of the investigation, lasting two to three months, was concerned primarily with obtaining detailed psychiatric information on all cases reported in the first stage of the investigation while searching for additional psychiatric cases by consulting records of nearby public and private psychiatric hospitals, general hospitals, and health centers; it was carried out by two psychiatrists and a social worker or a psychiatric nurse.

In the final stage of the field work, every household was visited by a research team, consisting of a psychiatrist and a social worker or a psychiatric nurse, who conducted interviews with all members of each household. These interviews were carried out in a friendly atmosphere enhanced by the presence of a community leader. The latter would introduce the research team to the head of the family and explain the purpose of the visit as a health inquiry. As a rule, it was prearranged that all the adult members of a household stayed at home for the visit, and the research team interviewed them first in a group. Conversation started usually by asking about the main occupation of the family and the education and health of each member of the family. Every detail of personal data obtained from census records— age, sex, family relationship, date of migration, occupation, work situation, school attendance and religion—was checked; meanwhile their behavior, attitude, and content of conversation were scrutinized systematically. Any member of a household was singled out for an individual interview if he belonged to one of the following categories: (1) Those recorded through the first and second stages of the investigation as suffering or possibly suffering from some kind of mental disorder. (2) Those discovered to have a poor work record, a poor school record, a poor health record, or a police record. (3) Those manifesting abnormal behavior during the interviews.

The intensive individual psychiatric screening took the form of general psychiatric examination including history taking. Persons who were judged in accordance with prescribed criteria to be in need of psychiatric treatment were identified. These cases were referred to the principal investigator for final examination, and a clinical diagnosis was given. In a number of cases when two diagnoses did not agree, only a provisional diagnosis was given at this stage, waiting until a follow-up study before making the final diagnosis.

A brief description of the organization of the research and the preparation of the research team for the field work is in order. The senior psychiatrists, in collaboration with the principal investigator, took an active part in all research preparations, namely, preparation of family data sheets, a manual for obtaining and recording the social data, and a manual for psychiatric screening and diagnosis. They also visited the community, together with the principal investigator, to initiate the field investigation and took charge of it to the final stage. The preparation of field workers—including psychiatrists, psychiatric residents, social workers, and nurses—for the third stage of investigation was carried out by the senior psychiatrists, the epidemiologist, and the principal investigator. In this preparation, lasting for a month, emphasis was laid on acquainting the workers with the community and, more important, training them in the prescribed research procedures and uniform recording. The use of the manuals was rehearsed in actual interviews with psychiatric patients of the clinic and their families.

Social and Demographic Data

The total number of Taiwanese inhabitants in the three communities studied increased from 19,931 in 1946–48 to 29,184 in 1961–63, a 46.4 per cent rise in 15 years, averaging 2.6 per cent annually. This figure is somewhat lower than the overall 3.0 per cent rate of population increase in Taiwan; the difference presumably is caused by migration. The combined excess of out-migration to large cities or new industrial areas from all three communities was estimated to have averaged 7.0 per cent. This tendency was noted in all the three communities but was somewhat more marked than elsewhere in Simpo, a small town which is a market center amidst a rural population. Baksa was originally an exclusively rural area of five villages; while the population increased less markedly in three villages, it almost doubled in the other two villages which together have become one of Taipei's expanding suburbs containing residences, offices, and schools. The population increase in Amping was slightly less than that in most cities in Taiwan and also lower than that in the rest of Tainan City, for two main reasons: Firstly, the trade of the seaport of Amping has been in a continuous decline; and, secondly, Amping, located on a narrow strip between the sea and the main body of the city of Tainan, has no space for expansion to accommodate new industries.

As shown in Fig. 1, the age distributions in the populations of the three communities surveyed changed between the 1946–48 and 1961–63 studies. The age group 10–19 was significantly smaller in 1961–63 than in 1946–48 ($p < .01$). This drop may well be related to the low birth rate and the high infant mortality rate observed in Taiwan during and immediately after World War II. Probably because of the war losses of able-bodied youths, the age group 20–29 was significantly smaller in 1946–48 than in 1961–63 ($p < .05$). By contrast, the age group 40–49 was significantly smaller in 1961–63 than in 1946–48 ($p < .01$). Two factors may have contributed to this drop: Firstly, the relative shortage of the corresponding 20–29 age group in the 1946–48 population; and, secondly, the excess of out-migration of this age group. In addition, there was a significant increase ($p < .01$) in the age group 70 and over, probably paralleling the prolonged life expectancy of the Taiwanese population after World War II. While the whole population has increased by 46.4 per cent, the members aged 70 and over have increased by 74.7 per cent.

Fig. 2 gives the distribution of the educational background in 1946–48 and 1961–63. The dramatic fall in the illiterate proportion of the population ($p < .01$) was accompanied by a considerable increase ($p < .01$)

Figure 1: Percentage Age Distribution in 1946–1948 and 1961–1963 Surveys

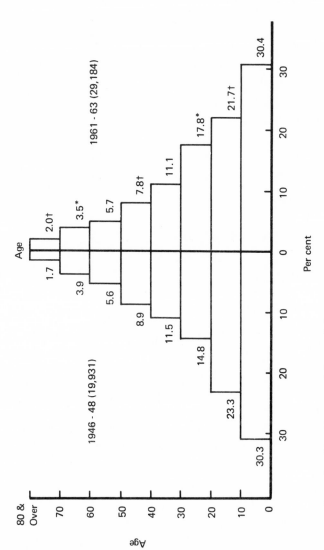

Comparisons between two populations studied:

* p < .05

† p < .01

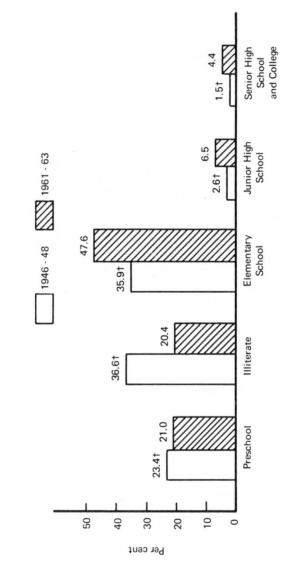

Figure 2: Percentage Distribution of Educational Level in 1946–1948 and 1961–1963 Surveys

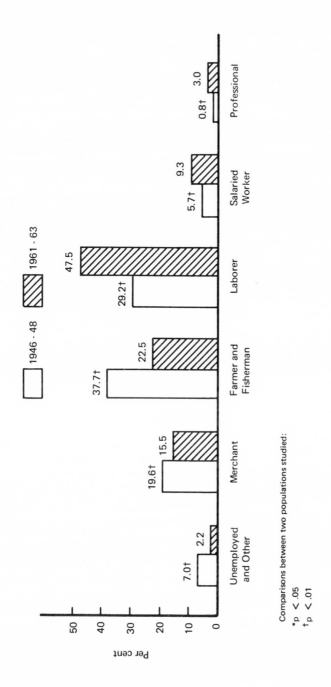

Figure 3: Percentage Distribution of Family Occupation in 1946–1948 and 1961–1963 Surveys

Per cent

1946 - 48   1961 - 63

Unemployed and Other: 7.0† / 2.2
Merchant: 19.6† / 15.5
Farmer and Fisherman: 37.7† / 22.5
Laborer: 29.2† / 47.5
Salaried Worker: 5.7† / 9.3
Professional: 0.8† / 3.0

Comparisons between two populations studied:
*p < .05
†p < .01

in the number receiving elementary, secondary, and higher schooling, a phenomenon consistent with the rapid educational development in Taiwan.

Fig. 3 illustrates the changes in the distribution of family occupation in the two studies. The marked increase of laborers ($p < .01$) in contrast to the significant decrease of farmers and fishermen ($p < .01$) is attributed to the rapid industrialization of the country. The decrease in unemployment reflects the relative prosperity of recent times compared to the immediate postwar period. The decrease in the number of traders may result from absorption of some of the small traders into factories and also into the salaried workers category. On the whole, the occupational distribution of the population in 1961–63 appears to reflect the social change in Taiwan over the preceding 15 years.

Psychiatric Findings

As illustrated in Fig. 4 and shown in Table 1, there was a significant increase ($p < 0.1$) from 9.4/1,000 in 1946–48 to 17.2/1,000 in 1961–63 in the prevalence of all mental disorders. Those in the 41–50 age group in 1961–63 were aged 26–35 in 1946–48. They were about 20–29 during World War II and, after bearing the brunt of war, had to readjust to changing patterns of life. The chief increase seems to have been among persons who were already adult at the beginning of the war; there was less change among those who have grown up under different circumstances since the war. Fig. 5 shows that this general pattern was observed in all three communities in 1961–63. Within the overall pattern, however, it was noted that the rates for older people were low in Baksa, which is still partly rural, and high in Amping, where trade has declined and healthy persons may have moved elsewhere in search of employment leaving a more vulnerable population.

In Table 2 the numbers and rates of mental disorders per 1,000 population in 1961–63 are given for each age group and sex. The prevalence rates for all mental disorders of all age groups showed no significant difference by sex (males 16.1/1,000; females 18.3/1,000). The high rates observed in 1961–63 at ages 41–50 were accounted for largely by the very high female rate; there also was a marked difference at ages 51–60.

As given in Table 3, the males showed a high rate of 6.3/1,000 of mental deficiency and 2.3/1,000 of psychopathic personality, compared to 3.5/1,000 and 0.4/1,000 of the respective female groups ($p < .01$ in both instances). These differences were noted in most age groups. Females showed an 11.3/1,000 rate of psychoneuroses, significantly higher than that of 4.3/1,000 in males ($p < .01$). The highest rates of female psychoneuroses were observed in age groups 31–40, 41–50, and 51–60, particularly in the middle group.

As illustrated in Fig. 4 and shown in Table 4, there was a significant increase ($p < .01$) in the prevalence of all mental disorders from 9.4/1,000 in 1946–48 to 17.2/1,000 in 1961–63. The two studies showed no significant changes, however, in psychoses as a general category: 3.6/1,000 in the first study and 3.1/1,000 in the second study. There was even a significant drop (p < .05) of schizophrenia from 2.2/1,000 to 1.4/1,000 for the total population. This drop was observed in almost all age groups. The marked overall increase in the prevalence rate was caused by the nonpsychotic group of disorders, notably mental deficiency and psychoneurosis. In the case of mental deficiency, the rate of 3.4/1,000 in 1946–48 increased to 4.9/1,000 (p < .05) in 1961–63, and psychoneurosis rose from 1.2/1,000 to 7.8/1,000 (p < .01). The age groups 31–40, 41–50, 51–60, and 61–70 showed the greatest increase in psychoneuroses, particularly among females.

Table 5 shows the rates of different types of mental disorders in various social classes in both studies. The drop in the rate of schizophrenia in the second study was significant in the lower class (p < .05), while the increase in that of psychoneuroses was observed in all three classes (p < .01). The prevalence of schizophrenia in the lower class in the second study, however, was still significantly higher than in the middle class. Similarly, the prevalence rate of mental deficiency was still greater in the lower class than in the middle and upper classes. The distribution of psychoneuroses differed: the upper class had the highest rate, the lower class the second highest, and the middle class the lowest.

Table 6 shows the differential prevalence rates of mental disorders in various educational groups. Clearly the group of people who received no formal education had the highest rates of almost all types of mental disorders in 1961–63. In comparison with the 1946–48 figures, the increase in prevalence was also marked in this uneducated group, especially in mental deficiency (p < .05), and psychoneuroses (p < .01). The other group showing a significant increase in prevalence consisted of the people who received an elementary school education.

The prevalence rates of mental disorders in different occupational groups in the two studies are shown in Table 7. The rate of total mental disorders showed a significant increase (p < .01) in all occupational groups except professionals and merchants. The increase in psychoneurosis was the single major contributing factor. The decrease in the rate of schizophrenia among merchants also was significant (p < .05).

In relating mental disorders and the area of residence, the residents in business areas showed a lower rate of total mental disorders than did the rest (p < .01) in 1961–63. As compared with the findings of the first study (1946–48), the concentration of schizophrenia in the densely populated central part of the community is no longer apparent. The higher prevalence rate of mental deficiency in farm and hill areas and the higher rate of psychoneuroses in residential areas observed in 1961–63, as presented in Table 8, were in line with the 1946–48 findings.

Table 9 shows the rates of mental disorders in different population groups according to the length of residence in the community and also the

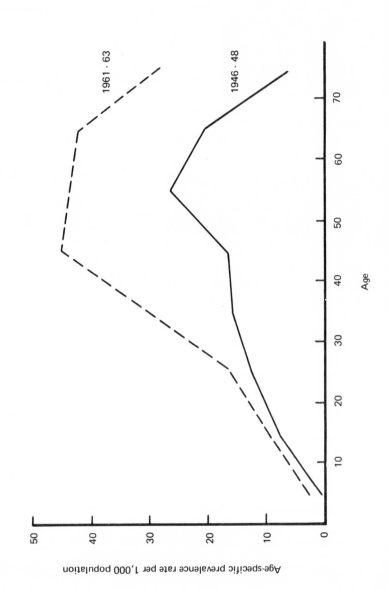

Figure 4: Prevalence Rate per 1,000 Population of Mental Disorders by Age in 1946–1948 and 1961–1963 Surveys

Figure 5: Prevalence Rate per 1,000 Population of Mental Disorders by Age in Three Communities in 1961–1963 Survey

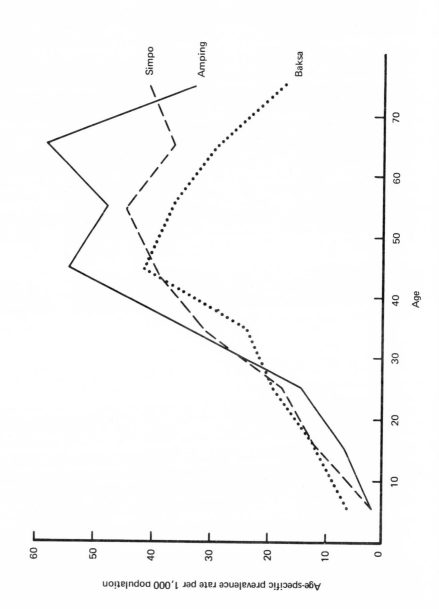

Table 1: Prevalence Rate per 1,000 Population of Mental Disorders by Age Group in 1946–1948 and 1961–1963 Surveys

Survey	Age Group								
	1–10	11–20	21–30	31–40	41–50	51–60	61–70	71 and Over	All Ages
1946–48	0.3	7.7	12.5	15.7	16.4	26.8	20.7	5.9	9.4
1961–63	2.8†	9.8	16.1	30.0†	45.0†	43.5†	42.4†	28.6†	17.2†

Comparisons between two populations studied:
* p < .05
† p < .01

Table 2: Frequency and Prevalence Rate per 1,000 Population of Mental Disorders by Sex and Age Group in 1961–1963 Survey

Frequency and Rate	Age Group								
	1–10	11–20	21–30	31–40	41–50	51–60	61–70	71 and Over	All Ages
Frequency									
Male	17	36	46	47	35	29	22	5	237
Female	8	26	38	50	67	43	21	12	265
Rate									
Male	3.7	10.9	17.9	28.7	31.4	36.0	44.4	20.1	16.1
Female	1.8	8.6	14.4	31.4	58.3†	50.9†	40.7	34.8	18.3

Comparisons between male and female:
* p < .05
† p < .01

Table 3: Prevalence Rate per 1,000 Population by Age, Sex, and Diagnostic Group in 1961–1963 Survey

Diagnostic Group	Age Group and Sex									
	1–10		11–20		21–30		31–40		All Ages	
	M	F	M	F	M	F	M	F	M	F
Schizophrenia	—	—	0.3	—	1.6	1.1	3.7	3.8	1.2	1.6
Manic-depressive psychoses	—	—	0.3	—	1.2	0.4	0.6	0.6	0.8	0.4
Senile psychoses	—	—	—	—	—	—	—	—	0.3	0.5
Other psychoses	—	—	0.6	0.6	1.2	—	1.2	2.5	1.0	0.6
Mental deficiency	3.7	1.8	6.7	5.9	6.2	3.4	12.8	3.1†	6.3	3.5†
Psychopathic personality	—	—	0.6	0.3	3.1	—	3.1	—	2.3	0.4†
Psychoneuroses	—	—	2.4	1.6	4.7	9.5*	7.3	21.3†	4.3	11.3†

Diagnostic Group	41–50		51–60		61–70		71 and Over	
	M	F	M	F	M	F	M	F
Schizophrenia	3.6	1.7	2.5	7.1	2.0	7.8	—	5.8
Manic-depressive psychoses	2.7	2.6	1.2	1.2	2.0	—	—	—
Senile psychoses	—	—	—	—	—	5.8	16.1	11.6
Other psychoses	1.8	0.9	6.2	1.2	2.0	—	—	2.9
Mental deficiency	2.7	7.0	7.4	2.4	14.1	—	4.0	—
Psychopathic personality	7.2	0.9	5.0	1.2	14.1	1.9	—	5.8
Psychoneuroses	13.4	45.2†	13.6	37.8†	10.1	25.2	—	8.7

Comparisons of male and female rates within diagnostic groupings:
* p < .05
† p < .01

Table 4: Prevalence Rate per 1,000 Population by Age Group and Diagnostic Group in 1946–1948 and 1961–1963 Surveys

Diagnostic Group	Age Group							
	1–10		11–20		21–30		31–40	
	1946–48	1961–63	1946–48	1961–63	1946–48	1961–63	1946–48	1961–63
Schizophrenia	—	—	0.9	0.2	2.0	1.3	6.1	3.7
Manic-depressive psychoses	—	—	—	0.2	1.0	0.8	1.3	0.6
Senile psychoses	—	—	—	—	—	—	—	—
Other psychoses	—	—	—	0.6	0.7	0.6	0.9	1.8
Mental deficiency	0.3	2.8†	6.7	6.3	4.1	4.8	3.5	8.0*
Psychopathic personality	—	—	0.2	0.5	2.4	1.5	0.9	1.5
Psychoneuroses	—	—	—	2.0	2.4	7.1†	3.0	14.2†
All diagnoses	0.3	2.8†	7.8	9.8	12.6	16.1	15.7	29.8†
Total population	6,045	8,883	4,647	6,338	2,953	5,203	2,288	3,232

Table 4: (Continued)

	Age Group									
	41–50		51–60		61–70		71 and Over		All Ages	
Diagnostic Group	1946–48	1961–63	1946–48	1961–63	1946–48	1961–63	1946–48	1961–63	1946–48	1961–63
Schizophrenia	4.0	2.6	7.2	4.8	5.2	4.9	–	3.4	2.2	1.4*
Manic-depressive psychoses	1.7	2.6	2.7	1.2	1.3	1.0	–	–	0.6	0.5
Senile psychoses	–	–	–	–	6.5	3.0	2.9	13.5	0.3	0.4
Other psychoses	2.3	1.3	3.6	3.6	2.6	1.0	–	1.7	0.7	0.8
Mental deficiency	2.3	4.8	7.2	4.8	3.9	6.9	–	1.7	3.4	4.9*
Psychopathic personality	2.8	4.0	2.7	3.0	1.3	7.9	2.9	3.4	1.0	1.4
Psychoneuroses	3.4	29.6†	3.6	26.0†	–	17.8†	–	5.0	1.2	7.8†
All diagnoses	16.5	44.9†	27.0	43.4†	20.8	42.5†	5.8	28.7†	9.4	17.2†
Total population	1,768	2,267	1,117	1,654	773	1,013	340	594	19,931	29,184

Comparisons between two populations studied:
* p < .05
† p < .01

Table 5: Prevalence Rate per 1,000 Population by Diagnostic Group and Social Class in 1946–1948 and 1961–1963 Surveys

| | Social Class | | | | | | | |
| | Upper Class | | Middle Class | | Lower Class | | Total | |
Diagnostic Group	1946-48	1961-63	1946-48	1961-63	1946-48	1961-63	1946-48	1961-63
Schizophrenia	3.5	0.8	1.2	1.1	4.5	2.1*	2.2	1.4*
Manic-depressive psychoses	1.1	–	0.6	0.7	0.6	0.3	0.7	0.5
Senile psychoses	–	–	0.1	0.4	0.9	0.4	0.3	0.4
Other psychoses	0.6	2.5	0.5	0.9	1.3	0.4	0.7	0.8
Mental deficiency	1.1	0.8	2.6	3.0	6.6	9.4†	3.4	4.9*
Psychopathic personality	1.1	–	0.7	0.7	1.9	2.9	1.0	1.4
Psychoneuroses	2.9	13.1†	0.9	7.0†	1.5	8.7†	1.2	7.8†
All diagnoses	10.3	17.2	6.6	13.8†	17.3	24.2†	9.5	17.2†
Total population	1,727	1,218	13,501	18,998	4,703	8,968	19,931	29,184

Comparisons between two populations studied:
* p < .05
† p < .01

place of origin in 1961–63. There was no significant variation in the prevalence rates of schizophrenia, manic-depressive psychoses, and other psychoses among the original inhabitants and the migrant Taiwanese. It is worth noting that senile psychoses were found only among the original inhabitants. Mental deficiency was significantly higher among the original inhabitants than among the migrant Taiwanese. The most striking difference was observed in the rates of psychoneuroses. Among the original inhabitants, the rate was 6.9/1,000, which was already five times higher than the figure in the previous study and yet represented only half of the figure of 12.1/1,000 for the group of migrant Taiwanese (p < .01). It was in this group of mental disorders that a most significant difference (p < .01) was observed between the Chinese mainlanders and the Taiwanese: the rate of the former was 16.1/1,000, more than double that of the original inhabitants and nearly 30 per cent higher than that of the migrant Taiwanese. The 2.9/1,000 rate of mental deficiency among Chinese mainlanders was significantly lower (p < .01) than that among the original inhabitants, comparable to that of the migrant Taiwanese. There was no significant difference between Taiwanese and Chinese mainlanders in the crude rates of schizophrenia and other psychoses.

Conclusions

Comparison of mental disorders between two or more population groups with different characteristics probably has been one of the most interesting subjects in psychiatry, and literature on it has abounded since the time of Kraepelin. When strict scientific criteria are applied to evaluate the comparability of such studies, however, few apparently can stand the test, a situation which seems unavoidable at the present stage of scientific development of psychiatry and social science. Several major factors contribute to the difficulty of comparative study of mental disorders.

The concept of mental disorder varies extremely among different cultures and also among certain population subgroups within one culture. In the absence of clearcut etiology for most mental disorders, social criteria usually play a dominant role in identifying a psychiatric case and hence make comparative study difficult.

In addition to cultural variation in the concept of mental disorder, the divergent views of different schools of psychiatry on the etiology of mental disorder is the single major factor barring a uniform classification of psychiatric disorders. The lack of uniformity even extends to the descriptive terms of individual psychiatric symptoms, syndromes, or deviant behaviors.

Furthermore, the method of identification of a case varies according to several factors. The purposes of studies—e.g., to estimate the number of psychiatric patients in need of hospital care or to count the number of people mentally disqualified for military service—require different diagnostic criteria and techniques for case identification in different samples. The choice

Table 6: Prevalence Rate per 1,000 Population by Diagnostic Group and Education in 1946–1948 and 1961–1963 Surveys

	Education					
	No Formal Education		Preschool		Elementary	
Diagnostic Group	1946–48	1961–63	1946–48	1961–63	1946–48	1961–63
Schizophrenia	3.8	3.7	—	—	1.1	1.2
Manic-depressive psychoses	0.7	0.5	—	—	0.7	0.9
Senile psychoses	0.5	1.8	—	—	0.3	—
Other psychoses	1.1	0.7	—	—	0.6	0.8
Mental deficiency	5.8	10.4*	0.2	1.3	3.5	5.0
Psychopathic personality	1.8	2.9	—	—	0.8	1.5
Psychoneuroses	1.2	20.4†	—	—	1.5	5.5†
All diagnoses	14.9	40.4†	0.2	1.3	8.5	14.9†
Total population	7,287	5,940	4,674	6,140	7,162	13,904

Table 6: (Continued)

| | Education | | | | | | | |
Diagnostic Group	Junior High		Senior High		College		Total	
	1946–48	1961–63	1946–48	1961–63	1946–48	1961–63	1946–48	1961–63
Schizophrenia	5.7	—	13.0	1.9	18.2	—	2.2	1.4*
Manic-depressive psychoses	3.8	—	4.3	—	—	—	0.6	0.5
Senile psychoses	—	—	—	—	—	—	0.3	0.4
Other psychoses	3.8	3.1	—	1.0	—	8.0	0.7	0.8
Mental deficiency	—	1.6	—	—	—	—	3.4	4.9*
Psychopathic personality	1.9	0.5	—	1.0	—	—	1.0	1.4
Psychoneuroses	3.8	7.3	8.7	12.5	—	12.0	1.2	7.8†
All diagnoses	19.0	12.5	26.0	16.4	18.2	20.0	9.4	17.2†
Total population	522	1,910	231	1,039	55	251	19,931	29,184

Comparisons between two populations studied:
* p ∨ .05
† p ∨ .01

Table 7: Prevalence Rate per 1,000 Population by Diagnostic Group and Family Occupation in 1946–1948 and 1961–1963 Surveys

	Family Occupation							
	Professional		Salaried Worker		Merchant		Farmer and Fisherman	
Diagnostic Group	1946–48	1961–63	1946–48	1961–63	1946–48	1961–63	1946–48	1961–63
Schizophrenia	—	—	0.9	0.4	3.6	0.9†	1.7	1.1
Manic-depressive psychoses	6.4	—	0.9	1.5	1.3	0.4	0.4	0.3
Senile psychoses	—	2.3	—	—	0.3	—	0.5	0.6
Other psychoses	—	3.4	0.9	1.5	0.8	0.2	0.5	0.6
Mental deficiency	—	3.4	0.9	3.3	1.3	2.9	4.1	6.2
Psychopathic personality	6.4	1.1	0.9	0.7	0.5	1.5	0.4	1.1
Psychoneuroses	12.8	13.8	0.9	11.8†	1.3	6.4†	0.9	5.5†
All diagnoses	25.6	24.0	5.4	19.2†	9.1	12.3	8.5	15.4†
Total population	156	871	1,138	2,710	3,912	4,526	7,512	6,569

Table 7: (Continued)

Diagnostic Group	Family Occupation							
	Laborer		Unemployed		Other		Total	
	1946–48	1961–63	1946–48	1961–63	1946–48	1961–63	1946–48	1961–63
Schizophrenia	1.7	1.9	3.8	5.5	—	—	2.2	1.4*
Manic-depressive psychoses	0.3	0.6	0.8	—	—	—	0.6	0.5
Senile psychoses	0.2	0.4	—	—	—	—	0.3	0.4
Other psychoses	0.7	0.8	1.5	1.8	—	—	0.7	0.8
Mental deficiency	3.3	5.0	9.1	9.1	—	18.7	3.4	4.9*
Psychopathic personality	1.9	1.4	1.5	7.3	—	—	1.0	1.4
Psychoneuroses	1.4	7.4†	—	23.7†	11.6	28.0	1.2	7.8†
All diagnoses	9.5	17.5†	16.7	47.4†	11.6	46.7†	9.4	17.2†
Total population	5,813	13,853	1,314	548	86	107	19,931	29,184

Comparisons between two populations studied:
* p < .05
† p < .01

of method for case identification, e.g., questionnaires, interviews, psychological testing, or combinations of these, also greatly influences the results. Professional background and special training in research methodology of the research workers also greatly influence the results. When more than one investigator is involved, consistency and reliability in the use of screening techniques are of great importance for judging the quality of data produced.

Measurement of the degree of psychiatric impairment also presents a serious problem in a comparative study. The difficulty inherent in quantifying normal and deviant human behavior, especially when the observer himself is an intimate participant in the process under study, makes a precise comparison hard to achieve. The multiplicity of dynamic factors interacting in mental illness makes exact reproduction of the situation under study impossible. This problem is complicated further by the chronicity of mental illness, a factor which introduces the element of change in time.

In the second study of the three communities in 1961–63, care was taken to insure maximum comparability to the best ability of the investigators. As mentioned previously, the repeated use of the same research technique by the same investigators provided a reasonable foundation for comparability. The specific psychiatric and sociological questions and the instruction manuals for investigators used in the first study were reproduced

Table 8: Prevalence Rate per 1,000 Population by Diagnostic Group and Living Area in 1961–1963 Survey

Diagnostic Group	Living Area			
	Business	Residential	Farm	Hill
Schizophrenia	1.2	1.4	1.8	1.0
Manic-depressive psychoses	0.5	0.6	0.2	1.4
Senile psychoses	0.3	0.2	0.7	0.5
Other psychoses	1.3	0.3	1.2	1.9
Mental deficiency*	3.2	4.6	7.0	6.3
Psychopathic personality	1.0	1.8	0.5	1.4
Psychoneuroses[†]	5.2	9.1	8.0	4.8
All diagnoses[††]	12.6	18.1	19.5	17.5
Total population	6,007	15,526	5,591	2,060

* Comparison between business + residential area and farm + hill area, p <.01.
[†] Comparison between residential area and business area, p <.05.
[††] Comparison between business area and residential area, p <.01; between business area and farm area, p <.01.

after careful study and confirmation of their relevance for use in the second study. In training investigators for the second study, the main concerns were to acquaint them with details and, more importantly, to teach them to perform and record investigations uniformly with the least possible observer's error. Cross-validation techniques were used for testing the reliability of observations as well as for assessing the quality of the investigators in training. Concern for the stability of diagnostic criteria used in the two studies was so strong that a test was given to assess agreement in this regard. The case histories of the first study, without diagnostic labels, were given to two psychiatrists, a senior psychiatrist who had participated in the previous study and a psychiatrist with six years of psychiatric training and experience. Each made an independent diagnosis of each case including subclassifying psychosis or neurosis wherever possible. The extent of agreement turned out to be very high: 96.2 per cent between the diagnosis of Dr. A and the previous diagnosis; 92 per cent between the diagnosis of Dr. B and the previous diagnosis; and 91.5 per cent between diagnoses of the two psychiatrists.

Table 9: Number and Prevalence Rate per 1,000 Population by Diagnostic Group and Cultural Group in 1961–1963 Survey

	Cultural Group					
	Taiwanese				Mainlanders	
	Original Inhabitants (Residence ≥15 Years)		Migrants (Residence <15 Years)		(Residence <15 Years)	
Diagnostic Group	Number	Rate	Number	Rate	Number	Rate
Schizophrenia	35	1.4	6	1.2	19	1.9
Manic-depressive psychoses	15	0.6	1	0.2	1	0.1
Senile psychoses	11	0.5	–	–	–	–
Other psychoses	20	0.8	4	0.8	9	0.9
Mental deficiency*	125	5.1	18	3.7	29	2.9
Psychopathic personality†	37	1.5	3	0.6	19	1.9
Psychoneuroses††	168	6.9	59	12.1	158	16.1
All diagnoses§	411	16.9	91	18.7	235	23.9

* Comparison between Taiwanese original inhabitants and mainlanders, p <.01.
† Comparison between Taiwanese migrants and original inhabitants, p<.05;
  between Taiwanese migrants and mainlanders, p<.05.
†† Comparisons between all pairs among the three groups, p<.01.
§ Comparison between Taiwanese original inhabitants and mainlanders, p<.01;
  between Taiwanese migrants and mainlanders, p<.01.

On the strength of the above precautions taken to insure a maximum degree of uniformity of criteria and methodology in the two studies, I will proceed to comment on some of the major findings.

The fact that no increase was observed in psychotic disorders in the three communities over the 15-year period from 1946–48 to 1961–63 constituted a striking contrast to the significant increase in nonpsychotic disorders, especially psychoneuroses. Though it may be possible that the diagnostic criteria were maintained better and applied more uniformly by the investigators to psychotic disorders than to nonpsychotic disorders, the marked difference between the two groups of disorders is more real than apparent. Psychotic disorders seem to be affected less by environmental changes than are nonpsychotic disorders. It also is possible that the span of 15 years was too short a period for environmental factors to provoke a psychotic process in a sufficient number of persons within a population to affect the prevalence rate. This finding also may be taken to support the fairly widespread view that some innate genetic or organic factors play a more important role in the etiology of psychotic disorders than in that of neurotic disorders, but the preliminary data presented in this paper are insufficient to warrant further discussion on this finding.

The significant decrease of schizophrenia in the second study, especially in the lower class and among merchants, deserves attention. Since no special age group, sex, or educational level was found to be associated with this finding, further analysis of data is needed for a plausible explanation.

The most interesting findings concerned psychoneuroses. While the prevalence rate of psychoneuroses for the whole investigated population increased significantly ($p < .01$), several population subgroups particularly contributed to this phenomenon. Regardless of social class, the middle age groups (31–40, 41–50, 51–60) with elementary education or no formal education showed the most significant increase in psychoneuroses, particularly females and people who had moved into the communities investigated since the first study. The differences in prevalence rates of psychoneuroses among original inhabitants, migrant Taiwanese, and Chinese mainlanders suggest a positive correlation between psychoneurotic manifestation and degree of stress accompanying in-migration. For mental deficiency, on the contrary, a higher prevalence rate was noted among the original inhabitants than among the other groups. This finding may be attributable to low mobility of mental defectives.

ACKNOWLEDGMENT

This investigation was aided by a grant from the Foundations' Fund for Research in Psychiatry (FFRP Grant 62-257).

REFERENCES

Lin, T. 1953. A study of incidence of mental disorders in Chinese and other cultures. Psychiatry 16:313–36.

————. 1961. Evolution of mental health program in Taiwan. American Journal of Psychiatry 117:961–71.

Rin, H., and T. Lin. 1962. Mental illness among Formosan aborigines as compared with the Chinese in Taiwan. Journal of Mental Science 108:134–46.

Rin, H., H. M. Chu, and T. Lin. 1966. Psychophysiological reactions of a rural and suburban population in Taiwan. Acta Psychiatrica Scandinavica 42:410–73.

6. Psychiatric Epidemiological Surveys in Japan:
    The Problem of Case Finding

MASAAKI KATO, M.D.
National Institute of Mental Health
Konodai, Ichikawa-shi
Chiba-ken, Japan

Nationwide Epidemiological Surveys

Between 1954 and 1963, the Japanese Ministry of Health and Welfare carried out five nationwide epidemiological surveys on mental disorders: The First Nationwide Prevalence Survey of Mental Disorders in 1954; the Nationwide Survey of Hospitalized Mental Disorders in 1956; the Nationwide Survey of Attitudes toward Mental Disorders in 1960; Follow-up Study of Newly Treated Mental Disorders in 1960–61; and The Second Nationwide Prevalence Survey in 1963. Accounts of these studies have been published by the Japanese Ministry of Health and Welfare (1955, 1957, 1965), and the author (Kato, 1962).

In this chapter I will review these national surveys and also a number of regional studies, particularly with reference to the problem of case finding. Prevalence surveys before World War II in Japan were limited to specific regional populations, i.e., isolated islands, some rural districts, or certain districts in a metropolis. The survey carried out in 1954 was the first nationwide survey attempted in Japan. Both the 1954 and 1963 surveys were made in order to estimate the number of persons needing treatment for mental disorders, to obtain basic data for promoting mental health programs, and to afford a basis for comparison.

In order to obtain stratified random samples in the two nationwide surveys, the Statistical Bureau of the Ministry of Health and Welfare selected 100 out of 3,690 national census areas in 1954 and 203 out of 2,792 national census areas in 1963. The selection of sample census areas in 1954 was based on whether the area was predominantly urban or rural and on the predominant type of occupation (fishing, farming, clerical work, factory work, and so on) followed by householders in the area. This process resulted in stratifying the selection of census areas in 1954 into 14 different types of sample areas (e.g., urban and rural factory areas, urban and rural fishing areas). In 1963 the criteria for selection of sample areas were somewhat different. The first criterion was whether the area was predominantly metropolitan, suburban, or rural. The second criterion again was the predominant occupation of householders in the area. This process resulted in stratifying the selection of sample areas into 18 different types. The total number of households surveyed in 1954 was 4,895, and these households contained 23,993 persons. In the 1963 survey, the total number of households was 11,853, and these included 44,092 persons.

The choice of leading psychiatrists, psychologists, sociologists, and statisticians to serve on a committee for each national prevalence survey was referred by the Minister of Health and Welfare to the National Council for Mental Health. Drs. Hayashi, Okada, and Kato were appointed the supervising inspectors for all the national surveys from 1954 to 1963. Pilot surveys first were carried out in some districts near Tokyo in order to review and revise the survey items to be used in subsequent surveys. July 1 was selected as the day on which one-day point prevalence rates were scored in each survey. Indirect information on mental cases was gained from local authorities, social welfare officers, public health nurses, and similar sources in the districts surveyed. Each district was investigated by a team of one or two psychiatrists, a public health nurse or a psychiatric social worker or both, and an examiner of basic data in public health. Accordingly, more than 300 personnel in 1954 and more than 650 personnel in 1963 co-operated as the investigators. In order to lessen the diagnostic differences, the supervising inspectors selected carefully 100 psychiatrists in 1954 and 203 psychiatrists in 1963 who were in close agreement on diagnostic standards.

Active cases detected in these surveys numbered 355 in 1954 and 569 in 1963. Among these cases, 66.2 per cent in 1954 and 68.9 per cent in 1963 were detected through indirect information, and the remaining cases were discovered by the investigators in their direct interviews. "Active cases," according to the definition employed, were persons who had shown schizophrenic symptoms within the preceding one-year period; those who had shown manic-depressive symptoms within the preceding six months; those who had had epileptic fits within the prior six months or one year (the latter applying to persons taking anticonvulsive drugs continuously); and those who had shown any other psychiatric symptoms within the preceding year. Only imbeciles and idiots were included as cases of mental deficiency in

Table 1: Prevalence Rate of Mental Disorders
per 100 Population by Diagnostic Group
in 1954 and 1963 Surveys

Diagnostic Group	1954	1963
Schizophrenia	0.23	0.23
Affective psychoses	0.02	0.02
Epilepsy	0.14	0.10
General paresis	0.02	0.01
Organic psychoses	0.10	0.23
Mental deficiency	0.70	0.42
Other nonpsychotic disorders (including neuroses)	0.30	0.28
All diagnoses	1.51	1.29

Table 2: Prevalence Rate of Mental Deficiency
per 100 Population by Age Group
in 1954 and 1963 Surveys

Age Group	1954	1963
Under 19	0.80	0.64
19 to 59	0.63	0.38
60 and over	0.10	0.12

Table 3: Percentage Classification of Mental
Disorders Due to Organic Brain Disease
in 1954 and 1963 Surveys

Organic Brain Disease	1954 (N=36)	1963 (N=95)
Cerebrovascular disease	52	52
Brain injury	4	17
Syphilis - caused	20	6
Senile dementia	20	16
Other	4	9
Total	100	100

these surveys. "Neurotics" were defined as those who could not work or go to school on account of psychogenic disorders; "psychopathy" covered those who showed abnormal behavior patterns that were harmful to others.

Relying on analysis of the detected active cases, the results of the two surveys showed that the prevalence rates of mental disorders were 1.5 per cent in 1954 and 1.3 per cent in 1963; the estimated numbers of mental disorders in the nation were 1,300,000 in the former and 1,240,000 in the latter survey. The prevalence rates for psychoses were 0.5 per cent in 1954 and 0.6 per cent in 1963 (the estimated numbers were 450,000 and 570,000); the rates of mental deficiency were 0.7 per cent in 1954 and 0.4 per cent in 1963 (the estimated numbers were 580,000 and 400,000); and rates of "other mental disorders" were in both years 0.3 per cent (estimated to number 270,000 in both surveys). In 1954 the total population of Japan was 88 million and in 1963 it was 95 million.

The prevalence rates for the mental disorders detected in the two nationwide prevalence surveys by diagnostic classification appear in Table 1. Although both surveys were carried out by the Ministry of Health and Welfare, using almost the same methods and definitions, the results obtained from the data were somewhat different.

The prevalence rate for mental deficiency obtained in the 1963 survey was 0.42 per cent, much lower than the rate of 0.70 per cent in 1954. The rate of mental deficiency for persons under 19 years of age in 1963 was remarkably lower than the respective rates in 1954, as Table 2 shows. Of course, a factor in lessening the overall prevalence rate of mental deficiency in 1963 might be the difference in economic conditions, that is to say, it might be more difficult to detect mental deficiency in relatively affluent times when even the mentally handicapped could get jobs.

As also shown in Table 1, the prevalence rate of mental disorders due to organic psychoses more than doubled from 0.10 per cent in 1954 to 0.23 per cent in 1963. Table 3 shows that approximately one-half of these mental disorders were caused by cerebrovascular disease in both studies. Mental disorders resulting from brain injuries increased remarkably in 1963. The real reason for the overall increase in mental disorders due to organic brain disease in 1963 is difficult to identify. An increase in traffic accidents could be an explanation; another might be improvement in detecting elderly psychotics.

In this connection, it is noteworthy that detected psychoses among the population 60 years old and over increased from 1.0 per cent in 1954 to 1.42 per cent in 1963. As Table 4 shows, however, the prevalence rate for psychoses among the aged remains lower than that in Western countries.

As to distribution by sex, the prevalence rate in the male population was somewhat higher than that in the female population, i.e., 1.6 per cent for males and 1.4 per cent for females in 1954 and 1.4 per cent for males and 1.1 per cent for females in 1963. Both surveys showed that the rate of organic psychoses was highest in the age group 60 years old and over and

Table 4: Prevalence Rate of Mental Disorders per 100 Population by Diagnostic Group and Age Group in 1963 Survey

Diagnostic Group	Age Group							
	0—9	10—19	20—29	30—39	40—49	50—59	60 and Over	Tot
Psychoses	0.20	0.34	0.36	0.87	0.73	0.87	1.42	0.!
Mental deficiency	0.52	0.70	0.29	0.35	0.52	0.15	0.12	0.4
Other nonpsychotic disorders	0.20	0.10	0.13	0.35	0.68	0.62	0.45	0.:
Total	0.92	1.14	0.78	1.57	1.93	1.64	1.99	1.

Table 5: Percentage Distribution of Mental Disorders by Diagnostic Group and Age Group in 1963 Survey

Age Group	Psychoses (excluding organic psychoses)	Organic Psychoses	Mental Deficiency	Neuroses and Others	All Mental Disorders
10 - 19 (N=105)	22	8	61	10	101
30 - 39 (N=104)	48	8	22	22	100
60 and over (N=84)	12	60	6	23	101

Table 6: Prevalence Rate of Mental Disorders per 100 Population by Monthly Expenditure per Person in 1963 Survey

Mental Disorders	Monthly Expenditure (in yen)					
	0— 1,999	2,000— 3,999	4,000— 6,999	7,000— 9,999	10,000— 19,000	20,000 and Over
Psychoses*	1.22	0.78	0.62	0.57	0.24	0.36
Mental deficiency	0.88	0.84	0.44	0.23	0.11	—
Other disorders	0.48	0.31	0.32	0.20	0.20	0.22
Total disorders	2.58	1.93	1.38	1.00	0.55	0.58

* This general category combines the classifications of schizophrenia, affective psychoses, epilepsy, general paresis, and organic psychoses.

that mental deficiency was greatest in the age group under 19. Table 5 shows the differences by diagnostic classification in three age groups in 1963.

In relation to living areas, both surveys showed that the prevalence rates in agricultural and fishing areas were higher than in commercial and industrial areas. Metropolitan living areas had the lowest rate. In the 1963 survey, the rates were 0.8 per cent in metropolitan areas, 1.2 per cent in urban areas, and 1.7 per cent in rural areas. These differences may be related to problems of detection, population mobility, permissiveness toward psychiatric patients, and so on.

As far as the economic status of the detected patient is concerned, the two surveys showed that the lower the income, the higher the rate, and the higher the income, the lower the rate. Table 6 shows these findings very clearly in the data from the 1963 survey. These results coincide with those of Lemkau, Tietze, and Cooper (1943) in Baltimore and of Hollingshead and Redlich (1958) in New Haven.

In the 1956 Nationwide Survey of Hospitalized Mental Disorders, the proportion of admitted patients 60 years old and over was only 4.9 per cent and that of discharged patients 60 years old and over was 5.7 per cent. The rates of the admitted patients by age and sex in the 1956 survey are shown in Table 7. One of the reasons for the apparently low rate of psychoses among the population 60 years old and over may be the difficulty in detecting

Table 7: Rate of Hospitalized Patients
per 10,000 Population by Age
Group and Sex in 1956 Survey

Age Group	Male	Female
0-9	0.1	—
10-14	0.7	0.8
15-19	6.4	5.0
20-24	19.6	11.2
25-29	32.4	14.8
30-34	33.5	16.7
35-39	26.6	15.9
40-44	22.1	14.6
45-49	19.4	12.5
50-54	15.4	10.6
55-59	12.4	8.4
60-64	9.5	6.6
65-69	6.3	5.5
70 and over	5.2	4.4

these cases, for reasons closely connected with the code of the traditional family. The family code itself has changed rapidly since World War II, however, particularly in urban and metropolitan areas. In recent years there has been a visible increase in the detection and admittance of psychiatric patients 60 years of age and over.

The Nationwide Survey of Hospitalized Mental Disorders in 1956 was carried out to gain detailed information concerning age, sex, marital status, diagnosis, and a variety of other factors, such as communication with

Table 8: Percentage Distribution of Mental Disorders by Diagnostic Group in 1954, 1956, and 1960–1961 Surveys

Diagnostic Group	Newly Treated Patients in 1960-61 Survey (N=4,625)	Hospitalized Patients in 1956 Survey (N=9,066)	Prevalence in 1954 Survey (N=355)
Schizophrenia	24.8	70.0	15.5
Affective psychoses	8.4	3.7	1.1
Epilepsy	9.4	3.8	9.6
Mental disorders due to syphilis	1.7	8.3	1.4
Alcoholic psychoses and alcoholism	2.1 ⎤	1.0 ⎤	⎤
Narcotic dependence	0.6 ⎥	0.1 ⎥	⎥ 7.0
Amphetamine dependence	0.1 ⎥	0.6 ⎥	⎥
Other drug dependence	0.4 ⎦	– ⎦	⎦
Psychosis due to organic brain disease	1.9 ⎤	0.8 ⎤	⎤
Psychosis with cerebral arteriosclerosis	2.6 ⎥	0.7 ⎥	⎥
Psychosis due to other physical condition	0.6 ⎥	0.1 ⎥	⎥ 7.3
Presenile psychosis	1.5 ⎥	1.0 ⎥	⎥
Senile psychosis	1.9 ⎥	1.7 ⎥	⎥
Other psychoses	0.6 ⎦	– ⎦	⎦
Mental deficiency	3.5	3.0	44.5
Psychopathy	2.6 ⎤	1.4 ⎤	⎤
Neuroses	29.3 ⎥	2.9 ⎥	⎥ 13.5
Other	6.1 ⎦	0.5 ⎦	⎦
Total	100.0	100.0	99.9

family, the means of paying costs of hospitalization, the duration of hospital stay, the length of time between the appearance of symptoms and the patient's admittance, the effect of treatment, the accuracy of prognosis, the reasons for discharge, and so on. Sixty of the 301 mental hospitals in existence at the time were sampled randomly, and information was obtained on 9,066 inpatients as of July 15, 1956, and 4,651 patients discharged between January 1 and June 30, 1956. Although the number of psychiatric beds in Japan increased rapidly from 54,866 in 1956 to 136,387 in 1963, or from 6.08 to 14.18 per 10,000 population, the findings of this early survey still are important because four psychiatric research workers visited each hospital to inspect hospital records and three psychiatrists jointly took part in diagnoses based on hospital records. Diagnostic classification of the hospitalized patients showed that 70.0 per cent were schizophrenic, while 15.5 per cent of the patients detected in the prevalence survey in 1954 and 24.8 per cent of the newly treated patients surveyed in 1960–61 were schizophrenic. Thus there seems to have been a concentration on schizophrenic patients in the hospitals. On the other hand, mental defectives and neurotics seem to have been underrepresented in hospitals: 44.5 per cent of the patients in the prevalence survey of 1954, 3.0 per cent of the hospitalized patients in 1956, and 3.5 per cent of the patients in the newly treated patients survey of 1960–61 were mentally defective; neurosis was diagnosed for 29.3 per cent of the newly treated patients but only for 2.9 per cent of the hospitalized patients. These and other findings appear in Table 8.

The Follow-up Study of Newly Treated Psychiatric Patients in 1960–61 established that approximately 255,000 new psychiatric patients were treated annually in all psychiatric facilities in Japan. Thirty-five per cent of the newly treated patients were hospitalized within a month of their first consultations; another 35 per cent continued treatment as outpatients; and the remaining 30 per cent were considered to have lost contact with their particular hospitals, for they were not seen during the month following initial contact. Because 34 per cent of the mental hospitals were located within a 30-minute walk (one way) of the patients' homes and about 86 per cent in total were within two hours' distance (one way), only 14 per cent of the patients were unable to make a visit to the hospital within the period of a day. About 56 per cent of the outpatient clinics were located within 30 minutes' distance (one way) of the patients' homes and about 93 per cent in total were within two hours.

Regional Surveys of Mental Disorders

As mentioned earlier in this chapter, all epidemiological surveys in Japan before 1954 were regional. I shall review some of these surveys, especially those which make certain comparisons possible or confirm other findings.

The first regional surveys of mental disorders in Japan were carried out in 1940 by the Neuropsychiatric Department of Tokyo University, under Professor Yushi Uchimura on Hachijō Island and then on Miyake Island, both south of Tokyo (*see* Uchimura, 1940, 1942). In 1941 the same group carried out two surveys in urban and rural areas, one in a part of the Ikebukuro area in Tokyo and one in the small town of Komoro in Nagano Prefecture (*see* Tsugawa, 1942; Akimoto *et al.*, 1943). Comparative analysis of these four surveys shows some interesting differences.

Hachijō Island is one of the Izu Islands located about 300 kilometers from Tokyo. The population at the time of the survey was 8,318, and the 20–49 age group constituted 31.4 per cent, although the same age group in the entire Japanese population totaled 38.3 per cent. The difference was accounted for by the out-migration of the labor force of the island. A strange characteristic of this island in 1940 was the high prevalence rate of schizophrenia, particularly in the specific villages B and D, as shown in Table 9. When Hachijō Island was resurveyed in 1961, almost the same rates prevailed as in 1940, although the population had increased to 12,027 (*see* Tables 9 and 10).

The survey of Miyake Island was notable for the high prevalence rate of mental deficiency, approximately three times the average rate in the four regional surveys. The main reason for this difference may have been the intensive investigation of school children in this survey.

Following these two surveys, Tokyo University carried out the Ikebukuro urban survey and the Komoro rural survey in 1941. Ikebukuro is a crowded residential area, located in the northwestern part of the city of Tokyo. The survey was carried out under the leadership of a psychiatrist who had lived in the district and was well acquainted with the area. The prevalence rate for mental disorders found in the survey was relatively high, especially for schizophrenia. At the time of the survey of Komoro, its population was 13,339. The town was typical of a locality with a decreasing population. Approximately 40 per cent of the population was surveyed, i.e., 5,207 persons. The survey showed a comparatively high rate of manic-depressive psychosis, higher than schizophrenia, especially among the highly educated members of the population. Not surprisingly, the highly educated section of the population had a lower rate of mental deficiency (and epilepsy also) than did the less educated segment of the population.

The most distinctive feature of these four surveys was that they were carried out from the genetic point of view; that is, the investigators were searching for evidence of hereditary factors in mental disorders and were strongly influenced by German biogeneticists, such as Ruedin and Luxenburger.

Among postwar regional surveys, I shall mention only the Chichibu Survey by Tōhō Medical University, led by Professor Arai; the Tokyo Survey by the Tokyo City Association for Mental Health; the Chiba Survey by the National Institute of Mental Health, conducted by the writer; and the Chōshi Survey made by Dr. Sato.

The Chichibu Survey was carried out in 1957 in two agricultural villages in Chichibu County in Saitama Prefecture, near Tokyo (*see* Arai *et al.*, 1958). The results showed that the prevalence rate for psychoses in the poor, nonurbanized village A was higher than in the rich, urbanized village B, although the size of the two populations was almost identical. The rate for neuroses, however, was higher in village B than in village A. An analysis of population mobility is needed to explain these differences.

The prevalence survey of Tokyo City (Tokyo Mental Health Association, 1962) was carried out in three stages. The first stage was part of a survey of the mentally and physically handicapped in April, 1961, by untrained staff members of public health centers. The randomly sampled 30,923 households surveyed included 92,769 persons. Only 73 cases (i.e., 0.079 per cent) of mental disorder were found in this survey, in which the case finding relied

Table 9: Prevalence Rate of Schizophrenia
per 100 Population in
Five Villages of Hachijō Island
in 1940 and 1961 Surveys

Village	1940	1961
A	0.78	0.88
B	1.30	1.26
C	0.30	1.16
D	1.41	1.31
E	–	0.19

Table 10: Prevalence Rate of Main Mental Disorders per 100
Population of Hachijō Island in 1940 and 1961 Surveys and
Nationwide in 1954 Survey

Mental Disorder	Hachijō 1940	Hachijō 1961	Nationwide 1954
Schizophrenia	0.38	0.47	0.23
Affective psychoses	0.10	0.08	0.02
Epilepsy	0.06	0.14	0.14
General paresis	0.04	–	0.02

only on information supplied by the public health nurses of district public health centers. In the second stage, a random selection was made of one-tenth of the aforementioned households, and these sample 3,107 households were surveyed by 59 university students trained as enumerators and inter-viewers by the special investigators. There were 102 cases of mental disorder found in this survey, approximately 1.2 per 100 population. The third stage of the survey was carried out by 40 well-trained psychiatrists who found that 66 per cent of the cases diagnosed as mental disorders by the students were correctly diagnosed. The differences in the findings in the three stages are believed to reflect the differences in the enumerators and interviewers—from untrained public health officers to trained university students to well-trained psychiatrists—as well as the variations in the number of households sur-veyed. Apparently the better trained the interviewers and the smaller the segment of the population surveyed, the higher and the more accurate is the prevalence rate.

The Chiba Survey was carried out in Ichikawa City and Awa County in 1954 (*see* Kato, 1955). Through inspection of the inpatient data of the psychiatric institutions in and around both areas from 1946 to 1953, the annual admission rates per 100,000 population were determined; they were 99.9 in Ichikawa City and 50.2 in Awa County. Awa County had a generally lower rate than Ichikawa City for each type of illness, a difference which was especially marked for neuroses. A curve to determine the annual average rate of mental disorders per 100,000 population revealed that ages

Table 11: Number and Prevalence Rate of Mental Disorders per 100 Population by Diagnostic Group in Chōshi City, 1954–1959, and Nationwide Prevalence Rate in 1954 Survey

Diagnostic Group	Chōshi City, 1954-1959 Number	Rate	Nationwide 1954 Survey Rate
Schizophrenia	253	0.28	0.23
Affective psychoses	115	0.13	0.02
Epilepsy	111	0.12	0.14
General paresis	35	0.04	0.02
Organic psychoses	68	0.07	0.10
Mental deficiency	49	0.05	0.70
Neuroses	376	0.41	
Psychopathy	12	0.01	0.30
Other nonpsychotic disorders	135	0.15	
Total	1,154	1.26	1.51

20 to 30 were high in general and that the figures for Ichikawa City generally were higher than the corresponding ones for Awa County. Intensive case studies in five small areas in Ichikawa City showed that 39.7 per cent of the mentally ill were living in their previous places of residence after discharge from hospitals. It was difficult to determine whether the differences between admission rates in Ichikawa City and Awa County were based on actual differences in the occurrence of mental disorder or whether they were connected with the degree of utilization of mental hospitals.

As an example of a recent community-centered epidemiological survey, I should like to call attention to the mental health work of the Department of Neuropsychiatry, Chōshi City Hospital, conducted by Dr. I. Sato (*see* Sato, 1966). Chōshi is a provincial city relying on fishing and agriculture, located 100 kilometers east of Tokyo, with a stable population of 90,000. The City Hospital is a general hospital with 254 beds, including 106 psychiatric beds. The psychiatric department of this hospital treated 1,154 new patients on an in- and out-patient basis during the five years from 1954 to 1959, i.e., 1.3 per cent of the city population. The detected patients were classified diagnostically as shown in Table 11.

Table 11 shows that the rate of affective psychoses was higher, and that of mental deficiency was lower than the rates in the nationwide preva· lence survey in 1954. As regards the proportion of mania and depression in affective psychoses, the detected patients in Chōshi City showed a ratio of 1:2 compared with a ratio of 1:7 found by the Neuropsychiatric Department of Tokyo University. Although Dr. Sato did not speculate on the reason why the rate of mania was very high in Chōshi City, this figure is interesting for both cultural and epidemiological reasons.

Conclusions

In analyzing the data gained in several nationwide and regional surveys of mental disorders in Japan, it was observed that case finding was more difficult in urban than in rural areas, in residential than in agricultural areas, with females than with males, with old people than with young people, with paranoid schizophrenic cases than with hebephrenic and deteriorated schizophrenic cases, and with obsessive-compulsive neurotic cases than with hypochondriacal and hysterical state cases.

These observations bring me to my concluding point. Once again, I want to stress the belief that in order to overcome the difficulties in the detection of psychiatric cases it is necessary to promote the activities of community-centered clinics and hospitals and to win the confidence of the inhabitants. In a country changing as rapidly as is Japan, analytic and dynamic epidemiology of mental disorders is required instead of static and descriptive epidemiology.

REFERENCES

Akimoto, H., T. Shimazaki, K. Okada, and M. Tatetsu. 1943. Chihō shōtoshi ni okeru minseigaku-teki oyobi seishinigaku-teki chōsa. Seishin Shinkei Gaku Zasshi 47:1-24.

Arai, N., Y. Shibata, Y. Iijima, A. Akabane, Y. Toda, and T. Maruyama. 1958. Chichibu sanson ni okeru issei chōsa ni yoru seishinigaku-teki kōsatsu narabi ni ta-nōson tono hikaku, Seishin Shinkei Igaku Zasshi 60:1-12.

Hollingshead, A. B., and F. C. Redlich. 1958. Social class and mental illness. New York, Wiley.

Japanese Ministry of Health and Welfare. 1955. Nationwide prevalence survey of mental disorders in 1954. Tokyo, Japanese Ministry of Health and Welfare. Mimeographed.

————. 1957. Nationwide survey of hospitalized mental disorders in 1956. Tokyo, Japanese Ministry of Health and Welfare. Mimeographed.

————. 1965. Wagakuni ni okeru seishin-shōgai no genjō. Tokyo, Kōsei-shō Kōshū Eisei Kyoku.

Kato, M. 1955. Shōtoshi ni okeru seishin-shōgaisha no seitaigaku-teki kenkyū. Iryō 9:41-49.

————. 1962. Seishin-eisei narabi ni seishin-shōgai ni taisuru ninshiki oyobi chiryō-teki taido ni kansuru kenkyū. Seishin Eisei Kenkyū No. 10:1-15.

Lemkau, P. V., C. Tietze, and M. Cooper. 1943. A summary of statistical studies on the prevalence and incidence of mental disorders in sample populations. Public Health Report, Vol. 5, No. 53.

Sato, I. 1966. Seishin-byōin no tachiba kara. Seishin Igaku 8:6-10.

Tokyo Mental Health Association. 1962. Tokyo-to seishin-shōgaisha jittai chōsa. Tokyo, Tokyo-to Eisei Kyoku.

Tsugawa, B. 1942. Daitoshi ni okeru seishin-shikkan no hassei-hindo ni kansuru kenkyū. Seishin Shinkei Gaku Zasshi 47:204 ff.

Uchimura, Y. 1940. Hachijō-jima ni okeru seishin-shikkan no shutsugen-hindo ni kansuru kenkyū. Seishin Shinkei Gaku Zasshi 44:745 ff.

————. 1942. Miyake-jima ni okeru seishin-shikkan no hassei-hindo ni kansuru kenkyū. Minzoku Eisei 10:1 ff.

7. Sibling Rank, Culture, and Mental Disorders

HSIEN RIN, M.D.

Department of Neurology and Psychiatry
National Taiwan University Hospital
Taipei, Taiwan

THIS CHAPTER is concerned, first, with data on the relation of sibling rank and mental disorder among Chinese in Taiwan and, second, with certain theoretical and methodological issues relating to cross-cultural studies of sibling rank.

It is widely recognized that different cultures show variance in family expectations of the role of a child according to sex and sibling rank. In some cultures, for example, the eldest child may be oriented to the exercise of power and authority as a leader in the family, but he also may be pampered by his parents during early childhood and thus grow up lacking in ego strength. The youngest child, having no followers, also may be pampered in some cultures, although in others he equally may be rejected by his parents as unwanted. Sibling rank and the composition of the family thus may have direct effects on socialization, personality development, and occurrence of mental disorders. Since each child encounters parental expectations that are deeply predetermined by their society and culture, his personality is likely to be influenced within this framework.

Two Types of Sibling Rank Studies in Taiwan

Stimulated by the work of Caudill (1963) and Schooler (1961, 1964) in the United States and Japan, I attempted to study the relation of sibling rank and mental disorders among Chinese in Taiwan. For this purpose, use was made of two different sets of data obtained by the writer and his colleagues in their previous studies:

1) The information obtained on sibling rank and sex on all 158 psychotic patients admitted to the National Taiwan University Hospital during 1958–59 (*see* Rin, 1965).

2) The information obtained on sibling rank and sex on all 488 persons who were selected as an age-stratified random sample of the population of Musan, a suburban community of Taipei, a sample originally used for an epidemiological study of psychophysiological reactions (Rin, Chu, and Lin, 1966).

In the sibling rank study of schizophrenics and other psychotics, the sample consisted of 85 schizophrenics (46 males and 39 females) and 73 nonschizophrenic functional psychotics with paranoid, manic-depressive, and involutional disorders (40 males and 33 females) who were admitted to the psychiatric ward of the National Taiwan University Hospital in 1958–59. All siblings born alive were taken into consideration. Table 1 shows the frequency of eldest and youngest siblings of both sexes in the schizophrenic and nonschizophrenic groups. Of total-born siblings, there were 14 first-born and 3 last-born among 46 male schizophrenics (p < .01), but the difference between the 7 first-born and 10 last-born female schizophrenics was not significant. Among nonschizophrenic psychotics, the findings were not significant for males or females. For both schizophrenic and nonschizophrenic psychotics, there were more first-born males (p < .01), but there was no difference for females. In rank among same-sex siblings

Table 1: Frequencies of Eldest and Youngest Siblings among 158 Psychotics Admitted to the Department of Psychiatry National Taiwan University Hospital in 1958–1959

Sibling Rank	Schizophrenics		Other Psychotics		Total Psychotics	
	Male (46)	Female (39)	Male (40)	Female (33)	Male (86)	Female (72)
Among total-born siblings						
Eldest	14	7	14	7	28	14
Youngest	3*	10	7	7	10*	17
Among same-sex siblings						
Eldest	13	12	13	7	26	19
Youngest	8	14	6	8	14	22

* p <.01; significance level determined by chi-square, df= 1.

only, eldest males were again in the majority, but the differences did not reach statistical significance for either males or females in any of the groups.

Of the 488 age-stratified sample randomly chosen from the general population of Musan, 206 (42 percent) were suffering from psychophysiological reactions of varying degrees. Sibling rank was analyzed in order to explore the relation between the prevalence rates of psychophysiological reactions and family role patterns in Chinese families. As presented in Table 2, the prevalence rate of psychophysiological reaction was significantly higher for youngest-born females among both total-born siblings ($p < .01$) and same-sex siblings ($p < .01$). Although the number of cases was too small for a statistical check, close inspection of the data indicates that in this sample there were no apparent differences by age, marital status, date of migration, education, or social class. When the data on all eldest and youngest members were further broken down by size of family and social class, the higher prevalence rate among youngest females occurred in all family sizes and classes. Since rates of psychophysiological reactions may be related to the amount of human stress, this study suggests that youngest females are under considerable emotional stress owing to their position in the Chinese family.

To summarize, results from the two Chinese studies showed that eldest males were overrepresented among psychotics compared with youngest males but not among patients with psychophysiological reactions, and that youngest females were overrepresented among patients with psychophysiological reactions.

The first question to be asked about these results is: why should there be so many eldest sons among hospitalized psychotic patients? We do not understand this finding fully at present and intend to carry out further research on it, but one cannot rule out the possible selective factor that because the eldest son is the most important son for the Chinese family the family may seek treatment more often for the eldest than for other sons. In addition, because eldest sons in Chinese families are frequently overprotected by their mothers and grandmothers during childhood, they may be more disposed to mental conflict when the time comes for them to assume their responsibilities as eldest sons.

The second question is: why are there more youngest females than others with psychophysiological reactions? Traditional families provide less privileged circumstances for girls, and Chinese mothers who grew up in such families tend to become nagging and aggressive. Contrary to the situation reported by Caudill (1963) for small-business families in Japan, Chinese mothers customarily do not encourage the youngest daughter to serve her father or allow her to be pampered as a child. Instead, the youngest daughter is often the object of intrafamilial tension and aggression and even may be put up for adoption if the family needs to curtail expenses.

Adoption of daughters, practiced particularly by the native Taiwanese families, must be described here because of its cultural significance

Table 2: Psychophysiological Reactions by Sibling Rank for 488-Person, Age-stratified Random Sample in Musan Village in 1963–1964

Sibling Rank	Among Total-born Siblings							
	Male				Female			
	Pp N	Not Pp N	Total N	Rate %	Pp N	Not Pp N	Total N	Rate %
Only	4	6	10	40	4	4	8	50
Eldest	29	47	76	38	25	40	65	39
Youngest	18	23	41	44	23	9	32	72
Intermediate	51	69	120	43	51	82	133	38
Significance of difference between only, eldest, youngest, and intermediate (df = 3)		n.s.				$X^2 = 12.6$ p < .01		
Significance of difference between eldest and youngest (df = 1)		n.s.				$X^2 = 9.6$ p < .01		

Table 2: (Continued)

Sibling Rank	Among Same-sex Siblings							
	Male				Female			
	Pp N	Not Pp N	Total N	Rate %	Pp N	Not Pp N	Total N	Rate %
Only	13	15	28	46	12	15	27	44
Eldest	33	56	89	37	35	53	88	40
Youngest	19	24	43	44	27	15	42	64
Intermediate	37	50	87	43	28	54	82	34
Significance of difference between only, eldest, youngest, and intermediate (df = 3)		n.s.				$X^2 = 10.8$ p < .02		
Significance of difference between eldest and youngest (df = 1)		n.s.				$X^2 = 6.8$ p < .01		

Note: Pp = psychophysiological cases.

for the status of youngest daughters. Among the Musan random sample from the study of psychophysiological reactions, there were 16 adopted females, all but 1 from native Taiwanese families. Of these 15 adopted daughters, 10 were suffering from psychophysiological reactions or other mental disorders. Although not of statistical significance, it is noteworthy that 6 of the 15 adopted daughters were originally the youngest children in their birth ranks in terms of either both-sex or same-sex siblings. Moreover, 4 of the 6 youngest daughters came from very large families having 10 or more children.

Adoption of a daughter usually occurs in one of the following situations: a family wants to reduce the number of children in consequence of economic hardship; a mother wants to reduce the physical and emotional burden of rearing children; a family superstitiously regards the existence of a baby girl as the cause of family misfortunes; or a family gives away or exchanges a girl with another family for marital reasons. Depending upon the motivation in these situations, the status of the adopted girl may vary from that of a mere domestic servant to that of the future bride of a son of her foster parents.

Intercultural Comparisons

Caudill (1963) analyzed sibling rank and social characteristics of all 717 patients admitted to four psychiatric hospitals in the Tokyo area in 1958. In this study of Japanese patients, Caudill found an overrepresentation among same-sex living sibs of eldest sons and youngest daughters among psychotic patients, but there were no findings among neurotic patients of either sex. When data on Japanese schizophrenic patients only were analyzed, eldest sons and youngest daughters again were overrepresented among same-sex living birth ranks (but *see also* Caudill and Schooler, Chapter 8).

Caudill's data indicate that eldest psychotic sons were concentrated in small-business families in contrast to families in which the principal earner worked in a large corporate business or in government. Among daughters there was no clearcut difference by sibling position and family type. When, however, the additional variable of marital status was introduced, it became clear that, among psychotic female patients, single, youngest daughters from small-business families were overrepresented.

Yamaguchi *et al.* (1964) reported on an analysis of sibling rank among 601 schizophrenics and 904 neurotics seen during the period from 1959 to 1962 at Nihon University in Tokyo. There was a trend for females born in the last half of their total sibships to be significantly overrepresented among schizophrenics, but no difference was found among males. Among siblings of the same sex, schizophrenic youngest daughters were overrepresented. When the case material was divided into large (five or more sibs) and small (less than five sibs) families, more eldest sons than youngest sons in small families were in both schizophrenic and neurotic groups.

The above results suggest that interpersonal relations centering around the roles of eldest son and youngest daughter in Japan carry more than their share of psychological problems, particularly in small-business families which tend to be more traditional in Japan.

Findings somewhat similar to those in Japan emerged from a preliminary analysis of data on Chinese samples in Taiwan concerning the emotional difficulties and psychiatric problems of eldest sons (among psychotic patients) and youngest daughters (among persons with psychophysiological reactions). Emphasis upon the position and duties of the eldest son remains strong in traditional families in both cultures. In the present observations, however, the youngest daughter's position in the traditional Chinese family and the nature of her emotional conflicts seem to differ from those of the youngest daughter in the traditional Japanese family.

Several studies in North America have supported the hypothesis that last-borns are more likely to be hospitalized in mental hospitals than first-borns. Malzburg's (1940) data on first admissions with dementia praecox between 1930 and 1935 at Manhattan State Hospital showed more last-born than first-born patients of families with four or more children. Gregory's (1959) family data on 1,000 patients admitted to Ontario Hospital between 1954 and 1958 also showed more last-born than first-born patients in this population. Schooler (1961) collected data on a sample of hospitalized female schizophrenics in Springfield State Hospital during 1959 and found that significantly more patients came from the last half of their sibship than from the first half. He examined, in addition, records of all patients admitted to Spring Grove State Hospital between 1942 and 1949 and also found a significant relation between birth order and hospitalization for schizophrenia among female patients (Schooler, 1964). In this study no significant overall relation between birth order and hospitalization for schizophrenia was found among males either in terms of disproportionate numbers of first-born, last-born, or middle-born patients or of position in the first or last half of sibship. Among female patients, however, there was a highly significant overrepresentation of last-born sibs.

The above studies support Schachter's (1959) finding of a relation between birth order and affiliative tendency in normal females in a series of experimental studies in which subjects who were first-born or only children tended to be more affiliative than others in an anxiety-provoking experimental situation. Schooler and Scarr (1962), using a modification of Schachter's technique, found that female chronic schizophrenics born in the first half of their sibship were significantly more sociable than those born in the second half of their sibship, even after an average of 11 years in the hospital for all patients in the study.

From these studies on American patient populations, birth order seems to have a definite effect on the rate of hospitalization for schizophrenia among females but not among males, indicating similarities with the data on birth rank for female patients in Tokyo and Taipei. Of special interest in the findings in Asian cultures, however, is the overrepresentation of eldest sons among hospitalized patients. Moreover, prevalence data for Taiwan indicate that the overrepresentation of hospitalized eldest sons and youngest daughters with psychotic reactions within their same-sex birth rank may exist in the general population as well.[1]

The traditional families in the Orient are those in which extended kinship values, interpersonal and intrafamilial decorum, and family role differences by age and sex are emphasized strongly. In the years since World War II a contrasting life style has developed in the families of professional and salaried employees who belong to a growing new middle class in the Asian countries. The co-existing "traditional" and "modern" families represent dual family life styles in these changing societies. In the majority of the modern families in Asian countries, just as in middle-class American families (*see* Kohn, 1963), parental values stress self-direction rather than passive obedience to parental commands. Also, the differential roles of children by sex are stressed less in modern than in traditional families, so that the role differences previously attached to sibling positions have abated to a great extent. The emotional difficulties of the eldest son and youngest daughter discussed in this chapter thus pertain to the conflict situation within traditional families. Although the emphasis on the role of the eldest son seems to be universal in developing countries, particular conflicts for youngest females appear to vary among cultures. These ideas need to be clarified and tested by further research. I and my colleagues already have made plans to collect additional data on a large sample (about 1,000 cases in each culture) of Chinese, Japanese, and American patients to analyze further sibling position in relation to family role patterns and psychological problems. Although there are many methodological difficulties in sibling rank studies, a cross-cultural study using proper samples and survey techniques will greatly contribute to understanding the sociocultural background of mental disorders.

NOTE

1.   From the data in a not yet completely analyzed follow-up survey of mental disorders in three communities in Taiwan (*see* Lin *et al.*, Chapter 5), there is an interesting finding concerning birth order and the prevalence rate of psychoses among same-sex birth rank: the rates of all psychoses per 1,000 population for first, second, third, fourth, and fifth or more birth ranks are for males 3.6, 1.7, 2.6, 2.8, and 1.1; and the rates for females are 3.0, 5.0, 3.5, 0, and 5.7. There thus appears to be a tendency for psychotic reactions to be more prevalent in first-rank males and in fifth-or-more rank females. This finding again seems to support the tendency for an overrepresentation of psychoses among first-born males and last-born females in the Chinese culture. In the follow-up survey, no such tendencies were observed in the categories of neuroses, character disorders, or other psychiatric illnesses.

REFERENCES

Caudill, W. 1963. Sibling rank and style of life among Japanese psychiatric patients. *In* Proceedings of the Joint Meeting of the Japanese Society of Psychiatry and Neurology and the American Psychiatric Association, Tokyo, H. Akimoto, ed. Supplement No. 7 of Folia Psychiatria et Neurologia Japonica. Tokyo, Japanese Society of Psychiatry and Neurology.

Gregory, I. 1959. An analysis of family data on 1,000 patients admitted to a Canadian mental hospital. Acta Genetica et Statistica Medica 9:54–96.

Kohn, M. L. 1963. Social class and parent-child relationships: an interpretation. American Journal of Sociology 68:471–80.

Malzburg, B. 1940. Social and biological aspects of mental disease. Utica, State Hospitals Press.

Rin, H. 1965. A family study of Chinese schizophrenic patients: loss of parents, sibling rank, parental attitude and short-term prognosis. Transcultural Psychiatric Research 2:24–26.

Rin, H., H. M. Chu, and T. Lin. 1966. Psychophysiological reactions of a rural and suburban population in Taiwan. Acta Psychiatrica Scandinavica 42:410–73.

Schachter, S. 1959. The psychology of affiliation. Stanford, Stanford University Press.

Schooler, C. 1961. Birth order and schizophrenia. Archives of General Psychiatry 4:91–97.

————. 1964. Birth order and hospitalization for schizophrenia. Journal of Abnormal and Social Psychology 69:574–79.

Schooler, C., and S. Scarr. 1962. Affiliation among chronic schizophrenics: relation to intrapersonal and birth order factors. Journal of Personality 30:178–92.

Yamaguchi, T., H. Makihara, H. Nagai, N. Hagiwara, T. Ishikawa, U. Anazawa, S. Yano, and T. Kobayashi. 1964. Bunretsubyō oyobi shinkeishō no dōhōjun'i. Seishinigaku 6:578–86.

8.   Symptom Patterns and Background Characteristics of Japanese Psychiatric Patients

WILLIAM CAUDILL, Ph.D.
Laboratory of Socio-environmental Studies
National Institute of Mental Health
Bethesda, Maryland

CARMI SCHOOLER, Ph.D.
Laboratory of Socio-environmental Studies
National Institute of Mental Health
Bethesda, Maryland

THIS CHAPTER is concerned with results from a further analysis of data on a sample of 717 Japanese psychiatric patients representing all admissions in 1958 to four representative psychiatric hospitals in Tokyo.[1] Earlier analyses of these data have presented findings relating both to the birth rank of patients (Caudill, 1963) and to the symptoms shown by patients diagnosed as schizophrenic (Schooler and Caudill, 1964).

Our earlier findings on birth rank indicated that among Japanese psychotic patients in general, and among schizophrenic patients in particular, eldest sons and youngest daughters were overrepresented. This finding was not true among Japanese neurotic patients. In arriving at these conclusions, we considered birth rank in four different ways. The finding for psychotic patients was most clear and statistically significant when birth rank was considered in relation to the position of the patient among living same-sex sibs, and the finding was least clear and not statistically significant when birth rank was considered in relation to the position of the patient among living and dead sibs of both sexes—that is, the biological birth order.[2] Since the finding was clearest when we considered the social status of being an eldest son or youngest daughter among same-sex sibs who were living at the time of admission to the hospital, we will refer to sibling position as a social structural or cultural variable and not as a biological variable.[3]

Our earlier findings on the symptoms of schizophrenic patients indicated that, compared to American patients, both male and female Japanese schizophrenic patients had been more physically violent (especially toward family members, particularly the mother) and more emotionally impulsive in the year prior to their current admission to the hospital (Schooler and Caudill, 1964). Phillips and his colleagues (*see* Draguns *et al.*, in press; Phillips and Draguns, Chapter 2) have validated this finding by comparing our Japanese data with a separate sample of American schizophrenic patients, and the finding also has been confirmed in the work of Katz and his colleagues (Katz, Gudeman, and Sanborn, Chapter 9), who used a sample of Japanese schizophrenic patients residing in Hawaii in comparison with a sample of American schizophrenic patients residing in mainland United States. In this chapter we will explore the problem further, paying particular heed to indications of physical violence and emotional impulsivity among Japanese schizophrenic patients.

The earlier findings were arrived at by first grouping patients according to diagnosis and then analyzing the data in terms of birth rank and symptoms. Each symptom was considered singly as a variable. This procedure has at least two difficulties: (1) diagnosis is subject to the individual interpretation of the psychiatrist plus the cultural bias that he may share with other psychiatrists in his country in interpreting symptoms; and (2) analysis in terms of symptoms considered singly is less powerful than analysis in terms of a grouping of symptoms into meaningful clusters.

In an attempt to avoid these difficulties, we will present data by means of a factor analysis of symptoms. This analysis is independent of diagnosis and results in five clusters (or factors) of symptoms for males and five for females. We first will give the composition of these factors and then consider them in relation to a series of social and cultural background variables. Thus the central approach of this chapter is to examine our sample of Japanese patients in a fresh way, using meaningful and empirically derived clusters of symptoms. In this approach diagnosis itself is one of the background variables investigated.[4]

The Patterning of Symptoms in the Sample

Of the total of 717 patients admitted in 1958 to the four hospitals in Tokyo, we excluded 49 patients diagnosed as having organic brain disorders or mental deficiency and 10 additional patients on whom there were no symptom data. For the remaining 658 patients, (411 males, 247 females), the case history of each was examined according to a slightly modified version of the symptom check list developed by Phillips and Rabinovitch (1958). Each record was coded for the presence or absence of each of 62 symptoms during a period which covered the year prior to the present admission and the early phase of hospitalization leading to the first staff conference on the patient's case.

We next examined the frequency of symptom occurrence by sex. In order to meet the requirements for factor analysis, we included only symptoms which occurred in at least 8 per cent of the male or the female cases, respectively. This method resulted in a list of 24 symptoms for males and 26 symptoms for females. Using these data on symptoms by sex, we made an orthogonal principal component factor analysis. Before rotation, we extracted nine factors for each sex and then ran a series of rotations to simple structure involving different numbers of factors, finally settling on a basically four-factor rotation for both males and females. All other rotations in the series, however, were generally similar.

For both males and females, one of the factors in the four-factor rotation split very cleanly in half in further rotations and was particularly clear in the six-factor rotation. We therefore decided to use, for both sexes, the original three factors (from the four-factor rotation) plus the two that derived from the splitting of the fourth factor. Thus we have five factors for each sex. On four of the five factors, the factor structure for both sexes was sufficiently similar to give the factors the same names; one factor was unique for each sex.[5] Tables 1 and 2 present the factors for each sex and the way the individual symptoms load on them. In the tables positive or negative loadings of less than .30 are omitted. The total amount of variance accounted for (h^2) in the different analyses hovers around 45 per cent.

The names we have given these factors are fairly self-explanatory in terms of the symptoms on which they have heavy loadings. For example, the depressed factor for males (*see* Table 1) has a loading, i.e., a correlation, of .65 on depressed, .46 on irritated, .33 on no appetite, .44 on suicidal attempts, and .65 on sleep disturbances. The symptoms for the other factors can be read off the tables.[6] We used Japanese words in naming two factors. *Shinkeishitsu* means "nervous temperament"; its importance to us is the sharp characterization of the factor by tense interpersonal relations and phobias. *Wagamama* in Japanese means "self-indulgence" or "take me as I am"; its importance to us is the characterization of the factor by behavior which is childish, negative, apathetic, irresponsible, and punctuated with emotional outbursts. It is not that these sorts of behavior do not occur in the West but that they conform very closely to commonly recognized ordinary patterns of Japanese behavior; in addition, clinically, *shinkeishitsushō* ("nervous temperament illness") is used as a diagnosis by Morita therapists (for discussion of Morita therapy, *see* Caudill and Doi, 1963).

One of the hospitals we used—Kōseiin—specializes in treating *shinkeishitsu* patients. In order to eliminate the possibility that this patterning of symptoms was the result of the clinical views of the medical staff at Kōseiin, we performed a separate factor analysis using only the data from the other three hospitals. At the other three hospitals the diagnosis of *shinkeishitsushō* seldom is used. Even in this separate analysis of the symptoms of patients at the other three hospitals, the *shinkeishitsu* factor appeared essentially unaltered.

In summary, the patterning of symptoms in Japan seems generally similar to what might be expected in a Western psychiatric population. Indeed, one might expect to find depressed, reality break, manic, and acting out symptom patterns in any psychiatric population. This attribute of the data seems to point to certain probably universal ways in which human beings behave in their attempts to handle emotional problems. Two symptom patterns, however—*shinkeishitsu* and *wagamama*—are more characteristically Japanese than Western. The next question is: How do all these symptom patterns relate to other variables, such as the diagnoses and background characteristics of the patients? Before we could begin to answer this question, we had to design a method for assigning each patient a score on each factor.

Assignment of Factor Scores to Individual Patients

The scoring system was determined by examining the loadings of the symptoms on each factor. Symptoms with loadings of .30 to .44 were given a weight of one, .45 to .59 a weight of two, .60 to .74 a weight of three, .75 to .89 a weight of four, and negative loadings (where they occur appropriately within a group of positive loadings) similarly were given negative weights. Thus the score of a patient on a factor consists of the sum of the weights for the symptoms he had which are relevant to that factor.[7] For example, a male patient could have a maximum score of 10 on depressed, but, in fact, a particular patient has, let us say, a score of 9 because he lacked the symptom of "suicide attempts" but showed all the other relevant symptoms. This same male patient also logically could have a maximum score of 16 on acting out but, in fact, has a score of 2 since he only showed the symptom of "irritated" among the relevant symptoms. In this way, a factor score on each factor was determined for each patient, and the array of scores over the factors for a particular patient results in a clear picture of the patterning of symptoms for that patient.

Relation of Factor Scores to Diagnostic Groupings

We now can begin to answer the question of how the picture of a patient derived from his factor scores fits with his clinical diagnosis. Table 3 shows, first, a very significant relation (determined by a one-way analysis of variance) [8] between diagnosis and a high factor score on the most likely factor. For example, for males, schizophrenic patients had a significantly higher mean factor than did other diagnostic groups on reality break (as expected) and also on manic (which was less expected and presents an interesting problem to which we will return shortly). Male patients with a diagnosis among the other psychoses (which are predominantly manic-depressive and involutional psychoses) had a higher score on depressed than on other factors. Male neurotic patients score higher on *shinkeishitsu* and lower on reality break and acting out. Finally, male sociopathic patients had

Table 1: Major Rotated Factors in a Factor Analysis of Symptoms of Male Patients

Male Symptoms	Major Rotated Factors				
	Depressed*	Shinkei-shitsu*	Reality Break*	Manic†	Acting Out†
Delusions			-.66		
Phobias		.67			
Hallucinations			-.74		
Self-deprecative		.32			
Depressed	.65				
Euphoric				.44	.40
Apathetic					
Tense		.42			
Emotionally labile			-.45	.65	
Irritated	.46				.46
Physically violent			-.32		.53
Negative behavior					.52
Irresponsible behavior					.48
Impulsive behavior			-.46	.62	.32
Talking to self			-.35	.55	
Restless					.45
Drinking				-.44	.50
Tense interpersonal relations		.73			
Withdrawn		.40			
No appetite	.33		-.30	.32	
Suicidal attempts	.44				
Bodily complaints		.47			-.37
Sleep disturbances	.65				
Psychosomatic disorders					-.33

* From four-rotated factor analysis.
† From six-rotated factor analysis.

Table 2: Major Rotated Factors in a Factor Analysis of Symptoms of
Female Patients

	Major Rotated Factors				
Female Symptoms	Depressed*	Shinkei-shitsu*	Reality Break*	Manic[†]	Wagamama[†]
Delusions			.63		
Phobias		-.61			
Hallucinations			.48		
Self-deprecative	−.56				
Depressed	−.64				
Euphoric				.61	
Mood swings					
Apathetic	−.35				.58
Tense		−.44	−.36		
Emotionally labile				.46	
Irritated					
Physically violent			.33		
Emotional outbursts					.55
Negative behavior					.58
Irresponsible behavior					.55
Impulsive behavior			.43	.50	
Talking to self	.34			.60	
Restless			-.30	.65	
Childish, regressive					.61
Tense interpersonal relations		−.75			
Withdrawn	−.37				
No appetite	−.51				
Suicidal attempts	−.53				
Bodily complaints		−.47	−.42	−.40	
Sleep disturbances			−.53		
Psychosomatic disorders					

* From four-rotated factor analysis.
[†] From six-rotated factor analysis.

Table 3: Relation of Diagnostic Groups to Weighted Factor Scores by Sex of Patient

	Mean Factor Scores									
	Male (N=406)					Female (N=243)				
Diagnostic Group	Depressed	Shinkei-shitsu	Reality Break	Manic	Acting Out	Depressed	Shinkei-shitsu	Reality Break	Manic	Wagamama
Schizophrenia (♂N=132, ♀N=115)	3.0	3.1	5.3	4.4	4.8	3.2	1.9	6.8	4.7	1.8
Other psychoses (♂N=22, ♀N=19)	4.5	2.9	2.2	2.6	4.0	5.4	2.1	3.6	2.6	1.7
Neuroses (♂N=228, ♀N=109)	3.1	5.1	.7	1.5	2.4	4.5	3.5	3.0	1.5	1.6
Sociopathic illness (♂N=24, ♀N=0)	1.6	1.7	2.5	2.2	5.8	—	—	—	—	—
F Ratio	4.1	25.9	130.1	52.1	32.9	8.0	16.0	90.9	32.9	.3
Degrees of freedom	3/402	3/402	3/402	3/402	3/402	2/240	2/240	2/240	2/240	2/240
Probability <	.01	.001	.001	.001	.001	.001	.001	.001	.001	n.s.

the highest mean score on acting out, but they did not differ significantly in this respect from patients diagnosed as having schizophrenia or an "other psychosis." [9] Perhaps the most general statement that can be made concerning the factor of acting out is that among male patients in Japan there seems to be a rather high level of acting out regardless of diagnosis, except for patients labeled neurotics.[10]

The overall patterning for female patients in Table 3 is very similar to that for males. Female schizophrenic patients also had a significantly higher mean factor than did other diagnostic groups on the reality break and manic factors. Female patients with a diagnosis among the other psychoses or the neuroses did not differ significantly in their mean scores on the depressed factor, but these two groups combined were more depressed than were schizophrenic patients. Both female and male neurotic patients scored higher on the *shinkeishitsu* factor than did other diagnostic groups. None of the diagnostic groups for female patients had a significant relation to the *wagamama* factor. As can be seen from the symptoms making up this factor (*see* Table 2), *wagamama* can be considered the female equivalent of the acting out factor for males which, like *wagamama,* is not limited to any particular diagnostic group.

In general, then, Table 3 shows a significant relation for both males and females between diagnosis and the most likely symptom pattern, a result which perhaps was to have been expected in view of the clinical experience of psychiatrists. The relation, however, is by no means perfect, and it should not be forgotten that after a "correct" diagnosis had been made the patient still had symptoms other than those predominantly related to his diagnosis.

The latter issue is particularly clear in Table 3, for both male and female patients with a diagnosis of schizophrenia had a high score on the reality break factor and also on the manic factor. This is, we believe, the most unusual finding in Table 3. This finding again directs our attention to the physical violence and emotional impulsivity of Japanese schizophrenic patients. If we look back to the symptoms which make up the reality break factor, which is defined primarily by the presence of delusions and hallucinations, we find that the symptoms of physical violence and impulsive behavior have meaningful loadings for both sexes. Furthermore, the manic factor, to which the diagnosis of schizophrenia also is related, contains meaningful loadings on emotional lability and impulsivity for both sexes. We will return to the question of "explosiveness" in the prehospitalization histories of Japanese schizophrenic patients when we consider the factors of reality break and manic in relation to the background characteristics of the patients.

Relation of Factor Scores to Social and Familial Background Variables

We next examined the factor scores in a series of analyses of variance in which the independent variables were derived from the patient's social and familial background. The independent variables used were grouped under seven headings as follows:

1)   Age of patient
2)   Birth order
    a)   Both-sex living sibling rank
    b)   Same-sex living sibling rank
3)   Education of patient
4)   Marital status of patient
5)   Size of business (or more conceptually, style of life) [11]
    a)   In which patient's father was employed
    b)   In which patient was employed
    c)   In which principal earner in family was employed [12]
6)   Supervisory level of job (owner or manager, employee, or unpaid family worker)
    a)   Of patient's father
    b)   Of patient
    c)   Of principal earner in family
7)   Social class [13]
    a)   Of patient's father
    b)   Of patient
    c)   Of principal earner in family

For each sex separate one-way analyses of variance were performed relating each of the background variables to each of the factor scores. Possible interactions were explored through a series of two-way analyses of variance, which examined the joint effects of the pairings of the seven types of independent variables. All significant results of the one-way analyses are reported. Of the two-way analyses, main effects which were not significant in the appropriate one-way analyses are not reported, because of the loss of cases in the two-way analyses, for not all patients' records contained all the data necessary to classify them on both independent variables. This loss reduces the representativeness of the samples contained in the two-way analyses. Also excluded from the presentation are six interactions for which no credible interpretations exist and which, since they were either not significant at below the .01 level or had very few cases in critical categories, are quite probably chance findings. All other findings are reported.

Male Patients: Relation of Factor Scores to Background Variables

Depressed Factor.   Overall, it can be generalized from the findings on the depressed factor among male patients that the higher the social status on a background variable, the greater the degree of depressive symptoms. As can be seen in Table 4, male patients showed a linear trend in which depressive symptoms increased with age in a culture which conventionally assigns higher status as a person grows older. Similarly, the position of the eldest son in a Japanese family has higher status, and in Table 4 it can be seen that among both-sex living sibs first-born males were more depressed than were intermediate- and last-born males.[14] In the same way, married and divorced males were more depressed than were single males. Moreover, there was a linear trend in terms of the supervisory level of the patient's job—owners and managers had more depressive symptoms than did paid employees who, in turn, were more prone to depression than were unpaid family workers. The relation of higher status to increased depression is confirmed even more strongly by the data on the social class of both principal earner and patient: there was a linear trend from lower to upper social class in which the depressed factor scores increased with higher social class.

It should be understood that the above findings do not mean that higher social status inevitably leads to depression, just as being married does not necessarily make a man depressed; however, the relatively higher level of social competence shown in his managing to get married may go along with a tendency to show depression instead of other kinds of symptoms (on this idea, *see* Phillips and Draguns, Chapter 2). Another, though not necessarily contradictory, hypothesis which comes to mind, especially when we consider the ascribed rather than achieved status of eldest son, is that concern over failure to fulfill the increased responsibilities of higher social status may lead to the self-blame of depression.

Acting Out Factor. In terms of social class, the acting out factor tends to reverse the pattern of the depressed factor: acting out was greatest in the lowest social class (*see* Table 5). Looking at marital status, the finding was not so much a contrast between being single or married (as it was for male patients with depressive symptoms), as that acting out patients were most highly concentrated among divorced individuals—those who had not been able to maintain a marital relationship.

In general, the findings on birth rank for acting out were similar to those for the depressed factor in that, for both factors, first-born sons had higher scores among both-sex living sibs than did other sons. In addition, male patients who were the only sons in their families (i.e., only males in same-sex living sibships) were lowest in acting out symptoms. Of greatest interest, however, was the finding of an interaction between social class and same-sex living sibling rank. Among first-born sons there was a linear trend in that the lower the social class, the greater the acting out; among last-born sons the linear trend was in the opposite direction—the higher the social class, the greater the acting out. The trend among intermediate-born sons was similar to that of first-born sons, though it was not significant.

These data indicate that at higher social class levels the eldest son, perhaps influenced by the general cultural expectation that he will properly fulfill his responsibilities, acts out less. As social class becomes lower and the eldest son must try to meet his responsibilities with decreasing economic resources, he may become more inclined to shirk the obligations of his role and to use his greater command of the family's limited resources for his own ends—acting out by drinking and engaging in other irresponsible behavior.[15] In contrast, the youngest son, irrespective of social class, does not have any formally ascribed responsibilities and frequently is in the position of being the "baby" among his brothers. At higher class levels, where economic resources are plentiful, the youngest son is indulged and is able to spend the family's money in acting out. At lower class levels, where economic resources are scarce and the eldest son has priority, the youngest son is less likely to be indulged and to have access to money to be used in acting out.

Finally, we found that male patients whose fathers were employed in large businesses had more acting out symptoms than did those whose fathers were employed in small businesses. This difference may occur because fathers who work in small businesses are in more prolonged daily contact with family members and, hence, are more available to advise and control their sons than are fathers who work in large businesses, who usually leave home early in the morning and return quite late in the evening from businesses located a long distance from home.

Table 4: Relation between Background Variables and Depressed Factor Scores for Male Patients

Depressed Mean Factor Scores by:

	Age Group					
	≤ 24	25-34	35-44	45-54	55-64	65+
Number of cases	144	150	42	43	23	7
Mean score	2.5	2.7	3.0	4.0	5.7	6.7

F Ratio 10.0, df 5/403, p < .001

	Both-sex Living Sibling Rank		
	First-born	Intermediate-born	Last-born
Number of cases	95	132	77
Mean score	3.6	2.7	2.9

F Ratio 3.0, df 2/303, p < .05

	Marital Status		
	Single	Married	Divorced
Number of cases	258	122	9
Mean score	2.5	4.0	3.9

F Ratio 12.7, df 2/386, p < .001

Shinkeishitsu Factor. The tense, phobic, hypochondriacal male neurotic patients were those with high scores on the *shinkeishitsu* factor, and these patients differed on several background variables from patients with high scores on the depressed and acting out factors. First of all, as can be seen in Table 6, *shinkeishitsu* symptoms were especially intense among young male patients (24 years or less). Secondly, *shinkeishitsu* symptoms were higher for only sons and intermediate-born sons among same-sex living sibs.[16] Thirdly, such symptoms predominated among patients working in large businesses; and lastly, such symptoms occurred less among lower class patients than among other classes. Putting these findings together, it appears that male *shinkeishitsu* patients are most likely to be young, only or intermediate-born sons, and employed as white-collar or skilled-trade workers in large businesses.

Table 4: (Continued)

Depressed Mean Factor Scores by:

	Supervisory Job Level of Patient		
	Owner or Manager	Employee	Unpaid Family Worker
Number of cases	64	200	19
Mean score	4.3	3.0	2.2

F Ratio 6.8, df 2/280, p < .01

	Social Class of Principal Earner in Family				
	Upper	Upper-middle	Lower-middle	Working	Lower
Number of cases	30	84	110	103	28
Mean score	4.3	3.7	3.1	2.7	2.0

F Ratio 4.3, df 4/350, p < .01

	Social Class of Patient				
	Upper	Upper-middle	Lower-middle	Working	Lower
Number of cases	20	66	85	80	35
Mean score	5.4	3.8	3.3	2.5	2.2

F Ratio 6.4, df 4/281, p < .001

Reality Break and Manic Factors.   The most striking finding about the scores for males on the reality break and manic factors (the ones related most closely to a schizophrenic diagnosis) is that, with one exception, they related only to age among our background variables (*see* Table 7). High scores on both factors occurred most in the 25–44 year age range. The only other finding was that manic symptoms were concentrated in the lowest social class.

Since, as opposed to the other diagnoses, schizophrenia is related significantly to high mean scores in *two* of the symptom factors, reality break and manic, for both males and females, it seemed possible that a relation between these two factors and the background variables might be lacking because these orthogonal factors and their constituent symptoms

Table 5:   Relation between Background Variables and Acting Out Factor Scores for Male Patients

Acting Out Mean Factor Scores by:

| | Both-sex Living Sibling Rank | | |
	First-born	Intermediate-born	Last-born
Number of cases	95	132	77
Mean score	4.5	3.5	3.6
F Ratio 3.2 df 2/301, p <.05			

| | Same-sex Living Sibling Rank | | | | |
| | Only | First Half | | Middle | Last Half | |
		First-born	Other		Other	Last-born
Number of cases	101	101	11	25	7	57
Mean score	2.9	4.7	4.5	4.0	5.6	4.0
F Ratio 4.8, df 5/306, p<.005						

| | Same-sex Living Sibling Rank by Social Class of Patient | | | | | |
| | First-born | | Intermediate-born | | Last-born | |
	Number	Mean	Number	Mean	Number	Mean
Upper	7	3.3	1	1.0	2	10.0
Upper-middle	13	3.7	10	3.0	9	4.3
Lower-middle	18	5.5	8	4.5	15	3.3
Working	15	4.5	7	4.3	14	3.6
Lower	11	6.2	9	5.4	10	3.0
F Ratio 2.5, df 8/134, p < .025						

occurred in different combinations in schizophrenic patients with different backgrounds. We therefore divided the male schizophrenics into the four logical categories that occur in terms of the patient's position above or below the means for schizophrenia on the two factors (reality break = 5.3, manic = 4.4; *see* Table 3). These four logical categories are: (1) low reality break-high manic, (2) low reality break-low manic, (3) high reality break-high manic, and (4) high reality break-low manic.

Analysis of the relation between the background variables and these four logical categories revealed that patients in one of the categories had a distinctive background. Patients in the low reality break-low manic category were younger (24 years or less) and more likely to be students than were other patients; they also were rather quiet in the sense of not showing the

Table 5: (Continued)

Acting Out Mean Factor Scores by:

	Marital Status		
	Single	Married	Divorced
Number of cases	258	122	9
Mean score	3.6	3.2	5.9
F Ratio 4.1, df 2/386, p. $<$.025			

	Size of Business Employing Patient's Father	
	Large Business (30 + Employees)	Small Business ($<$ 30 Employees)
Number of cases	76	159
Mean score	4.5	3.7
F Ratio 4.0, df 1/233, p $<$.05		

	Social Class of Patient				
	Upper	Upper-middle	Lower-middle	Working	Lower
Number of cases	20	66	85	80	35
Mean score	3.7	3.0	3.7	3.2	4.7
F Ratio 2.6, df 4/281, p $<$.05					

Table 6: Relation between Background Variables and *Shinkeishitsu* Factor Scores for Male Patients

Shinkeishitsu Mean Factor Scores by:

	Age Group					
	≤ 24	25-34	35-44	45-54	55-64	65+
Number of cases	144	150	42	43	23	7
Mean score	4.7	3.9	3.0	4.3	3.6	4.0
F Ratio 2.7, df 5/403, p <.05						

	Same-sex Living Sibling Rank					
	Only	First Half		Middle	Last Half	
		First-born	Other		Other	Last-born
Number of cases	101	101	11	25	7	67
Mean score	4.7	3.2	3.6	4.1	3.7	3.1
F Ratio 3.9, df 5/306, p <.01						

	Size of Business Employing Patient	
	Large Business (30 + Employees)	Small Business (<30 Employees)
Number of cases	157	107
Mean score	4.4	3.5
F Ratio 8.1, df 1/262, p <.01		

	Social Class of Patient				
	Upper	Upper-middle	Lower-middle	Working	Lower
Number of cases	20	66	85	80	35
Mean score	4.0	4.7	3.8	4.3	2.5
F Ratio 3.9, df 4/281, p <.01					

symptom of physical violence particularly in contrast to patients in the high reality break-high manic category.[17] The possibility that there is a special subgroup among Japanese male schizophrenic patients who are young, quiet students who do not show a very high degree of either reality break or manic symptoms should be considered in future work.

The Major Effects on Background Characteristics on the Patterning of Symptoms among Male Patients

The most important background characteristics for male patients were social class, age, and, to a somewhat lesser extent, birth rank. The other characteristics examined appear to be relatively unimportant.

Table 7: Relation between Background Variables and Reality Break and Manic Factor Scores for Male Patients

Reality Break Mean Factor Scores by:

	Age Group					
	≤ 24	25-34	35-44	45-54	55-64	65+
Number of cases	144	150	42	43	23	7
Mean score	1.8	2.8	3.6	2.0	1.6	1.4
F Ratio 4.0, df 5/403, p <.01						

Manic Mean Factor Scores by:

	Age Group					
	≤ 24	25-34	35-44	45-54	55-64	65+
Number of cases	145	150	42	43	23	7
Mean score	2.2	2.9	2.9	1.9	2.1	2.6
F Ratio 2.2, df 5/404, p <.06						

	Social Class of Patient				
	Upper	Upper-middle	Lower-middle	Working	Lower
Number of cases	20	66	85	80	35
Mean score	2.6	2.3	2.7	2.3	3.6
F Ratio 1.9, df 4/281, p <.06					

Table 8: Relation between Background Variables and Depressed Factor Scores for Female Patients

Depressed Mean Factor Scores by:

	Age Group of Patient by Marital Status					
	≤ 24		25-34		35-44	
	N	Mean	N	Mean	N	Mean
Never married (single)	66	4.3	40	4.0	4	2.3
Ever married (married, divorced)	5	5.2	38	3.1	31	3.0

	45-54		55 +	
	N	Mean	N	Mean
Never married (single)	3	1.7	2	0.5
Ever married (married, divorced)	41	4.4	14	5.5

F Ratio 2.7, df 4/234, p $<$.05

	Same-sex Living Sibling Rank by Size of Business Employing Principal Earner in Family					
	First-born		Intermediate-born		Last-born	
	Number	Mean	Number	Mean	Number	Mean
Large business (30 + employees)	22	3.8	12	3.5	32	3.5
Small business (<30 employees)	17	2.1	12	4.8	18	5.0

F Ratio 3.9, df 2/107, p $<$.025

	Social Class of Principal Earner in Family				
	Upper	Upper-middle	Lower-middle	Working	Lower
Number of cases	28	34	66	53	11
Mean score	5.4	3.5	4.0	3.4	3.8

F Ratio 2.4, df 4/187, p $<$.05

Social class appeared as a meaningful background variable for all the factors except reality break. Lower class males showed more acting out and manic symptoms and less depressed and *shinkeishitsu* symptoms than did higher class patients. These findings were strikingly congruent with findings in other cultures on social class differences in symptomatology. For example, Phillips and his colleagues have found that higher class patients are more likely to have both "ideational" symptoms and those involving "turning against the self," while lower class patients are more likely to have "action-oriented" symptoms and those involving "turning against others" (*see* Phillips and Draguns, Chapter 2, for a review of these ideas). These tendencies for the locus of symptoms to be internal for higher class patients and external for lower class patients are paralled by findings in several cultures (*see* Kohn, 1963, for data on the United States; Pearlin and Kohn, 1966, for data on Italy) which have shown that higher class parents are more concerned with the inner reasons for their children's behavior while lower class parents are more concerned with the external consequences of their children's behavior.

Age appeared as a meaningful background variable for all the factors except acting out. Starting at the lower end of the age range, male patients aged 24 years or less were most prone to *shinkeishitsu* symptoms; moving into the 25–44 year age range, they were most prone to reality break and manic symptoms. Over the entire age range, depressed symptoms increased, rising steeply at 45 years of age. Thus among hospitalized male patients, except for acting out symptoms which appeared at a relatively constant level across the life span, the nature of the symptoms shifted with age.

Birth rank appeared as a meaningful background variable for the depressed, acting out, and *shinkeishitsu* factors but not for the other two factors analyzed. In terms of position in both-sex living birth rank, eldest sons were likely both to be more depressed and to act out more than were other sons. These findings seem to represent alternative solutions for eldest sons who have difficulty in meeting the requirements of their role: (1) either they accept the additional responsibilities of being an eldest son but feel they cannot fulfill them and hence become depressed, or (2) they reject their responsibilities and act out. The effect of social class on the alternative chosen by eldest sons is shown by the finding among same-sex living sibs that eldest sons in the lower social class levels acted out more than did those in higher social classes. On the other hand, youngest sons in higher social classes, where, presumedly, money is readily available for them to spend in the search for pleasure, acted out more than did those in lower social classes. Finally, to complete the picture, we found that in the same-sex living birth rank only and intermediate-born sons were more *shinkeishitsu*—that is, phobic and tense as patients rather than depressed or given to acting out.

In summary, symptom patterns for men seem to be most influenced by social class and age, which are the two variables most central to occupational careers. The interrelation between symptom pattern and occupational career very possibly is linked to Japan's rapidly changing economic structure and to the concomitant increase in the opportunity for social mobility.[18] The importance of age is evident in the nature of the symptoms which were most prevalent at different points in the occupational career. During the extremely competitive years of higher schooling and occupational training (24 years or less), within which the outcome of examinations to secure a beginning place in a university or major firm can determine a man's general path of life (Vogel, 1963), anxious, tense, *shinkeishitsu* symptoms predominated. During the period of 25–44 years obvious occupational failure becomes evident, and it was at this time that reality break and manic symptoms appeared strongest—either as a cause of, or a reaction to, occupational failure. Depression was greatest after 45 years of age, especially at higher class levels, possibly because of either failure in measuring up to high aspirations or the feeling that the actual rewards of success are hollow.

Female Patients: Relation of Factor Scores to Background Variables

Depressed Factor.   Among women, the effect of social class on depressive symptomatology was somewhat similar to that among men, the difference between the sexes being that for men there was a linear trend of increasing depression from lower to higher class levels, while for women only in the highest class was depression significantly increased (*see* Table 8). As opposed to men, among whom eldest sons were most depressed, there was no overall finding by birth rank. Among women an interaction existed between same-sex living sibling rank and principal earner's size of business such that first-born daughters in small-business families were less depressed than all other groups. Also in contrast to men, increasing age did *not* result in increasing depression. Among women there was an interaction between age and marital status; for women who had ever been married (currently married, widowed, or divorced), there was a U-shaped curve showing a definite decline in the degree of depression during the child-rearing years of 25–44. Apparently, child rearing acts as a buffer against depression, which was higher in the years generally preceding child birth and later in the years of the "empty nest" and the onset of menopause.[19] Among women who had never been married (i.e., single), a downward trend in depression was evidenced as age increased, although with the small number of cases in the upper age range significance was not reached.

Wagamama Factor.   In contrast to other forms of acting out behavior for both male and female patients in our data and also to the findings of other studies mentioned earlier, *wagamama* symptoms among women occurred more strongly at higher rather than lower social class levels, as indicated by the amount of education received and the prestige of the school attended (*see* Table 9). There was a linear trend on amount of education: the higher the education, the greater the *wagamama* symptoms, culminating in a sharp increase among women with graduate school training. There

Table 9: Relation between Background Variables and *Wagamama* Factor Scores for Female Patients

Wagamama Mean Factor Scores by :

Same-sex Living Sibling Rank by Size of Business Employing Principal Earner in Family

	First-born		Intermediate-born		Last-born	
	Number	Mean	Number	Mean	Number	Mean
Large business (30 + employees)	22	2.7	12	0.3	32	1.7
Small business (< 30 employees)	17	0.5	12	1.5	18	2.7

F Ratio 6.6, df 2/107, p < .005

Same-sex Living Sibling Rank by Size of Business Employing Patient's Father

	First-born		Intermediate-born		Last-born	
	Number	Mean	Number	Mean	Number	Mean
Large business (30 + employees)	12	3.3	7	0.3	12	1.3
Small business (< 30 employees)	16	0.4	11	0.9	30	2.1

F Ratio 6.6, df 2/82, p < .005

Education of Patient

	Elem.	Jr. High	Attended Sr. High	Graduated Sr. High	Attended College	Graduated College	Graduate School
Number of cases	19	31	29	99	18	12	5
Mean score	1.5	1.0	1.6	1.5	2.2	2.9	5.2

F Ratio 3.4, df 6/206, p < .01

Prestige of Senior High School or College from Which Patient Graduated

	Prestige School	Ordinary School
Number of cases	22	62
Mean score	3.7	1.8

F Ratio 10.3, df 1/82, p < .01

seems to be something peculiarly Japanese about the picture of a post-graduate, professionally trained woman who as a patient is emotional, negative, irresponsible, and childish.

There was no overall finding by birth rank for the *wagamama* factor. An interaction, however, existed between same-sex living sibling rank and size of business in which both the principal earner and the patient's father were employed. A linear trend existed among small-business families for increasing *wagamama* behavior in later birth ranks. Among large-business families *wagamama* behavior was less in the intermediate birth ranks than among first-born and last-born female sibs. In general, first-born daughters from large-business families and last-born daughters from small-business families were more *wagamama* than all other daughters.

Shinkeishitsu Factor. As for male patients, *shinkeishitsu* symptoms were higher for only and intermediate-born daughters among same-sex living sibs (*see* Table 10). Also if, parallel to the hypothesis for males, it is predicted that a higher degree of *shinkeishitsu* occurs among young female patients, then there is significantly more *shinkeishitsu* symptomatology in females under 35 years of age than occurs in patients in the 35–64 year age range. This finding, however, should be accepted with caution because the overall analysis of variance on which it is based was not significant and also because an upswing in *shinkeishitsu* symptoms occurred at age 65 or more.[20]

Thus, for both men and women, there is evidence that *shinkeishitsu* symptoms are more pronounced in young patients than in older ones and in those who are only or intermediate-born sibs among children of their own sex. Women, however, differed from men in that the occurrence of *shinkeishitsu* symptoms was not affected by social class.

Reality Break and Manic Factors. As among male patients, the reality break factor among female patients was not related to many of the background variables. There were only two findings (*see* Table 11).

Table 10: Relation between Background Variables and *Shinkeishitsu* Factor Scores for Female Patients

Shinkeishitsu Mean Factor Scores by:						
	Same-sex Living Sibling Rank					
	Only	First Half		Middle	Last Half	
		First-born	Other		Other	Last-born
Number of cases	58	44	8	14	7	67
Mean score	3.0	2.0	2.3	2.9	4.3	1.8
F Ratio 3.3, df 5/192, p < .01						

One was a highly significant—and to us rather puzzling—interaction between both-sex living birth rank and size of business in which the patient's father was employed such that intermediate-born daughters of fathers in large businesses showed less reality break symptoms than did first- or last-born daughters, while intermediate-born daughters of fathers in small businesses showed more reality break than did their sisters. The second finding indicated that single female patients showed more reality break than did married or divorced patients.

On the manic factor, however, in contrast to the relatively sparse findings among men, we can specify fairly precisely the conditions under which women will show manic behavior. As presented in the second part of Table 11, the combination of conditions most likely to produce manic behavior occurs when a woman is single, psychotic, and an unpaid family worker whose father owns or manages a small business.

Paralleling the analysis among men where we looked at the interrelation between the two factors, reality break and manic, on which schizophrenics had significantly higher scores, we also divided the female schizophrenic patients into the same four logical categories in terms of their positions above or below the means on the two factors (reality break = 6.8, manic = 4.7; *see* Table 3). Analysis of background differences of female schizophrenic patients in terms of these four categories revealed that patients in the high reality break-low manic group were more likely than others to have fathers in a higher social class. Similarly, female schizophrenic patients in this high reality break-low manic group showed a not quite significant tendency ($p < .10$) to be drawn disproportionately from those whose fathers were employed in large businesses. When a direct comparison was made between the two symptom groups who were high on one but not on the other of the factors (high reality break-low manic *vs.* low reality break-high manic), a significant difference ($p < .02$) emerged. Patients who were high on reality break and low on manic symptoms came from families in which the father was employed in a large business. In contrast, patients who were low on reality break and high on manic symptoms came from families in which the father was employed in a small business.[21] The latter female schizophrenic patients seem to have contributed substantially to our general finding among all female patients that manic behavior was more likely among single psychotic daughters of fathers who were owners or managers of small businesses.

The Major Effects of Background Characteristics on the Patterning of Symptoms among Female Patients

The most important background characteristic for female patients was the size of business in which the principal earner or the patient's father was employed; it was related to all the symptom factors except *shinkeishitsu*. As noted earlier (*see* Note 11), this variable is used to differentiate two

Table 11: Relation between Background Variables and Reality Break and Manic Factor Scores for Female Patients

Reality Break Mean Factor Scores by:

	Both-sex Living Sibling Rank by Size of Business Employing Patient's Father					
	First-born		Intermediate-born		Last-born	
	Number	Mean	Number	Mean	Number	Mean
Large business (30 + employees)	12	5.7	19	3.7	14	6.6
Small business (< 30 employees)	16	4.8	31	5.7	19	4.7
F Ratio 6.3, df 2/105, p < .005						

	Marital Status		
	Single	Married	Divorced
Number of cases	115	119	10
Mean score	5.5	4.3	4.4
F Ratio 6.0, df 2/241, p < .01			

Manic Mean Factor Scores by:

	Marital Status		
	Single	Married	Divorced
Number of cases	115	119	10
Mean score	3.8	2.6	1.9
F Ratio 4.7, df 2/241, p < .05			

	Marital Status by Diagnostic Group			
	Never Married (Single)		Ever Married (Married, Divorced)	
	Number	Mean	Number	Mean
Other psychoses	3	4.7	16	2.3
Schizophrenia	72	5.3	42	3.8
Neuroses	38	1.1	68	1.8
F Ratio 3.9, df 2/233, p < .025				

(Continued)

Table 11: (Continued)

Manic Mean Factor Scores by:

	Marital Status by Size of Business			
	Employing Principal Earner in Family			
	Never Married (Single)		Ever Married (Married, Divorced)	
	Number	Mean	Number	Mean
Large business (30 + employees)	49	2.9	55	2.9
Small business (<30 employees)	40	4.7	38	2.8

F Ratio 3.7, df 1/178, p <.07

| | Supervisory Job Level of Patient | | |
	Owner or Manager	Employee	Unpaid Family Worker
Number of cases	10	39	7
Mean score	1.5	2.9	5.9

F Ratio 3.8, df 2/53, p <.05

| | Supervisory Job Level of Patient's Father | |
	Owner or Manager	Employee
Number of cases	88	46
Mean score	3.5	2.2

F Ratio 5.1, df 1/132, p <.05

styles of life: the first is the world of the "salaryman," in which the husband or father works in a large business or governmental organization and spends most of his waking hours away from his wife and children, who usually do not contribute directly to the economic resources of the family; the second is the world of "small business," in which the husband or father either owns or works in a small commercial shop or tiny factory which is located in or near his home, where his wife and children frequently work along with him to contribute to the livelihood of the family.[22]

The great amount of personal and economic interdependence in the small-business family heightens the importance of familial variables, such as birth rank and marital status, in determining the behavior patterns of family members. In three of the four instances where style of life was related to factor scores it was in interaction with birth rank, and the effects were particularly strong in small-business families.

Eldest daughters in small-business families showed less depression than did daughters in any other position. Similarly, for *wagamama* symptoms there was a linear trend in small-business families such that eldest daughters showed the least *wagamama* symptoms and youngest daughters the most. In terms of reality break, intermediate-born daughters in small-business families showed more symptoms than did eldest or youngest daughters. On none of these three factors did eldest daughters in small-business families show more symptoms than other daughters did. Furthermore, these findings do not result from preferential concern over the eldest daughter so that she is hospitalized with less severe symptoms than are other daughters. Actually, if anything, in our sample of patients more youngest than eldest daughters were hospitalized from both small- and large-business families.[23]

The effects of a small-business style of life on manic behavior also were evident in interaction with another familial variable—marital status. Single female patients from families in which the principal earner was employed in a small business showed significantly more manic symptoms than did all other women. The effects of a small-business style of life were evidenced further in the linear trend toward increasing manic behavior as the female patient's job level decreased from that of an owner or manager, through an employee, to an unpaid family worker, as well as in the greater manic behavior displayed by female patients whose fathers were owners or managers as opposed to those whose fathers were employees.

In large-business families with a salaryman style of life, the effects of familial variables were less pronounced. The only findings were that intermediate-born daughters among same-sex living sibs showed the least *wagamama* symptoms; that intermediate-born daughters among both-sex living sibs showed the least reality break; and that eldest daughters in large-business families (when compared with youngest daughters in small-business families) showed the most *wagamama* symptoms.

The only finding among female patients relating birth order to the symptom factors which was not moderated by style of life was that only and intermediate-born daughters showed the most *shinkeishitsu* symptoms—a pattern which is identical to that found among men.

Considering the overall effects of birth rank on hospitalized female patients, it would seem that eldest daughters in small-business families have the least severe symptomology, as indicated by their scores on the different factors. An explanation of this finding should take into account the cultural role of the eldest daughter in Japan, particularly within the small-business family. In general, in Japan the eldest daughter's role is similar to that of the eldest son in that it carries with it responsibilities and privileges. It differs, however, from that of the eldest son in that it is carried out almost totally within the confines of the family in helping the mother to maintain a satisfactory equilibrium among the household members, while the eldest son shares responsibility with the father both for being the official representative of the family in the outside world and for maintaining the family's economic viability. Thus in the world of the small-business family with its complex interdependent interpersonal relations involving both emotional satisfactions and economic functions, the role of eldest daughter carries more prestige, meaning, and satisfaction than does the same formal role in the less complex interpersonal environment of the salaryman's family. At the same time, the eldest daughter in the small-business family does not have to contend with the economic responsibilities confronting the eldest son.

It also appears possible that intermediate-born daughters in large-business families have less severe symptomatology since they scored significantly low on two of the three factors showing an interaction between style of life and birth rank. On the whole, however, intermediate-born daughters together with only daughters scored high on the *shinkeishitsu* factor.

In addition to the already mentioned effect on manic behavior in small-business families, marital status had a more general relation to symptom patterns. For both of the factors—reality break and manic—which are related to a diagnosis of schizophrenia, single women scored higher than did married or divorced women. At the present time, however, the causal pattern implicit in these findings is by no means clear. A clearcut causal relation can be surmised from the interaction of marital status and age in producing depressive symptoms in that among women who had ever been married a definite decline in depressive symptoms during the years of 25–44 seemed to indicate that in Japan child rearing acts as a buffer against depression. This finding is particularly relevant in the light of the almost exclusively child-centered interpersonal and affective life of the Japanese mother, resulting in very intense, long-enduring relations with her children (*see* Vogel, 1963; Caudill and Plath, 1966).

Although the findings for symptom patterns in terms of the background variables of social class and education were relatively sparse, they are important in that they serve to emphasize both the overall effect of social structure on symptoms and the necessity for examining the differential effects of culture. The finding that upper class female patients had more depressive symptoms than did other females and the general picture of greater manic behavior among daughters who were unpaid family workers in small businesses agree with the cross-cultural findings previously discussed in the summary of the effects of background variables on men. As mentioned in that summary, higher social class tends to be associated with "ideational" symptoms and self-punitive behavior, and lower social class position with "action-oriented" symptoms and "turning against others." An examination of the effects of education on female patients revealed, however, a linear trend toward increasing *wagamama* behavior with increasing education. A similar relation between *wagamama* behavior and social status also was evident in the great amount of *wagamama* behavior among graduates of prestige schools. Thus, among female patients in Japan, higher social status appears to be related to a particular form of acting out—one which involves negative, irresponsible, childish behavior and emotional outbursts.

While among men the patterning of symptoms seems to focus on problems of occupational career, among women the importance of birth rank, marital status, child rearing, and the effects of living in a highly inter-dependent small-business family all seem to point to the formal roles in family life as central determinants of symptomatology. While relative status in the family probably is an influence on the patterning of symptoms in women in most societies, several of the tendencies which have emerged are related particularly to Japanese culture.

Conclusions

Several cautions about generalizing from our data should be stressed. Since the data are based on hospitalized patients, we do not know the extent to which similar trends occur in the general population. It is quite probable that the conditions leading to hospitalization vary in different countries, social classes, and styles of life. Furthermore, since the present data come primarily from hospital records, they are subject to both the individual and cultural biases of the psychiatrists and nurses who initially collected the information. Finally, because the primary data were obtained in the foregoing manner, a certain amount of relevant information was missing, and since we cannot assume that these omissions occurred randomly we cannot be sure that all our results would remain the same if we had complete information on all cases in our sample. A second sample of data which we have collected but not yet analyzed (*see* Note 4) avoids many of these pitfalls. In any case, the present data are based on consecutive admissions to four representative psychiatric hospitals in the Tokyo area, and, despite the above cautions, it seems likely that our findings are applicable to a reasonable extent to the patterning of psychiatric symptoms and emotional problems in the general Japanese population.

When considered cross-culturally, most of the factors which emerged from our analysis of symptoms seem markedly similar to what we would expect to find in other cultures. Two of the factors, however, *shinkeishitsu* and *wagamama*, exactly fit specific behavior patterns which generally are identified by these same terms in ordinary speech. These symptom patterns may well occur to some degree in other cultures, but in Japan they are commonly recognized as distinct character types which have concomitant interpersonal roles in ordinary social life.

Another finding which seems characteristic of Japan is that schizophrenics had high scores not only on the reality break factor but also on the manic factor. Furthermore, even the reality break factor had a meaningful loading on physical violence. As noted, this finding of greater violence and emotional impulsivity among Japanese schizophrenics than among others is in agreement with the findings of Katz, Gudeman, and Sanborn (Chapter 9) concerning the prehospitalized behavior of schizophrenics of Japanese ancestry in Hawaii.

Evidence that social structure can have similar effects in different cultural contexts was shown by the relation between higher social class and depression and between lower social class and manic and acting out behavior. The importance of the cultural context, however, cannot be neglected. For example, a particularly Japanese form of acting out—*wagamama* behavior— occurred most strongly among higher rather than lower status women. Also, the powerful effects on the patterning of behavior of a small-business versus a salaryman style of life suggest that this distinction is particularly significant in the changing society of present-day Japan. Finally, the importance of the cultural context can be seen in the existence of such significant interactions as the one between birth rank, style of life, and *wagamama* behavior, in which all three variables have special meaning in Japan. In conclusion, we believe our findings serve to emphasize the need to consider not only the effects of the present social structure in a country but also the cultural context derived from the country's past history.

NOTES

1. Three of the hospitals—Seiwa, Kōseiin, and Hiyoshi—are small private hospitals, while the fourth hospital—Matsuzawa—is a large public institution operated by the city of Tokyo. Excluding a few Chinese and Korean patients, the number of admissions of Japanese patients to each of these hospitals in 1958 was quite similar: Seiwa, 107 males, 80 females; Kōseiin, 137 males, 51 females; Hiyoshi, 120 males, 73 females; and Matsuzawa, 84 males, 65 females. The data were collected early in 1959 by means of a schedule which was completed for each patient by the psychiatrist in charge of the patient and the nurse on the ward, supplementing the patient's case record by knowledge from direct work with the patient.

2. The finding of an overrepresentation of eldest sons and youngest daughters was, as indicated, statistically true among living same-sex sibs, but the data were in the same direction in all three of the other ways of considering birth rank. The four ways in which the position of a patient in a birth rank was analyzed are: (1) the patient's position among living and dead sibs of both sexes, (2) the patient's position among living sibs of both sexes, (3) the patient's position among living and dead sibs of the same sex as the patient, and (4) the patient's position among living sibs of the same sex as the patient (*see* Caudill, 1963).

3. In studies of comparative data on birth rank in the United States, the best evidence is that youngest daughters are overrepresented among hospitalized schizophrenic patients and that the overall finding for sons is not significant. In these studies, birth rank was considered in terms of the patient's position among living and dead sibs of both sexes (*see* Schooler, 1961, 1964).

4. In a future paper we will report on an analysis of the symptoms and background characteristics of a comparable sample of American patients. The American data will be analyzed in the same way that the Japanese data are handled in this paper. We then can make a direct comparison of the symptom clusters found in the two cultures. In addition, we also have an opportunity to replicate the Japanese study reported here. We already have collected data from five hospitals in Tokyo (three of which were used in the present study) on all admissions during a 12-month period in 1963–64. There are approximately 1,000 patients in this second Japanese sample.

5. The correlations across the total patient population between the factors, derived from the male and female subgroups, which are given the same names are: depressed, .66; *shinkeishitsu*, .97; reality break, .79; and manic, .85. The correlation between the male factor of acting out and the female factor of *wagamama* is .53.

6. The reader should note that negative loadings that occur within a group of positive loadings should be read in the negative. For example, among the loadings on acting out for males, − .37 on bodily complaints and − .33 on psychosomatic disorders should be read as "no bodily complaints" and "no psychosomatic disorders." On the other hand, in a factor where all, or most, of the loadings are negative, the signs should be reversed in reading. Thus, on reality break for males, all loadings should be read as positive; and on depressed for females, .34 on "talking

to self" should be read as "not talking to self," whereas all the negative loadings should be read in the positive.

7.   In order to determine the score of a patient on a factor, the computer was programmed to ascertain the presence or absence (1 or 0) of a relevant symptom and then to compute a factor score using the following rules: (1) if a 1 occurs and the weighting is positive, the increment to be added equals the amount of the weighting; (2) if a 0 occurs and the weighting is positive, no increment is to be added to the factor score; (3) if a 1 occurs and the weighting is negative, no increment is to be added to the factor score because the weighting is to be used only for the *absence* of the symptom; and (4) if a 0 occurs and the weighting is negative, the positive increment to be added equals the amount of the negative weighting because the symptom is appropriately absent. The use of this system results in all factor scores being positive while, at the same time, accounting for negative weightings.

8.   From this point on, we will present our results in terms of one-way and two-way analyses of variance. The tables show the means for each cell. All a posteriori comparisons between cells were checked with the Newman-Keuls or Scheffé procedures. Linear trends among cells were tested by procedures suggested by Edwards (1960). Analyses of interacting effects were tested by methods suggested by Winer (1962). In addition to these procedures, several times we have made a priori predicted comparisons between cells which were tested by the t-test procedures suggested by Winer (1962). Predicted comparisons occur in the following places in the tables: (1) Table 4, involving the prediction of higher depressed factor scores for first-born males among both-sex living sibs, (2) Table 5, predicting higher acting out factor scores for lower social class male patients, (3) Table 7, predicting higher manic scores among lower social class male patients, (4) Tables 6 and 10, predicting differences among both men and women in the *shinkeishitsu* factor scores of the different birth ranks in same-sex living sibships (*see* Note 16), and (5) Table 6, predicting higher *shinkeishitsu* scores for younger males. All reported results, unless otherwise specified in the text, are significant at at least the .05 level using a two-tailed test.

9.   It should be noted that conventionally in Japan, as in the United States, women are not given the diagnosis of sociopathic illness, since this category is reserved largely for men.

10.   Even among neurotics we found a high level of acting out when we excluded the Kōseiin patients. The latter patients, on the whole, were rather quiet *shinkeishitsu* patients who came to Kōseiin because they had heard of its special method of treatment which requires, among other things, that the patient spend the first week resting in bed (Caudill and Doi, 1963). The neurotic patients in the three other hospitals were significantly less quiet and more given to acting out prior to their hospitalization. The point that emerges, therefore, is that, leaving out the Kōseiin patients, acting out is a general characteristic of male Japanese patients regardless of diagnosis.

11.   "Size of business," or more conceptually "style of life," relates to whether a person worked in a large corporate structure, either in business or government, or in a small business. For purposes of counting, we con-

sidered an enterprise having 30 or more employees a large business, and an enterprise having less than 30 employees a small business. The question of style of life is conceptually separate from that of social class and is discussed at length in Vogel (1963) and Caudill and Plath (1966).

12.   The "principal earner in the family" is the person in the family in which the patient was living who provided the main income for the family. If the patient was young, this usually was the patient's father or sometimes the patient's mother or other relative. If the patient was an adult male, this person usually was the patient himself; if the patient was an adult female, this person usually was the patient's spouse or father.

13.   Social class was determined by the interactive position on two 7-point scales for level of occupation and amount of education resulting in five social class divisions. The method follows that of Hollingshead and Redlich (1958) and is supplemented for particular Japanese occupational statuses by the work of the Nihon Shakai Gakkai Chōsa Iinkai (1958), and by the work of Odaka (1964, 1965). On social class, also see Inkeles and Rossi (1956) and Ramsey and Smith (1960).

14.   In this paper, as indicated earlier, we think of sibling position as a social structural or cultural variable and not as a biological variable. Our findings, therefore, are presented only in terms of position among living siblings of both sexes and among living siblings of the same sex. All findings discussed, however, were checked against the other ways of considering sibling position (*see* Note 2), and no substantial disagreement was found. Findings are reported both in terms of extended and condensed birth orders. The extended birth order contains the categories of: only child, first-born, first half but not first-born, middle child, last half but not last-born, and last-born. The condensed birth order ignores the only child and contains the categories of: first-born, intermediate-born (which includes first half but not first-born, middle child, and last half but not last-born), and last-born.

15.   The symptoms comprising the acting out factor in Table 1 indicate that, in the context of Japanese society, this cluster of symptoms involves irresponsible self-indulgence, which, for men in Japan, usually means spending money on drinking, entertaining at restaurants and bars, and playing with women.

16.   Using the stringent a posteriori Scheffé test, the only significant difference among the male same-sex living birth ranks was the greater amount of *shinkeishitsu* in only versus first-born and last-born sibs. Data for females showed that the intermediate-born sibs were similar to the only sibs in their high scores on the *shinkeishitsu* factor (*see* Table 10). Since a similar tendency existed among male sibs, the two sets of data were seen as predictive of each other, and a priori t-test statistics were used. With such statistics, the difference among males in the comparison of only and intermediate-born sibs versus first- and last-born sibs was significant at $p < .02$; among females the same comparison was significant at $p < .001$.

17.   The frequency distributions for male schizophrenic patients among the four logical symptom groups on which these findings are based are:

	Symptom Group			
	Low Reality Break		High Reality Break	
Background Variable	High Manic	Low Manic	High Manic	Low Manic
A. Age Group of Patient				
$\leq$ 24	5	28	7	6
25-44	9	28	19	20
45+	0	2	4	4
X^2 = 26.4, df = 6, p < .001				
B. Level of Job of Patient				
Owner/manager	1	1	4	1
Employee	5	25	14	23
Family worker	2	4	1	0
Student	3	20	5	3
X^2 = 20.6, df = 9, p < .02				
C. Occurrence of Symptom of Physical Violence				
Present	2	11	19	10
Absent	12	47	11	20
X^2 = 20.2, df = 3, p < .001				

18.   Opportunities for social mobility in Japan are, at present, greater in small and medium-sized businesses; for owners, managers, and executives at high levels; and for skilled workers at low levels. Lack of opportunity for mobility is most evident in large businesses and for the middle range of white-collar workers (*see* Tominaga, 1962).

19.   For an interesting related sidelight on this issue, see the analysis of sleeping arrangements in the urban Japanese family over the course of the family cycle in Caudill and Plath (1966).

20.   The date for this finding on *shinkeishitsu* factor scores for females by age group are:

	$\leq$ 24	25-34	35-44	45-54	55-64	65+
Number of cases	71	82	35	44	11	5
Mean score	2.8	2.9	2.1	2.3	2.1	2.8

F Ratio 1.1, df 5/242, not significant.

21.   The frequency distributions for female schizophrenic patients among the four logical symptom groups on which these findings are based are:

	Symptom Group			
	Low Reality Break		High Reality Break	
Background Variable	High Manic	Low Manic	High Manic	Low Manic
A. Social Class of Father				
Upper and upper-middle	3	2	3	11
Lower-middle and working	12	12	11	9
X^2 = 7.9, df = 3, p < .05				
B. Size of Business Employing Father				
Large business				
(30 + employees)	2	5	6	11
Small business				
(< 30 employees)	13	9	8	9

1) Comparison among all four groups: X^2 = 6.5, df = 3, p < .10
2) Comparison of high reality break-low manic *vs.* low reality break-high manic: X^2 = 6.3, df = 1, p < .02

22.   Salarymen have been in the ascendency in Japan during the spectacular economic recovery of the country since World War II, but a substantial proportion of urban families still engage in small businesses. Moreover, the two styles of life did not suddenly become differentiated in the post-war development of Japan but rather have a long history—in terms of the roles of the bureaucrat and the tradesman—extending back to the Meiji Period and even beyond with some roots in the distinctive way of life of the governmental functionary or *samurai*, on the one hand, and in the way of life developed by merchants and other townsmen, on the other (Vogel, 1963; Dore, 1958).

23.   Among same-sex living female sibs from families in which the principal earner worked in a small business, there were 19 eldest and 28 youngest daughters. Among those coming from families in which the principal earner worked in a large business, there were 22 eldest and 32 youngest daughters. The overall χ^2 for eldest *vs.* youngest daughters is 3.57, df = 1, p < .07.

REFERENCES

Caudill, W. 1963. Sibling rank and style of life among Japanese psychiatric patients. *In* Proceedings of the Joint Meeting of the Japanese Society of Psychiatry and Neurology and the American Psychiatric Association, Tokyo. H. Akimoto, ed. Supplement No. 7 of Folia Psychiatria et Neurologia Japonica. Tokyo, Japanese Society of Psychiatry and Neurology.

Caudill, W., and L. T. Doi. 1963. Interrelations of psychiatry, culture, and emotion in Japan. *In* Man's image in medicine and anthropology. I. Galdston, ed. New York, International Universities Press.

Caudill, W., and D. W. Plath. 1966. Who sleeps by whom? Parent-child involvement in urban Japanese families. Psychiatry 29:344–66.

Dore, R. 1958. City life in Japan. London, Routledge and Kegan Paul.

Draguns, J. G., L. Phillips, I. K. Broverman, and S. Nishimae. In press. Psychiatric symptoms in relation to social competence and culture: a study of Japanese psychiatric patients. *In* Proceedings of the Tenth Interamerican Congress of Psychology. C. F. Hereford, ed. Austin, University of Texas Press.

Edwards, A. L. 1960. Experimental design in psychological research. New York, Holt, Rinehart and Winston.

Hollingshead, A. B., and F. C. Redlich. 1958. Social class and mental illness. New York, Wiley.

Inkeles, A., and P. H. Rossi. 1956. National comparisons of occupational prestige. American Journal of Sociology. 61:329–39.

Kohn, M. L. 1963. Social class and parent-child relationships: an interpretation. American Journal of Sociology 68:471–80.

Nihon Shakai Gakkai Chōsa Iinkai, ed. 1958. Nihon shakai no kaisō-teki kōzō. Tokyo, Yūhikaku.

Odaka, K. 1964. The middle classes in Japan (part one). Contemporary Japan 28:10–32.

————. 1965. The middle classes in Japan (part two). Contemporary Japan 28:268–96.

Pearlin, L. I., and M. L. Kohn. 1966. Social class, occupation, and parental values: a cross-national survey. American Sociological Review 31:466–79.

Phillips, L., and M. Rabinovitch. 1958. Social role and patterns of symptomatic behavior. Journal of Abnormal and Social Psychology 57:181–86.

Ramsey, C. E., and R. J. Smith. 1960. Japanese and American perceptions of occupations. American Journal of Sociology 65:475–82.

Schooler, C. 1961. Birth order and schizophrenia. Archives of General Psychiatry 4:91–97.

————. 1964. Birth order and hospitalization for schizophrenia. Journal of Abnormal and Social Psychology 69:574–79.

Schooler, C., and W. Caudill. 1964. Symptomatology in Japanese and American schizophrenics. Ethnology 3:172–78.

Tominaga, K. 1962. Occupational mobility in Japanese society: analysis of labor market in Japan. The Journal of Economic Behavior 2:1–37.

Vogel, E. F. 1963. Japan's new middle class. Berkeley, University of California Press.

Winer, B. J. 1962. Statistical principles in experimental design. New York, McGraw-Hill.

9.   Characterising Differences in Psychopathology among
      Ethnic Groups: A Preliminary Report on Hawaii-Japanese
      and Mainland-American Schizophrenics

MARTIN M. KATZ, Ph.D.

Clinical Research Branch
National Institute of Mental Health
Bethesda, Maryland

HOWARD GUDEMAN, Ph.D.

Department of Psychological Services and Training
Hawaii State Hospital
Honolulu, Hawaii

KENNETH SANBORN, Ph.D.

Institute of Behavioral Sciences
Honolulu, Hawaii

AN EARLIER STUDY made at Hawaii State Hospital (Enright and Jaeckle, 1963) reported marked differences between the symptom patterns of patients of Japanese and Filipino ancestry who had been similarly diagnosed as paranoid schizophrenics. Since the pathology which characterized each group conformed to certain stereotypes or expectations about these ethnic groups, the results were viewed as still another example of the relation between ethnic background and the manner in which psychopathology is expressed. Such findings have important implications for persons interested in delineating the similarities and differences in modal behavioral patterns among cultures. In another context, they are highly relevant to researchers in psychopathology who are concerned with distinguishing the manifestations of illness which are shaped by culture from those which are supracultural or intrinsic to pathology.

As in much other research of this type, however, methodological problems—a small sample, inadequate case records, retrospective analysis of symptoms—restricted the conclusions. Clinical research since has developed more reliable techniques for describing and quantifying the disturbed behavior patients manifest in the hospital and in other settings. These techniques appear better suited to the task of delineating the overt psychopathology of ethnic groups.

At Hawaii State Hospital we have applied such new methods in an investigation of the characteristics of several ethnic groups in an attempt to develop a more comprehensive and definite picture of their similarities and differences in manifest psychopathology. Standardized techniques are being used to compare the modal behavior of patients in two settings: (1) in the community prior to hospitalization, and (2) in an intensive clinical interview shortly following hospital admission.

The hypotheses which grew out of the first Hawaii State Hospital study and which will be tested in the current one have to do with whether certain types of disturbed behavior (e.g., belligerent manic outbursts) are more prominent in Filipino than in Japanese psychotics and whether there is a different representation of certain patterns of disturbed behavior or subcategories of psychosis in the Filipino and Japanese samples.[1]

The current Hawaii State Hospital study will involve comparisons of samples of Japanese, Filipino, Hawaiian, and Caucasian patients. To exemplify the research approach and the manner in which hypotheses will be tested, we have done a preliminary comparison of a Japanese sample from Hawaii State Hospital and a cross-national sample of mainland-American schizophrenic patients from the National Institute of Mental Health-Psychopharmacology Service Center Collaborative Study of Drugs and Schizophrenia (NIMH-PSC, Collaborative Study Group, 1964). Hypotheses similar to those involved in the Japanese-Filipino study were tested in this preliminary investigation of the differences between American and Japanese samples.

Rationale of Methodology

In the current investigation we have used a descriptive or phenomenologic research approach. Before discussing the research methods used, we will present the rationale for this approach and consider its advantages and limitations for cross-cultural research.

MEASURING THE FACETS OF DISTURBED BEHAVIOR

The concept of psychopathology is so broad that it was necessary at the outset of the investigation to resolve several issues of definition and method. Because psychopathology is expressed at many levels of human functioning, we had to decide which level to study (e.g., the overt behavioral or the unconscious) and which aspects to investigate (e.g., the cognitive, perceptual, or behavioral manifestations). In other words, there were questions of content, research approach, and particular techniques to be used in investigating and measuring the pathology.

In attempting to deal with these issues, we noted that the definition of psychopathology and the selection of the appropriate methodology for its study are problems which are far from resolved in clinical research. The many theories which attempt to explain the bases of mental disorders emphasize different phenomena of human functioning which are critical for understanding the underlying mechanisms; thus they differ on how psychopathology should be defined and measured. Progress in developing appropriate methodology to test and extend these theories understandably has been slow.

In clinical research—where there is pressing need to describe accurately and objectively the nature of the various disorders, to predict their outcome, and to separate out the effects of various treatments—there has been a movement away from reliance on depth theory and a return to a more basic, descriptive approach. The descriptive approach is aimed at objectively delineating the overt behavioral and symptomatic manifestations of the various facets of mental disorder. Its advantages are that it introduces a set of methods which are standardized and provide quantitative indexes of the facets, thus permitting comparison between results of different studies and different populations. The techniques can involve the observation and systematic recording of the social behavior and symptomatology of patients in various settings, e.g., the community, the clinical interview, and the hospital ward, and by different types of observers, e.g., the relative, the clinician, the ward nurse. The procedures call for a minimum of judgment on the part of observers and thus are confined as closely as possible to a phenomenologic level of measurement. Psychometric analyses lead to the development of measures of the various facets of disturbed social behavior and symptomatology.

The limitation of the descriptive or phenomenologic method is its restriction to one level; it does not search below the surface of behavior for covert motives, underlying conflicts, or other possible causes of the disorder. It seeks simply to provide a systematic framework for the ordering of reliable information about overt behavior and manifest symptomatology. Although this approach may be viewed as overly restrictive, it can be argued that the pervasive influence which psychodynamic theory, with its particular focus on unconscious phenomena, has had on clinical research has resulted in an unfortunate neglect of the more immediate need to systematize the overt, observable phenomena of psychopathology. This neglect was reacted to from the methodological standpoint by Allport (1960), who criticized the increasing tendency among psychologists to rely almost exclusively on projective techniques in their study of personality, and from the theoretical standpoint by Sullivan (1945), who defined the subject matter of personality study as the individual's "pattern of interpersonal behavior," that behavior which is observable in his pattern of relating to others.

MEASURING PATTERNS OF DISTURBED BEHAVIOR

In addition to the theoretical and technical problems which appear to be intrinsic in clinical research, we noted that the conduct of cross-cultural inquiries in this area carries with it some special complications. Cross-cultural research which involves questions about the prevalence of

patterns of behavior or diagnoses within an ethnic group must take cogniz-
ance of the fact that the standard diagnostic nomenclature is probably too
unreliable and unspecific, even within the same culture, to be a very useful
framework in much of the research. In previous research we have found,
for example, that the diagnostic category paranoid schizophrenia, as currently used in the United States, is likely to include patients with markedly
different behavior patterns and symptomatology (Katz, Cole, and Lowery,
1964). Turning to the use of the standard nomenclature across cultures,
we found further complications. Statistics on diagnosis at Hawaii State
Hospital indicate a tendency for certain ethnic groups to be overrepresented
in a particular diagnostic category for reasons which are unclear and which
may not be at all related to symptomatology.

Preliminary research with samples of psychiatrists from different
ethnic backgrounds indicates that they may not only diagnose the same
patient very differently but that their perceptions of the specific symptomatology of the patient also may vary in some important respects (Katz, Cole,
and Lowery, 1966). In a study which compared the perceptions of symptomatology and the diagnoses of an American patient by samples of
American and British psychiatrists, the results indicated wide discrepancies
between the samples in both respects. Although one-third of some 40
experienced American psychiatrists diagnosed the study patient as schizophrenic, no one in a comparably sized British group of psychiatrists gave
this diagnosis. The perceptions of the two groups on the extent of various
symptoms also differed, but not as strikingly as in the area of diagnosis.

It is clear, then, that in cross-cultural studies controls have to
offset the tendency of psychiatrists of different ethnic backgrounds both
to diagnose the same patients differently and to perceive their symptomatology differently. These problems are complicated further when psychiatrists
of one nationality diagnose and describe the symptomatology of patients of
another nationality. Procedures have to be applied to minimize the effects
of stereotypes and, at the same time, to allow for the measurement of the
influence of these effects, so that the differences among patient groups can
be distinguished from the differences among psychiatrists. In the current
study we attempt to control the effects of such biases by two procedures: (1) standardizing the interview and the psychiatrists' and psychologists' symptom ratings, i.e., limiting the judgments in interviewing and
rating; and (2) going into the community to obtain behavioral and symptomatic data which are comparable to those obtained in the clinical setting.

The descriptive approach, in recent years, has gone beyond the
delineation of symptom factors to develop objective systems for classifying
disorders (Grinker *et al.*, 1961; Katz, 1966; Lorr, Klett, and McNair,
1963). These systems permit the assignment of patients to categories
on the basis of their quantitative similarity to previously identified behavioral
types. Where hypotheses concerning the similarity of patterns of disturbed
behavior between ethnic groups are at issue, the use of these objective systems

of classification will circumvent many, if not all, of the difficulties introduced by the standard nomenclature.

THE HYPOTHESES AND THE STUDY POPULATION

The intention in the current Hawaii State Hospital study is to assess the effectiveness of the descriptive research approach in testing hypotheses concerning expected differences in the pathology of several ethnic groups. The current study involves the application of several methods for describing and quantifying various facets of psychopathology to the study of Japanese, Filipino, Caucasian, and Hawaiian patients who enter the Hawaii State Hospital over the period of one year. The sampling includes all patients diagnosed as having functional disorders; it excludes organics, alcoholics, and the mentally deficient. Background data on all patients include socioeconomic status, education, length of illness, and family history. It is recognized that fairly large samples of patients are necessary in order to control for generation and socioeconomic factors and that the samples are by no means representative of Japanese and Filipinos. We will attempt, however, to separate the analyses of patients who have themselves migrated to Hawaii from those whose parents were immigrants. In this way it may be possible to indicate the results which apply more generally than to the Hawaiian groups alone. Since the early work on this problem at Hawaii State Hospital showed differences even when both groups were small and when relatively crude methodology was used, there is reason to believe that the basic ethnic differences do not disappear quickly following relocation.

The major hypotheses we intend to test are: (1) Filipino schizophrenic patients are more likely to be openly belligerent, violent, and expansive than are the Japanese; the Japanese are more likely to be withdrawn, apathetic, suicidal, and preoccupied than are the Filipinos. (2) When classified into behavioral subtypes of the psychoses, there will be proportionally more Filipinos in the "belligerent, manic" subcategory of psychosis than Japanese and proportionally more Japanese in the "withdrawn, helpless, suspicious," subcategory.

Methodology

We are aware from previous research (Katz, Lowery, and Cole, 1966) that the manner in which pathology actually is expressed by patients may be quite different in the community and in the hospital. The process of hospitalization itself appears to affect the level and the kinds of pathology manifested. The use of methods which describe the patient's behavior in the community prior to his entrance into the hospital permits an analysis of psychopathology in more than one setting and thus provides a comprehensive picture of the patient's social behavior and symptomatology.

The following methods are being used to compare the behavior and symptomatology of the two groups and to classify patients into behavioral subtypes: (1) Relative's Rating Inventory of Patient Symptoms and Social Behavior (Katz and Lyerly, 1963); (2) Mental Status Schedule (Spitzer *et al.*, 1964); and (3) Inpatient Multidimensional Psychiatric Rating Scale (Lorr *et al.*, 1962).

The Relative's Rating Inventory is administered to a close relative of the patient by a social worker who records the behaviors and symptoms (translated into lay language) which characterized the patient during the three-week period prior to hospital admission. Comparable data are available on very large numbers of psychiatric patients and normal controls in the United States. The inventory provides a quantified profile of 12 facets of social behavior, e.g., belligerence, withdrawal, suspiciousness, as presented in Table 1. An empirical system has been developed for classifying patients into six behavioral types (e.g., a "belligerent, manic" type), which has been validated both on a consensual basis (observers other than relatives independently have described similar behavior patterns among the patient types) and on a predictive basis (the patient types have been shown to respond differentially to treatment) (Katz, 1966).

The Mental Status Schedule interview form provides a standard set of questions fashioned after the traditional mental status interview. It is designed to cover manifest psychopathology comprehensively. An interviewer and an observer (a psychiatrist and a psychologist, respectively) administer the form sometime during the first week of a patient's hospitalization and record all pathological indications. The developers are in the process of refining the scoring system so that the various facets of pathology can be quantified. The standardized nature of the interview reduces the variability associated with different interviewers and insures that all symptoms are covered for all patients.

In administering the Inpatient Multidimensional Psychiatric Rating Scale, an interviewer and an observer rate some 70 behaviors and symptoms which occur during the interview. Latitude at the end of the standard interview allows them to ask additional questions which may be required to complete the ratings. The method provides quantified indexes of each of 10 symptom areas, e.g., excitement, hostile belligerence. The senior author of this chapter has developed a set of symptom patterns, so that patients can be classified into one of several types.

In the course of the study all patients admitted to the Hawaii State Hospital for approximately a one-year period who are diagnosed as functionally psychotic and who meet the other criteria described above are being interviewed and rated during the first week of their hospital stay, prior to the initiation of treatment. A trained social worker visits the family as soon thereafter as possible (within the first three weeks of hospitalization) to collect the necessary psychiatric history and demographic data and to administer the Relative's Rating Inventory. We plan to collect a total sample consisting of 80 Japanese, 40 Filipino, 80 Caucasian, and 40 Hawaiian patients.

Table 1: KAS* Form RI: Relatives' Ratings of Patient Symptoms and Social Behavior by Subtest Cluster†

(1) Belligerence

    28. Got angry and broke things
    50. Cursed at people
    45. Got into fights with people
    113. Threatened to tell people off

(2) Verbal Expansiveness

    100. Shouted or yelled for no reason
    106. Talked too much
    99. Spoke very loud
    105. Kept changing from one subject to another for no reason
    118. Bragged about how good he was

(3) Negativism

    46. Was not co-operative
    36. Acted as if he did not care about other people's feelings
    47. Did the opposite of what he was asked
    48. Stubborn
    56. Critical of other people
    51. Deliberately upset routine
    59. Lied
    37. Thought only of himself
    60. Got into trouble with law

(4) Helplessness

    93. Acted as if he could not make decisions
    74. Acted helpless
    92. Acted as if he could not concentrate on one thing
    3. Cried easily

(5) Suspiciousness

    40. Thought people were talking about him
    107. Said people were talking about him
    43. Acted as if he were suspicious of people
    108. Said that people were trying to make him do or think things he did not want to

(6) Anxiety

    19. Afraid something terrible was going to happen
    122. Said that something terrible was going to happen
    18. Had strange fears
    111. Talked about people or things he was afraid of
    23. Got suddenly frightened for no reason
    125. Talked about suicide

(7) Withdrawal and Retardation

    76. Moved about very slowly
    8. Just sat
    80. Very slow to react
    70. Quiet
    17. Needed to do things very slowly to do them right
    84. Would stay in one position for long period of time

(8) General Psychopathology

    5. Acted as if he had no interest in things
    12. Felt that people did not care about him
    30. Acted as if he had no control over his emotions
    31. Laughed or cried at strange times
    32. Had mood changes without reason
    33. Had temper tantrums
    34. Got very excited for no reason
    42. Bossy
    44. Argued
    52. Resentful
    55. Got annoyed easily
    67. Stayed away from people
    71. Preferred to be alone
    73. Behavior was childish
    79. Very quick to react to something said or done
    90. Acted as if he were confused about things; in a daze

(Continued)

Table 1: (Continued)

(8) General Psychopathology *(Continued)*

  91. Acted as if he could not get certain thoughts out of his mind

  94. Talked without making sense

  97. Refused to speak at all for periods of time

  98. Spoke so low you could not hear him

110. Talked about how angry he was at certain people

119. Said the same things over and over again

121. Talked about big plans he had for the future

127. Gave advice without being asked

(9) Nervousness

  20. Got nervous easily

  21. Jittery

  38. Showed his feelings

  22. Worried or fretted

(10) Confusion

  85. Lost track of day, month, or year

  86. Forgot his address or other places he knew well

  88. Acted as if he did not know where he was

(11) Bizarreness

116. Talked about strange things that were going on inside his body

  26. Did strange things without reason

  25. Acted as if he saw people or things that weren't there

124. Believed in strange things

  24. Had bad dreams

(12) Hyperactivity

  7. Had periods where he could not stop moving or doing something

  13. Did the same thing over and over again without reason

  6. Was restless

* Katz Adjustment Scales.

† Items within a cluster are listed in order of importance for interpretation of the cluster. Order is based on part-whole correlation of individual items with the cluster.

Results of Comparison of Hospitalized Hawaii-Japanese and Mainland-American Acute Schizophrenics

To exemplify the research approach and the analytic procedures to be used in the comparison of the Japanese, Filipino, Caucasian, and Hawaiian patients, we have carried out a preliminary analysis of the differences between a Hawaii-Japanese sample collected during the first six months of the Hawaii State Hospital study and a mainland-American sample of patients from the NIMH-PSC Collaborative Study of Drugs and Schizophrenia (NIMH-PSC Collaborative Study Group, 1964). The questions asked in this preliminary comparison were: (1) whether the sample of Hawaii-Japanese differs from a fairly representative mainland-American sample on certain behavioral factors, particularly belligerence, excitement, and withdrawal; and (2) whether these differences are reflected in their social behavior both prior to hospital admission and following hospitalization. Also of prime interest was whether the multimethod descriptive approach leads to a more comprehensive and more definitive picture of the pathology than do other approaches.

The American and Japanese samples differed somewhat in that the American patients all had been judged to be schizophrenic, while 27 of the 32 Japanese patients had been diagnosed as schizophrenic. All patients in both samples were newly admitted, but the Japanese had on the average been hospitalized more frequently than the more acute American sample. Interpretation of the results, therefore, must be tempered somewhat by the fact that the two samples were not strictly comparable.[2] The results of the comparison of psychopathology in the two groups are presented in two parts: (1) as manifested in the community prior to admission; and (2) as rated by psychiatrists and psychologists following hospital admission.

Table 2 presents a comparison (by means of t-tests) of the American and Japanese patients' social behavior and symptomatology in the community prior to hospitalization on each of the factors in the Relative's Rating Inventory. Of the 11 comparisons, 6 indicate significant differences between the rated behavior of the two samples, 3 of which are well beyond the .01 level of confidence. In all 3 of these cases it was the Japanese who exceeded the Americans. They exhibited significantly more negativism, general psychopathology, and nervousness. The Japanese also exceeded the Americans on all 3 factors which make up a second-order factor of social obstreperousness, i.e., the combined score on belligerence, verbal expansiveness, and negativism.

These findings indicate that the Japanese were significantly more socially obstreperous, nervous, and agitated (hyperactive) than were the Americans in the community prior to their entrance into the hospital. These findings conform partially to those reported by Schooler and Caudill (1964) on a comparison of Japanese and American state hospital patients and in their report in Chapter 8. Our findings, however, contradict the picture derived from the earlier study (Enright and Jaekle, 1963) of the stereotype of the Japanese psychotic as more preoccupied, schizoid, and compliant than his Filipino counterpart.

Turning now to the data on the behavior of these patients after admission to the hospital (the samples in the hospital include one additional Japanese case and sixty additional mainland cases), we found a different picture. As mentioned earlier, the hospital data are based on ratings made following a clinical interview. In the Hawaii study the standard Mental Status Schedule interview was used; in the NIMH-PSC study an unstructured interview was used. From the standpoint of content, however, the two types of interviews covered nearly the same ground. Whenever the interviewer in the Hawaii study found the structured interview incomplete for rating purposes, he was free to follow it with a brief unstructured interview. In practically all cases a follow-up interview was unnecessary. Thus there seems

Table 2: Social Behavior and Symptomatology in the Community (KAS*): Comparative Means for the Japanese (Hawaii State Hospital) and the NIMH-PSC Multihospital Samples of Acute Schizophrenics

KAS Cluster	Japanese (N=34)	NIMH (N=404)	t
Belligerence	1.41	0.91	2.500†
Verbal expansiveness	1.94	1.35	2.458†
Negativism	4.03	2.66	3.425††
Helplessness	2.18	1.87	1.409
Suspiciousness	2.59	2.11	1.920
Anxiety	2.24	2.51	0.843
Withdrawal and retardation	2.82	2.32	1.667
General psychopathology	13.65	11.06	3.237††
Nervousness	3.26	2.38	4.190††
Bizarreness	1.79	1.86	0.318
Hyperactivity	2.00	1.55	2.647†

* Katz Adjustment Scale.
† t-test of mean difference significant at .05 level.
†† t-test of mean difference significant at .01 level.

Table 3: Psychiatric Ratings of Symptomatology in the Hospital (IMPS*): Comparative Means for the Japanese (Hawaii State Hospital) and the NIMH-PSC Multihospital Samples of Acute Schizophrenics

IMPS Factor	Japanese (N=35)	NIMH (N=464)	t
Excitement	6.24	12.77	2.827††
Hostile belligerence	10.36	17.31	2.673†
Paranoid projection	8.91	19.36	4.180††
Grandiose expansiveness	2.40	5.10	1.837
Perceptual distortion	4.48	7.18	1.688
Anxious intropunitiveness	16.76	17.29	0.243
Retardation and apathy	13.83	15.61	0.788
Disorientation	2.40	0.86	5.310††
Motor disturbance	8.04	12.79	2.610†
Conceptual disorganization	4.68	6.00	1.20

* Inpatient Multidimensional Psychiatric Rating Scales.
† t-test of mean difference significant at the .05 level.
†† t-test of mean difference significant at the .01 level.

little reason to attribute the large differences in the two samples to the different types of interviews. Of the ten symptom factors in the Inpatient Multidimensional Psychiatric Rating Scale, the Americans significantly exceeded the Japanese on four factors and the Japanese exceeded the Americans on one, as presented in Table 3. On the basis of the symptomatology manifested in the clinical interview, the Americans were significantly more excited, exhibiting more paranoid projection, belligerence, and disturbance in the motor or postural area than did the Japanese. The Japanese were significantly more disoriented than were the Americans.

The results of the latter comparison are plotted in Fig. 1 to permit comparison of the types of symptoms which were prominent within an ethnic group with those which were present to lesser degrees. It can be seen that within the NIMH-PSC sample hostility and paranoid projection exceeded anxious intropunitiveness and apathy and retardation. The reverse pattern occurred for the Japanese; intropunitiveness and retardation far exceeded excitement, hostility, and paranoid projection.

What is most striking about the results in the two settings, the community and the hospital, is that they lead not only to different conclusions about the manifest psychopathology of the two ethnic groups but to conclusions which appear to be directly opposed. It therefore is important to consider the reasons for this diverse set of findings and some of its implications for cross-cultural research.

The indications are that both ethnic groups expressed their pathology in different ways in the community and in the hospital. The act of hospitalization in itself is apparently a factor influencing the manner of symptom expression. Its effects on the patients of Japanese ancestry may be to temper agitated, obstreperous behavior, and it may enhance these features in mainland-Americans who are not very obstreperous or agitated prior to entering the hospital. Which behavior is more characteristic of schizophrenia in either of these ethnic groups, however, is still open to question. The community data describe patients as they appear in their usual surroundings and may provide a more stable, dependable picture of the characteristic expressions of pathology in the culture. The picture presented in the clinical interview may be confounded by the influence of hospitalization and may reflect simply a temporary phase for the patient. We are aware that psychosis is a process, that patients go through various symptom stages, and that longitudinal studies of their course in the hospital ultimately will be necessary to identify the primary facets of the illness.

Where the interest is in cross-cultural differences in the expression of pathology, the results of this study point up the importance of investigating its expression in more than one setting (possibly, at several points in time) through the eyes of more than one type of observer. These results also clarify somewhat the reasons that different investigations of the same ethnic group sometimes have led to contradictory results. Since the results of cross-cultural studies usually have very significant implications for theories

Figure 1: Japanese Sample (Hawaii State Hospital) and the NIMH-PSC Multihospital Sample of Acute Schizophrenics (Psychiatric Ratings of Symptomatology Based on the Clinical Interview)

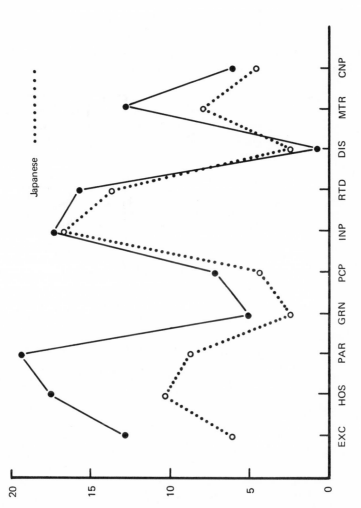

The IMPS factors are Excitement (EXC), Hostile Belligerence (HOS), Paranoid Projection (PAR), Grandiose Expansiveness (GRN), Perceptual Distortion (PCP), Anxious Intropunitiveness (INP), Apathy and Retardation (RTD), Disorientation (DIS), Motor Disturbances (MTR), and Conceptual Disorganization (CNP).

concerning the etiology of psychopathology, it is important that investigators in this field take seriously the significant influence that methodological and situational factors apparently play in determining their results.

If we want to make progress in the theory of personality and psychopathology, it seems that cross-cultural research should attach as much importance to identifying similarities as to uncovering differences between the ways two ethnic groups manifest disturbed behavior. In the community both of our samples exhibited relatively equal amounts of anxiety and bizarreness. The former measures extreme anxiety (in contrast to nervousness); and bizarreness, as can be seen from Table 1, measures delusional behavior. The two factors are related and have been interpreted on the basis of a second-order factor analysis of the 12 measures in the Relative's Rating Inventory, as "acute psychoticism."

The findings from the clinical interview after admission to the hospital indicate that the extent of anxious intropunitiveness, apathy and retardation, and conceptual disorganization was similar in the two samples. The levels of these factors are comparable to those obtained in a very large group of functional psychotics in the United States (Lorr, *et al.*, 1962). Thus the findings also reassure us that a common basis exists among these ethnic groups for the identification of psychosis, but it will take a more refined analysis of specific behaviors and more carefully matched samples than in our study to extend this line of inquiry.

Distinguishing among the elements which are common to psychosis across cultures from those which are shaped by a particular culture is a central concern of psychopathology. The identification of the common elements has obvious significance for etiological theories of mental disorders. Research in this area is complicated by the fact that subcategories of psychosis are identified not so much by the presence or absence of certain elements but by the manner in which these elements are patterned. When we refer to the likelihood that mental disorder is different from country to country, what is usually meant is that the *patterns* of behavior which characterize psychosis in one culture are different from those which characterize psychosis in another culture. Both the Filipino and the Japanese paranoid schizophrenics manifest paranoid symptoms *and* schizophrenic symptoms, but their overt symptomatic patterns are likely to be different, because of their close relation to the basic social behavior patterns of each culture. The hypothesis that the belligerent manic picture is likely to occur more frequently in the Filipino than in the Japanese culture will be tested in the Hawaii State Hospital study. With systems which permit reliable, valid measurement of social behavior patterns, however, other hypotheses—ones which grow out of theories about the social developmental patterns in a given culture—also can be tested. The descriptive, phenomenologic approach provides the framework and the methods to test such ideas, and it is hoped that this approach will provide a sounder base for more definitive research in this area.

Summary

In summary, the Hawaii State Hospital study is designed to provide a comprehensive picture of psychopathology in several ethnic groups. The research approach is descriptive or phenomenologic, with emphasis on the systematic delineation and quantification of the significant dimensions of social behavior and overt psychopathology. Psychopathology will be investigated as it appears in the patient's behavior both in his usual surroundings in the community and again following hospitalization. The methods for observing and recording will permit direct comparisons of symptom factors and also provide objective systems for classifying patients into behavioral subtypes. The extent to which symptom factors or behaviors are similar and the frequencies of particular behavioral patterns within groups then can be compared. The application of new, more objective systems of classification will avoid the necessity of relying on the standard psychiatric nomenclature. Several hypotheses concerning expected differences between the Japanese and the Filipino in the manifestations of psychosis will be tested.

A preliminary comparison of a sample of Hawaii-Japanese patients and a cross-national sample of American schizophrenic patients was described to exemplify the experimental approach. The results of this comparison indicate that the picture of psychopathology derived from a study of an ethnic group is influenced by the setting in which the patients are studied. The conclusions which were drawn from the community study about the comparative pathology of these two groups were diametrically opposed to those obtained from their comparison following hospitalization. This study points up the necessity for sampling behavior broadly in cross-cultural research.

ACKNOWLEDGMENT

This research and the preparation of this report were supported in part by a National Institute of Mental Health contract with the Institute of Behavioral Sciences, Honolulu, Hawaii (Contract No. PH 43-65-648).

NOTES

1.   For convenience, we refer throughout this paper to two of the Hawaiian ethnic groups as Japanese and Filipino. The large majority of the Japanese patients, however, are American and second- and third-generation residents of Hawaii, e.g., two-thirds are *Nisei*. When the ethnic designation is used, the reference is to patients of Japanese or Filipino ancestry rather than to nationals.

2.   The major criteria for patients selected in the NIMH-PSC Study were that they be newly admitted, acute, with evidence of symptomatology in two of seven major schizophrenic symptom areas, and between the ages of sixteen and forty-one. They should not have had a significant hospitalization within a period of 12 months prior to the current admission. The sample of 404 were drawn from nine hospitals in the United States, which included state institutions, university-teaching-acute treatment hospitals, and private treatment centers. Since the initial analysis, we have compared the Hawaii-Japanese sample with the norm group reported for the Inpatient Multidimensional Rating Scale (Lorr, *et al.*, 1962), a population which is more comparable than the NIMH-PSC sample to the Hawaii State Hospital sample (newly admitted and functionally psychotic but not necessarily schizophrenic). The results were similar in all major respects to those obtained from the comparison with the NIMH-PSC sample.

REFERENCES

Allport, G. W. 1960. Personality and social encounter: selected essays. Boston, Beacon Press.

Enright, J., and W. Jaeckle. 1963. Psychiatric symptoms and diagnoses in two subcultures. International Journal of Social Psychiatry 9:12–17.

Grinker, R. R., Sr., J. Miller, M. Sabshin, R. Nunn, and J. C. Nunnally. 1961. The phenomena of depressions. New York, Hoeber.

Katz, M. M. 1966. A typological approach to the problem of predicting treatment response. *In* Prediction of response to pharmacotherapy. J. R. Wittenborn and P. R. A. May, eds. Springfield, Thomas.

Katz, M. M., J. O. Cole, and H. A. Lowery. 1964. Nonspecificity of diagnosis of paranoid schizophrenia. Archives of General Psychiatry 11:197–202.

———. 1966. Studies on the diagnostic process. Paper presented at the American Psychiatric Association Meeting, May.

Katz, M. M., H. A. Lowery, and J. O. Cole. 1966. Patterns of schizophrenic behavior in the community. *In* Explorations in typing psychotics. M. Lorr, ed. Oxford, Pergamon Press.

Katz, M. M., and S. B. Lyerly. 1963. Methods of measuring adjustment and social behavior in the community. I. Rationale, description, discriminative validity and scale development. Psychological Reports 13:503–35.

Lorr, M., C. J. Klett, and D. M. McNair. 1963. Syndromes of psychosis. New York, Macmillan.

Lorr, M., C. J. Klett, D. M. McNair, and J. J. Lasky. 1962. Inpatient multidimensional psychiatric scale manual. Palo Alto, Consulting Psychologists Press.

NIMH-PSC Collaborative Study Group. 1964. Effectiveness of phenothiazine treatment of acute schizophrenic psychoses. Archives of General Psychiatry 10:246–61.

Schooler, C., and W. Caudill. 1964. Symptomatology in Japanese and American schizophrenics. Ethnology 3:172–78.

Spitzer, R. L., J. L. Fleiss, E. I. Burdock, and A. S. Hardesty. 1964. The mental status schedule: rationale, reliability and validity. Comprehensive Psychiatry 5:384–95.

Sullivan, H. S. 1945. Conceptions of modern psychiatry: the first William Alanson White Memorial Lecture. Washington, William Alanson White Psychiatric Foundation.

10. Psychopathology among Hawaii's Japanese:
     A Comparative Study

THOMAS MARETZKI, Ph.D.
Department of Anthropology
University of Hawaii
Honolulu, Hawaii

LINDA D. NELSON, M.A.
Department of Sociology
University of Hawaii
Honolulu, Hawaii

TESTING for basic psychological similarities and differences in populations of two societies without introducing cultural bias into the measuring devices continues to be a task of no small challenge to social scientists. In the anthropological literature comparisons of different populations frequently are linked to acculturation studies. Many anthropologists who have compared psychological characteristics of two populations at different acculturation stages have found projective tests useful. Depending on the level of analysis of personality characteristics, the Rorschach test and—where cultural differences are not too extreme and pictures can be designed for comparative analysis—the Thematic Apperception Test (T.A.T.) have been used with good results. We suggest that the study of mental illness may provide a simple index of the change in the psychological characteristics of populations undergoing acculturation and also that such study may provide new directions of inquiry.

Patient statistics contained in hospital records or available through interviews can be summarized for comparative purposes as is commonly done in epidemiological studies. Unlike projective tests, mental health statistics do not provide insights into personality dynamics unless information on patients is obtained in depth from the beginning of a research project. This was not the case in the present study. Nevertheless, even the examination of the cultural patterning in each population may provide a meaningful comparison. Methodological pitfalls in using mental health statistics from hospitals in different cultures as indexes for comparative purposes are well known and will not be elaborated on here.

The changing psychological characteristics of Japanese immigrants has been the subject of a number of studies. In a study of a Japanese population in Chicago, Caudill and DeVos demonstrated how the compatibility of value systems of immigrant and host cultures facilitated adjustment. Such adjustment, however, need not be based on similar basic personality structures (Caudill and DeVos, 1956). Adjustment can even reduce the pressure toward acculturation and psychological shifts in the direction of the host culture. According to Spindler (1955), such shifts in personality structure seem more likely to occur where cultural conflict is great between two societies which are in direct contact, as in the case of the Ojibwa and American whites. We do not know yet to what extent the basic personality structure of Japanese immigrants to the United States changes in the direction of Americans of similar social and economic status. Our own casual observation in Hawaii suggests that considerable psychological changes are taking place among those of Japanese descent who are now two and three generations removed from their immigrant forebears.

The Problem

The relation of mental illness to acculturation has been treated in terms of quantitative changes which show that as social disorganization increases psychiatric disorders rise concomitantly among individuals affected by cultural change (Kennedy, 1961). Much remains to be done in researching the cross-cultural comparability of mental disorders. We decided to make an investigation in this area by focusing on psychopathology manifested by Japanese in Hawaii, in particular, on whether acculturation was taking place in the patterns of mental disorder.

The work by Caudill and others gives a comparative basis for this study of psychopathology among Japanese immigrants and their descendants in Hawaii. A finding which we wished to examine in terms of our Hawaii group was the overrepresentation of eldest sons and youngest daughters, particularly when viewed in terms of position among same-sex siblings, among psychotic patients in Japanese hospitals (Caudill, 1963, MS). This sibling rank bias has been explained as a by-product of patterned family relations, specifically interactions between mothers and eldest sons and fathers and youngest daughters. Stresses resulting from these relations seem to engender mental disorders, especially where the economic base and the social fabric of families are affected by changes taking place in Japan.

In other work related to mental illness, Caudill and his associates have investigated the distribution of symptoms among Japanese mental

patients in Japan. Schooler and Caudill (1964) compared symptom distribution among patients in a Tokyo hospital with that of American patients
in a Maryland hospital. In the present study, using the same schedule for
symptom analysis that Caudill and Schooler used, we compared our data on
Japanese schizophrenic patients in Hawaii with the data available on schizophrenic patients in Tokyo and Maryland.

The focus of this chapter is on the psychopathology of a population
in cultural transition as a result of their descent from a Japanese immigrant
population. Because there is as yet an insufficient knowledge of family
relations and other relevant cultural patterns among the Japanese immigrant
population and their descendants in Hawaii, we state our hypotheses quite
generally: (1) Culturally patterned family relations of second-generation
Japanese (*Nisei*) and third-generation Japanese (*Sansei*) in Hawaii differ
sufficiently from the family dynamics of present-day Japanese in Japan as
a result of cultural drift so that overrepresentation of certain sibling ranks,
as reported by Caudill, need not hold in Hawaii. In fact, we expected from
the inception of this study that Japanese families in Hawaii exert pressure
toward economic improvement by nontraditional Japanese means even
though first-born *Nisei* in Hawaii probably were subjected to traditional
pressures to accept responsibilities toward their immigrant parents (referred
to as *Issei*) as well as toward younger siblings. We did not expect that
these pressures would be reflected in the same sibling rank bias which was
reported for Japan, nor did we think that the conflict of youngest daughters
would occur in Hawaii to the same extent. On the basis of casual observations, there is no evidence of the special emotional bonds between fathers
and their last-born daughters which have been described for Japan (Caudill,
MS). (2) The symptom distribution among Hawaii-Japanese mental patients
is not identical with or similar to the patterns reported for Japan. This
assumption reflects our general notion that acculturation of immigrants
modifies their psychological characteristics so that each succeeding generation approximates more the pattern of the host society. In line with a
widespread notion in Hawaii, we expected that *Issei* patients in Hawaii
would be more similar to Japanese patients in Japan than to their descendants
and that the acculturation gradient would operate on subsequent generations
of Japanese so that they increasingly would approach the symptom pattern
of other patients in hospitals on the continent of the United States.

Most Japanese in Hawaii are descended from residents of rural
regions in southern Honshū and the island of Kyūshū. It cannot be said
that culturally the *Issei* in Hawaii remained identical with their contem-
poraries who stayed behind in the home country. The changes affecting
the *Issei* in Hawaii after immigration match the changes which took place in
Japanese society before, during, and after World War II. We can only
speculate about the nature of divergences and about the psychological
factors which distinguished those who migrated from those who stayed
behind, thereby introducing basic distinctions even without cultural drift.

Methodology

In the original design, all psychiatric patients of Japanese background who were admitted for the first time at one of three institutions on Oahu—the Hawaii State Hospital at Kaneohe, the Hawaii State Convalescent Center, and the Queens Hospital—from December 1, 1963, to December 31, 1964, were to form our survey sample. At an early date it became apparent that the sample criteria would have to be modified, for the number of first admissions was much smaller than expected, and not all patients could be included because of the reluctance on the part of some physicians to make their patients and patient records accessible for study. The final sample of 190 consists of all patients of Japanese background who were admitted at the three institutions during the 13-month period, who had a functional illness, who were under 60 years of age at first admission, and for whom interview co-operation and records could be obtained. Fifty-nine per cent of the cases came from the State Hospital. There is an inherent economic bias in selecting cases from the two State institutions because their patients tend to come from lower socioeconomic strata than would be expected in a truly random sample of Hawaii's Japanese receiving psychiatric care.

Data were collected using a slightly modified version of the schedule Caudill used in his research in four Japanese hospitals (Caudill, MS; Caudill and Schooler, Chapter 8; Phillips and Rabinovitch, 1958). The schedule is a lengthy one which calls for basic background data, social history, description of symptoms, and a brief psychiatric history. The information was obtained from each patient in three ways: hospital records, an interview with the patient, and an interview with a relative (if at all possible) of the patient.

Table 1 presents the proportion of patients in each hospital and a percentage distribution of six background characteristics obtained from records and interviews of the 190 individuals. Since we considered generation in the United States a most important variable for analysis, the small number of the first or immigrant (*Issei*) generation, because of old age for this group as a whole, is a disappointment. The bulk of the sample are second- and third-generation patients and our analysis deals with these two groups only.

The symptom data came from hospital records describing the patient at the time of his first admission. Since patients fell into our sample without regard to the number of previous admissions, we controlled for the institutionalization variable by using hospital records concurrent with the patient's first psychiatric care. Almost all first admissions postdated World War II, and the majority were more recent than that. In a very few cases where first admission records were inadequate or missing altogether, records within five years after admission were used. Symptom data were secured for 152 of the 190 interviewed. A percentage distribution of the age and

Table 1: Percentage Distribution of Background Characteristics
of Hawaii-Japanese Psychiatric Patients

Characteristic	Male (N=97)	Female (N=93)	Total (N=190)
Hospital			
Hawaii State Hospital	63	56	59
Queens Hospital	12	24	18
State Convalescent Center	25	20	23
Generation			
Issei	3	6	5
Nisei	58	62	61
Sansei	22	19	21
Mixed	14	10	12
Marital Status			
Never married	74	42	59
Married	22	56	38
Residential Mobility			
Non-mobile: Oahu residence only	29	27	28
Mobile: inter-island	22	34	28
Mobile: outside Hawaii	48	38	43
Occupational Classification			
Professional	—	3	2
Proprietor and manager	—	—	—
Businessman	—	—	—
Clerk and kindred worker	9	23	16
Manual worker	59	16	38
Protective and service worker	18	38	27
Farmer	6	2	4
Student	4	6	5
Not working	2	12	7
Religion			
None	20	10	15
Buddhism	39	37	38
Shintō	1	—	1
Shamanism	—	1	1
Sōkagakkai and other new sects	—	1	1
Protestantism	31	40	35

(Continued)

Table 1: (Continued)

Characteristic	Male (N=97)	Female (N=93)	Total (N=190)
Religion *(Continued)*			
Catholicism	8	4	6
Other Western sects	1	3	2
Educational Attainment			
None	—	1	1
Some elementary school	4	9	6
Elementary school graduate	4	—	2
Some junior high school	8	11	9
Junior high school graduate	11	6	9
Some high school	19	8	13
High school graduate	24	37	31
Technical school	15	18	17
Some college	10	9	9
College graduate	3	—	2

diagnosis of these patients is shown in Table 2. Most of the 38 for whom no symptom information was obtained were patients of private physicians. Symptom records were evaluated according to a fairly exhaustive checklist of 174 symptoms prepared by Phillips (1965). Preferring to use symptoms exhibited prior to and on first admission, we had to leave uncontrolled some time-related factors, such as changes in medical staff, changes in hospital record keeping, and changing perceptions resulting from theoretical shifts in psychiatric orientation.

Findings

As mentioned, our inquiry was divided into two parts. The first part relates psychiatric disorder to sibling rank. The second part is a comparison of the frequency with which schizophrenic symptoms occurred among patients in Japan, Hawaii, and the continental United States.

Tables 3 and 4 describe the *Nisei* and *Sansei* patients according to birth order and sibship size. Our expectation was that disorders would occur randomly in terms of sibling rank position. Family size was eliminated as a variable since the sample was too small to control for a tendency of *Nisei* families to be larger than those of *Sansei;* in our patient sample

Nisei patients came from larger families than did *Sansei* patients. Our expectation concerning sibling rank position and disorder in Hawaii would contrast with Caudill's results in Japan which showed a sibling rank bias through overrepresentation of eldest sons and youngest daughters, as described earlier. Chi-square tests were run to determine whether the sibling positions represented in the Hawaii sample could be attributed to chance or whether cultural or other undefined factors might have played a part in the sampling distribution.

The *Nisei* appeared to be randomly distributed in terms of birth order. For the *Sansei*, however, we found an overrepresentation of first-born that is statistically significant at the .001 level. If the *Sansei* group is further classified by sex, then the overrepresentation of first-born patients is statistically significant only for males ($p < .01$). It can be stated, then, that eldest male *Sansei* more frequently become psychiatric patients than do those in other sibling positions and that this tendency also exists for female *Sansei,* although to a lesser degree.

We can only speculate on the meaning of these results. Since we found no overrepresentation of last-born *Nisei* or *Sansei,* we must assume that the dynamics which have been adduced to explain sibling rank distribution of patients in Japan do not operate in Hawaii in identical fashion. None of the chi-square tests showed any statistically significant results for the

Table 2: Percentage Distribution of Age and Diagnosis of Hawaii-Japanese Patients at First Admission for Psychiatric Care

Age and Diagnosis	Male (N=83)	Female (N=69)	Total (N=152)
Age			
10-19	25	23	24
20-29	41	45	43
30-39	24	17	21
40-49	6	7	7
50-59	4	7	5
Diagnosis			
Transient stress disorder	—	1	1
Personality disorder	4	4	4
Psychoneurotic disorder	7	4	6
Psychotic disorder			
Schizophrenic reaction	64	59	62
Affective psychotic reaction	2	7	5
No information	23	23	23

Table 3: Birth Order and Sibship Size (Total Sibling Rank) by Sex for *Nisei* Psychiatric Patients

Birth Order	Size of Sibship										Total
	1 M F	2 M F	3 M F	4 M F	5 M F	6 M F	7 M F	8 M F	9 M F	10 M F	M F
1	1 1	2 1	1 0	1 2	2 0	1 0	0 1	0 0	0 1	1 0	9 6
2		0 2	3 1	3 1	2 0	0 2	0 1	0 0	0 0	0 0	8 7
3			2 1	1 3	3 2	7 1	3 1	0 0	0 0	0 0	16 8
4				3 0	0 3	1 1	2 1	0 1	0 0	0 0	6 6
5					0 1	1 1	3 1	1 2	1 3	0 2	6 10
6						4 2	0 1	0 1	0 1	1 1	5 6
7							3 3	0 1	1 1	0 0	4 5
8								2 3	0 1	0 1	2 5
9									0 0	1 3	1 3
10										0 1	0 1
Total	1 1	2 3	6 2	8 6	7 6	14 7	11 9	3 8	2 7	3 8	57 57

Table 4: Birth Order and Sibship Size (Total Sibling Rank) by Sex for *Sansei* Psychiatric Patients

Birth Order	Size of Sibship							Total
	1 M F	2 M F	3 M F	4 M F	5 M F	6 M F	7 M F	M F
1	1 1	1 2	5 3	1 0	1 0	2 0	0 0	11 6
2		2 1	0 1	0 0	1 3	0 0	0 0	3 5
3			1 0	1 0	0 1	0 2	0 0	2 3
4				2 1	1 0	0 0	1 2	4 3
5					0 0	1 1	0 0	1 1
6						0 0	0 0	0 0
7							0 0	0 0
Total	1 1	3 3	6 4	4 1	3 4	3 3	1 2	21 18

Table 5: Percentage Distribution of Symptom Occurrence in Four Groups of Schizophrenic Patients from Tokyo Metropolitan Matsuzawa Hospital, Hawaii State Hospital, and Maryland Spring Grove State Hospital

Symptom	Male				Female				Total			
	Matsu-zawa	Hawaii Nisei	Hawaii Sansei	Spring Grove	Matsu-zawa	Hawaii Nisei	Hawaii Sansei	Spring Grove	Matsu-zawa	Hawaii Nisei	Hawaii Sansei	Spring Grove
Physically assaultive	53	29	14	11	42	35	10	8	48	31	12	9
Withdrawn	68	46	43	32	61	58	40	31	65	52	42	31
Euphoria	32	4	–	3	37	12	10	2	34	7	4	2
Sleep disturbance	38	21	36	8	46	19	50	13	42	20	42	11
Apathetic	30	14	21	3	15	27	–	3	23	20	12	3
Emotionally labile	17	11	7	7	39	19	20	13	27	15	12	10
Tense	34	36	14	19	–	42	30	–	–	39	21	–
Hallucinations	28	68	64	44	27	65	30	46	27	67	50	45
Bizarre ideas	–	29	14	11	–	19	20	11	–	24	17	11*
Perplexed	6	14	–	19	7	8	–	19	7	11	–	19
Number of cases	47	28	20	476	41	26	10	650	88	54	24	1,126

*We assume a printing error in Table 3 in Schooler and Caudill (1964) and have substituted the appropriate likely figure. (Maretzki and Nelson are correct in their assumption of a printing error in Schooler and Caudill (1964), and they have substituted the correct figure.—The editors of this volume.)

last-born. If the same family dynamics operated among Japanese in Hawaii as they apparently do in Japan or even if they continued to exist in a modified degree because of the weakening effect of acculturation, the tendency should have been greatest in *Issei* (inadequately represented in the sample for testing), less prevalent in *Nisei,* and least in *Sansei.*

There is no evidence for a tendency in this direction as far as *Nisei* are concerned. Hawaii *Nisei* may have been brought up by their immigrant parents in such a way that responsibility and achievement motivation were equally instilled in children regardless of birth order and sex, at least to such an extent that conflicts which might have resulted did not selectively emerge in the psychopathology of a particular sibship rank. This would mean that Japanese values favoring the eldest child or successor to family responsibilities (especially males) and actual child-rearing practices may not fully coincide. If *Nisei* first-born children were subjected to greater conflict about their responsibilities toward parents and the family in general than younger siblings, they seem to have been able to cope with problems arising from such pressures in such a way that the crude measure of sibling rank distribution used here did not reflect their existence.

How then should we explain the *Sansei* results? It is sometimes said that third-generation Japanese are more inclined to accept some of the cultural values of their immigrant ancestors because they are better established as Americans in the community and need not be as defensive about their Japanese background as their parents. This suggestion, however, lacks any empirical basis, and even if such a tendency exists it is unlikely to account for our findings. Instead, we suggest that *Nisei* parents continue to have expectations for their first-born, derived from traditional Japanese values, which differ for children born subsequently. *Sansei* children generally experienced less economic deprivation and, as a result, less parental pressure to contribute to the family welfare than did their parents. Because their *Nisei* parents had achieved so much more economic security and social respect than had the immigrant grandparents, *Sansei* children may have grown up with less consistent parental pressure toward responsibility and achievement than did their *Nisei* parents. At the same time *Sansei* children may have enjoyed greater indulgence in a more affluent environment than did their parents. The combination of less pressure toward responsible behavior, even though still valued and held up as ideal by parents, and an increased indulgence may have brought about more inconsistency in the training of *Sansei* children, particularly the eldest, than the *Nisei* had experienced in their childhood. If so, personality conflict may have increased among *Sansei* children, especially among eldest males, increasing their vulnerability to psychopathology. Only a careful study of child rearing of Japanese in Hawaii, in general, and of patients' childhood histories, in particular, can demonstrate the validity of such a *post hoc* attempt to account for the findings. Of course, another, though equally inconclusive *post hoc* suggestion is that the *Sansei* data reflect a general tendency toward overrepresentation of first-borns, as found in a number of studies related to personality, although, as Altus (1966) has pointed out, the findings linking mental disorder to birth order tend to be confusing and contradictory.

We now turn to the results of the symptom comparison of 78 schizophrenic patients in Hawaii with patients from Tokyo and Maryland hospitals. Table 5 compares the Hawaii data with those presented by Schooler and Caudill (1964) which we have reproduced for comparative purposes. Table 6 lists statistically significant differences when each of the four groups is compared with another using the t-test for differences between proportions. Of the ten symptoms, the Tokyo patients were significantly higher than the Maryland patients on six; on these same six symptoms, with only one exception, sleep disturbance, Hawaii *Nisei* and *Sansei* fell between the extremes of the Tokyo and Maryland patients, as predicted. For three symptoms on which Maryland patients were higher than Tokyo patients, the pattern was less clear for the Hawaii-Japanese.

The intermediate position of the Hawaii-Japanese was shown most strikingly for physical assault. The decrease in the amount of this symptom from Tokyo, to Hawaii, to Maryland, is in line with the findings reported by Katz and his associates (Chapter 9) concerning the preadmission behavior of Hawaii-Japanese and American schizophrenics. The hospital admission records which we used reflect the behavior of patients prior to the influence of hospitalization. The general decrease in assaultiveness from the Japanese high extreme to the Maryland low extreme also held when *Nisei* and *Sansei* were compared individually with the two other patient samples.

Several puzzling questions emerge from the symptom findings. Why did Hawaii *Nisei* and *Sansei* exhibit a higher frequency of hallucinations than would be expected if an acculturation gradient were operating uniformly? In order to search for possible explanations for such differences in symptom occurrence, four background factors—age, marital status, geographic mobility, and religion—were correlated with each of the symptoms. Hallucinations, however, appeared to be unrelated to any of these factors. It could be argued that religious conflicts might produce such symptoms. Perhaps our measurement of general religious identification rather than behavior or intensity of participation was too coarse to reveal religious conflicts. Still, in view of the negative findings from these correlations, explanations related to differences in the perception or actual occurrence of such symptoms, as these may vary between Japan and the United States, may be advanced. Either reports on hallucinations by patients in Japan and patients of Japanese descent in Hawaii, though similar, are evaluated differently by those who record these reports, or else patients indeed show significant differences in hallucinations, and we must assume that acculturation stresses have an effect on reality testing and produce such behavior in a context where it is culturally less likely to be tolerated. If the latter is the case, a similar explanation would apply to increased bizarre ideas among *Nisei* and *Sansei* in comparison with patients in Japan.

Table 6: Significant Differences* in Symptom Occurrence in Four Groups of Schizophrenic Patients from Tokyo Metropolitan Matsuzawa Hospital, Hawaii State Hospital, and Maryland Spring Grove State Hospital

Symptom	Matsuzawa and Hawaii Nisei			Matsuzawa and Hawaii Sansei			Hawaii Nisei and Sansei		
	M	F	Total	M	F	Total	M	F	Total
Physically assaultive	.05		.05	.01	.05	.001			.05
Withdrawn						.05			
Euphoria	.001	.05	.001	.001	.05	.001			
Sleep disturbance	.05	.05	.01						
Apathetic					.05			.01	
Emotionally labile									
Tense									
Hallucinations	.001	.01	.001	.05		.05			
Bizarre ideas	.01	.05	.001			.05			
Perplexed						.01	.05		.05

Symptom	Hawaii Nisei and Spring Grove			Hawaii Sansei and Spring Grove			Matsuzawa and Spring Grove		
	M	F	Total	M	F	Total	M	F	Total
Physically assaultive	.05	.01	.001				.01	.01	.01
Withdrawn		.01	.01				.01	.01	.01
Euphoria				.001			.01	.01	.01
Sleep disturbance		.05		.05	.05	.01	.01	.01	.01
Apathetic		.01	.01		.001		.01	.01	.01
Emotionally labile							.05	.01	.01
Tense							.01		
Hallucinations	.01	.05	.001				.05	.05	.01
Bizarre ideas	.05		.05				.05	.05	.05
Perplexed				.001	.001	.001			.05

Significance determined by two-tailed t-tests of differences between proportions.
Significant differences between Matsuzawa and Spring Grove taken from Schooler and Caudill (1964).

In general, it seems that our results on the intermediate position of Hawaii-Japanese have implications for the tentative explanations of the Tokyo and Maryland hospital findings which Schooler and Caudill have advanced. The results for sleeplessness are a case in point. If Schooler and Caudill's explanation is valid that sleep disturbance is high among Japanese patients because of sleeping patterns which reinforce parent-child conflicts, we would expect a higher incidence of sleep disturbance among *Nisei* than among *Sansei,* but such is not the case. Even though we suggested that parental conflicts may have more severe consequences for *Sansei* than for *Nisei,* sleeping patterns of *Nisei* approximated those of Japanese more than did sleeping patterns of *Sansei.* This possible discrepancy between theory and results is an example of the difficulty of reading cultural significance into mental illness statistics when cultural factors are inadequately known.

Conclusions

We have presented data based on a survey of patients of Japanese background in Hawaii from hospital records and interviews with patients and their relatives. We are fully aware of the problems in attempting cross-cultural comparisons of psychopathology by using statistics taken from hospital records. Our main purpose was to demonstrate that acculturation of immigrants may result in a gradual shift of personality patterns which ultimately is reflected in psychopathology measurable by our techniques. We believe that, in particular, the results of the symptom analysis support our general hypothesis that Japanese immigrants represent an intermediate position between representatives of the culture of their ancestors and those of the host country, whose general cultural pattern is likely to be the assimilation goal of future generations. This study has demonstrated that generational differences are meaningful for comparative purposes and that generation, as a variable, tends to discriminate even more than does sex.

ACKNOWLEDGMENT

This research was carried out with the help of a research grant (M.H. 08639) from the National Institute of Mental Health. Additional funds were made available by the University of Hawaii Research Council. The Social Science Research Institute at the University of Hawaii provided computer facilities. The burden of gathering information from hospital records and of interviewing was shared by a staff of interviewers under the competent guidance of Mrs. Mary Myers. All this support we acknowledge with gratitude. We also wish to express our appreciation to administrators and staff of hospitals who extended their co-operation and the private physicians who gave us their support.

REFERENCES

Altus, W. D. 1966. Birth order and its sequelae. Science 15:44–49.

Caudill, W. 1963. Sibling rank and style of life among Japanese psychiatric patients. *In* Proceedings of the Joint Meeting of the Japanese Society of Psychiatry and Neurology and the American Psychiatric Association, Tokyo. H. Akimoto, ed. Supplement 7 of Folia Psychiatria et Neurologia Japonica. Tokyo, Japanese Society of Psychiatry and Neurology.

————. MS. Social background and sibling rank among Japanese psychiatric patients.

Caudill, W., and G. DeVos. 1956. Achievement, culture, and personality: the case of Japanese Americans. American Anthropologist 58:1102–26.

Kennedy, D. 1961. Key issues in the cross-cultural study of mental disorders. *In* Studying personality cross-culturally. B. Kaplan, ed. Evanston: Row, Peterson.

Phillips, L. 1965. Maturity and psychopathology project: schedule of procedures. Worcester, Massachusetts, Research Institute of Life Sciences, Worcester State Hospital.

Phillips, L., and M. Rabinovitch. 1958. Social role and patterns of symptomatic behavior. Journal of Abnormal and Social Psychology 57:181–86.

Schooler, C., and W. Caudill. 1964. Symptomatology in Japanese and American schizophrenics. Ethnology 3:172–78.

Spindler, G. D. 1955. Sociocultural and psychological processes in Menomini acculturation. Berkeley, University of California Publications in Culture and Society, Vol. 5.

11.   A Mental Health Program at the Elementary School Level in Taiwan: A Six-year Review of the East-Gate Project

CHEN-CHIN HSU, M.D.
Taipei Children's Mental Health Center
National Taiwan University Hospital
Taipei, Taiwan

TSUNG-YI LIN, M.D.
Mental Health Unit
World Health Organization
Geneva, Switzerland

THE IMPORTANCE of early identification of maladjusted children and of adequate intervention has been well established, as has the strategic position of elementary schools and the need to involve classroom teachers in mental health work (Bower, 1960, 1963; Bower, Tashnovian, and Larson, 1958). In Taiwan certain practical considerations made it essential that we gain the active participation of classroom teachers in planning and implementing a mental health program at the elementary school level. For the 12 million population, with more than 96 per cent of its 2 million school age children attending public schools, the Taipei Children's Mental Health Center has been the only professional agency concerned with the mental health of children. Until 1962, not a single school had counselors or psychologists. The results of an epidemiological survey (Lin, 1953) indicated that the magnitude of mental health problems in Taiwan was no less than in other countries and more than the mental health profession alone could manage. In the first 25-year mental health plan (Lin, 1960), therefore, the participation of schoolteachers in mental health work was envisaged as one of the essentials. A search for effective ways of working with school teachers was initiated in 1954.

Accumulated experience gradually led to the initiation of an experimental mental health project, known in Taiwan as the East-Gate project.

In this chapter we recapitulate and examine some of the important points in the development of the pilot elementary school program.

Development of Elementary School Mental Health Program

Since the establishment in 1954 of the Chinese National Association for Mental Health, an increasing effort has been made to interest school-teachers in mental health. Lectures, panel discussions, and films initially were used as well as mass media, such as radio, newspapers, and later TV. Several years of such work, however, proved to be unrewarding in relation to the effort and time involved.

In 1959, in collaboration with the Provincial Public Health Nursing Training Center and as part of its training program, a mental health team, consisting of a child psychiatrist, a clinical psychologist, and a social worker, was sent to the health center in Tao-yuan, a town situated 20 miles south of Taipei, as a weekly mental health mobile clinic from the Taipei Children's Mental Health Center. The first of its sort in Taiwan, it was conceived more as a program to teach mental health to public health personnel than as a consultation service to solve problems related to mental health.

Soon after the initiation of the program, several teachers in the elementary schools of Tao-yuan became interested in the mental health program, presumably as a consequence of contacts with public health nurses who had visited the schools to talk with the teachers about children with behavior problems. The interested teachers asked to be allowed to join in the weekly conference. Soon the conference was split into two sections for the following reasons: (1) the size of the group had become too large to be effective because of the large number of interested teachers; and (2) the needs and background of teachers required a separate program. Thus, two volunteer teachers from each of the seven elementary schools of the town comprised a separate mental health conference for teachers.

These weekly conferences, lasting for two hours, reflected the needs of the participants, and became almost entirely problem-centered group discussions. The mental health team usually was requested to give a didactic lecture on a specific problem, such as truancy or intellectual inadequacy, which was followed by discussion of cases related to the problem presented by the participants. Although the conferences were welcomed by the teachers because they gained understanding of the factors involved in specific problems and help in working out better ways of dealing with children than before, it became clear that the program had some shortcomings. First, the case presentation without follow-up discussions and technical supervision was not sufficient to satisfy the actual needs of an individual teacher in his effort to help a particular child. Second, the unsystematic didactic lectures given upon the request of the participants combined with the unfeasibility in such a group of studying a specific case intensively failed to help the teachers acquire a comprehensive understanding of mental health. Third, the fact that the 14 teachers taking part in each conference came from seven different schools made it difficult to develop close working relations among the participants, and consequently the kind of *esprit de corps* and group leadership which is most advantageous for such a pioneering enterprise was missing. In addition, the distance of the town from the clinic tended to lessen the opportunities for informal contacts between the participants and the team members which are sometimes even more important than formal contacts in developing optimum working relations. Moreover, there was little time for contacts between the school principals and the team, although the leadership, understanding, and support of the school administration is essential.

Agreement was reached among the members of the team on a few principles and steps for formulating a program of increased effectiveness in promoting mental health in schools: (1) Instead of trying to reach many schools in different localities at one time, one school should be selected as the pilot project school. (2) The first and most important consideration in making this choice should be the principal—his ability, personality, leadership, and motivation toward collaboration with the mental health profession for the wholesome development of children. (3) The pilot school should be located in the vicinity of the clinic and preferably have high prestige in its community, in view of the leadership role it would be expected to play in future mental health work in elementary education. (4) The initial goal of the program should be to motivate and assist teachers in integrating mental health work into their daily teaching routine. (5) When the initial phase of the program proved to be a success, a counseling program should be established in the school which would be carried out by several teachers who would devote full time to mental health problems of the children. (6) After this stage, the leadership of various facets of the program should be transferred gradually from the mental health team to the counselors. (7) When a counselor's office in the school was firmly established and functioning effectively, the pilot school could be used as the training center for teachers from other schools, thus becoming the base of a school mental health program for the whole city.

Establishment of East-Gate Pilot Project

After an exploratory search, the East-Gate elementary school in Taipei, situated a few blocks from the clinic, was chosen as the experimental school because all members of the team felt that this school met the qualifications outlined above. Prior to designing an effective, practical program, it was felt necessary to assess objectively the teachers' concepts of and attitudes toward mental health in the school. All teachers in the school were surveyed by means of a standardized inquiry in 1960 to obtain answers to the following questions: (1) How many children are considered to have "problems"? (2) What types of "problems" are of special concern? (3) What are the characteristics of the children who are considered "problem children"? (4) How have the "problem children" been handled?

The results of this survey were published in a separate paper (Hsu, 1966), and only a brief résumé of the main points are presented here. The teachers of the East-Gate school designated only 3.5 per cent of the school population (291 of 8,329 pupils) as "problem children." The teachers were found to be more concerned with such categories of problems as acting out, inadequate learning attitudes, and intellectual inadequacy than with asocial behavior problems. Because Taiwan had at that time no provision for special education, the mentally subnormal children remained in the regular classes where the teachers found their presence raised serious educational and adjustment difficulties. It was found also that many of the reported "problem children" came from poor, lower-class parentage; were older than their classmates; and had histories of low academic achievement, repeating grades, and changing schools. Measures taken by the teachers for handling "problem children" ranged from scolding, punitive labor, and spanking to indifference ("leave him alone") and rejection ("encourage the parents to withdraw the child from school"). Only a few cases were handled through discussion with the parents. Only 3 of the 291 "problem children" had received professional care, although most of the teachers admitted the need for professional help in dealing with these children.

When the survey had been completed, a series of four lectures served as an orientation course for all teachers, with the aim of helping them to gain an understanding of the purpose and scope of the mental health program, for it was felt essential that such a pioneer program enjoy the support and co-operation of the entire school. An impressively large number of teachers responded with keen interest, some with enthusiasm, although a segment showed antipathy to the program. The orientation program succeeded at least in putting the term "mental health" in the minds of the latter group and also made conceivable the idea of a "mental health program" as a school activity.

The whole project was conceived as a six-year program in two major parts. The first part aimed to impart basic knowledge and skills in mental health to all teachers of the school by means of a mental health seminar for a group of 15 teachers each year. The second part aimed to train a nucleus of leadership personnel and to establish a counselor's office.

MENTAL HEALTH SEMINAR

Starting in September, 1960, a group of 13 to 15 teachers have attended the mental health seminar each year. The teachers have been recruited on a voluntary basis; in fact, 27 teachers asked to be allowed to attend the first year in response to the orientation course.

The objectives of the seminar have been: (1) To enable the teachers to acquire basic knowledge regarding the adjustment of a child in his intricate interaction with family, school, and social life, as well as to his own biological and psychological inner environment, and to apply this knowledge to their daily educational activities. (2) To acquaint the teachers with early signs and evidences òf maladjustment of children and to impart some skill in the early identification and management of such problems. (3) To enable the teachers to refer serious problems to proper professional agencies at an early stage and to collaborate with them in assisting the children.

The seminar has been held weekly throughout the academic year, allotting two hours per session. For the first two years it was held at the Taipei Children's Mental Health Center in the afternoon after school hours. The East-Gate school became the meeting place after the establishment of a counselor's office there.

The seminar has been divided into two consecutive parts: the first part has consisted of eight orientation sessions, and the second part has consisted of weekly discussions of casework done by the teachers. The survey of teachers served as a useful guide in planning and conducting the seminars so that the contents and methods are related to the needs of the teacher and the school. The topics of the orientation sessions have been:

1) What is a maladjusted child, and what are the signs and evidences of maladjustment?
2) Biological factors and the adjustment of children.
3) Emotional factors and the adjustment of children.
4) Intelligence and children's adjustment.
5) Family and social factors and the adjustment of children.
6) Group dynamics in the classroom.
7) Working with children.
8) Working with parents.

After completion of the eight orientation sessions, each participant has chosen one child with behavior problems from his class for case study and guidance under the supervision of the mental health team. Every week a teacher has presented one or two cases at the seminar for discussion, centering first around the possible factors involved in the manifestation of a child's problems. An effort has been made to assist the teacher to work out concrete ways of helping the child and the family. A progress report on each case has been given by the teacher to the seminar for assessment at an appropriate later time. Each participant has had at least three opportunities to present one of his cases to the seminar. Understandably, many unscheduled, informal contacts have occurred during each year between individual teachers and members of the mental health team. The team not only has supervised the case work of the teachers but also has provided technical assistance in medical and neurological examinations, psychological testing, and social work where needed.

As in evaluating the results of any educational or other program intended to change concepts, attitudes, and human behavior, ample time is required for objective assessment using refined evaluative research techniques. A detailed evaluative study of the present project will be published separately, and only a preliminary summary is given here.

As can be seen in Table 1, teachers, after completion of the 1961–63 seminars, identified an increased number of children (471 or 12 per cent as against 291 or 3.5 per cent before the seminar) who needed help and showed signs of maladjustment, especially in respect to asocial behavior, anxiety symptoms, and habit disorders.

Toward the end of the first academic year, the teachers almost unanimously expressed appreciation for rewarding experiences in the seminar. Most were aware of their own changed concepts of and attitudes toward a disturbing child. For instance, they were able to see that the truant child "does not play hooky without reasons." They now would try to search for the factors influencing the child's general adjustment in the class; thus instead of categorizing a child as "bad" and punishing him accordingly, they would try to help him modify and solve the underlying difficulties. In addition to reporting improvement in the behavior of the majority of children they had chosen for study in the seminar, most teachers reported that they

Table 1: Comparison of "Problem Children" Reported by Teachers* before and after Mental Health Seminars

Characteristic	Before Seminars (1960)	After Seminars (1961-63)
Number of children in classes	8,329	3,947
Number of "problem children" reported	291 (3.5%)	471 (12%)
Number of "problems" noted	603 (2.1 per child)	1,503 (3.2 per child)
Problems shown by "problem children" (in per cent)		
Acting-out disciplinary problems	78	95
Asocial behavior problems	19	63
Inadequate learning attitudes	45	40
Intellectual inadequacy	31	30
Anxiety syndromes	18	27
Habit disorders	14	20

* A total of 121 teachers at the East-Gate School were surveyed in 1960, and 58 of the same teachers participated in the seminars during 1961-63.

found themselves dealing differently with other children in the class.

By the end of the 1960–61 school year, 29 additional teachers wished to participate in the seminar the following year. Fourteen were chosen as the second group in the academic year 1961–62, and the same process has continued in succeeding years. Several seminar participants have been asked to help conduct the seminar during the following year as group leaders, and also to be trained to become school counselors later.

TRAINING OF COUNSELORS

Since not a single school in Taiwan had a school psychologist or counselor, it was deemed essential to train counseling teachers who would act first as the counterpart of the mental health team and gradually would take over the major responsibilities of the school mental health program. Several teachers participating in the mental health seminar, who increasingly recognized this need, volunteered to be trained as counselors. In September, 1962, and again in 1964, two teachers were selected for training, and they spent a full year at the Taipei Children's Mental Health Center. Still another two are being trained now, and thus by September, 1966, the East-Gate primary school will have one counselor for each of the six grades.

The first month of training in practical counseling, in the mornings, has been spent observing the clinical intake procedures of the social workers and child psychiatrists in order to learn how a mental health team handled a child and his family on their first clinic visit. In the following two months the teachers have worked as intake case workers under supervision. From the fourth month on, they have worked actively with cases (four selected sets of children and four parents per trainee) in intensive counseling. This training in intensive counseling, though it has in it a notion of therapeutic intervention, is not meant to make psychotherapists of the teachers but rather to help them apply some of the principles and techniques of mental health approaches in counseling "problem children" and their parents. It also is aimed at helping them to realize the limitations of a layman in dealing with severely disturbed children and children with possible organic pathologies and thus to assist them in referring such cases to appropriate institutions or clinics. Individual and group supervision by a child psychiatrist and a social worker have constituted the main training methods.

Theoretical training, given in the afternoons, has centered on such subjects as growth and development, child psychiatry, psychotherapy, psychiatric social work, interviewing techniques, general, clinical, and educational psychology, biological bases of behavior, and group dynamics. In view of the lack of school psychologists, it was considered essential for the counselors to acquire skills in assessing the intellectual potentialities of the children. Goodenough's Draw-A-Man test, the Bender-Gestalt test, and the WISC, all of which had been fairly well standardized for Chinese, were considered appropriate for school use. Theoretical training has been followed by observing, through a one-way screen, actual testing sessions conducted by the clinical psychologist. Then, under supervision, each of the two teachers in training has given tests to ten normal children and ten emotionally disturbed children. Of course, no teacher has been given the false idea of having been trained as a professional psychologist.

One more aspect of the counselors' training deserves special mention —the problem of professional jargon. It is necessary, of course, that the trainees acquire some understanding of psychiatric terms, but it is felt imperative that they translate these terms into everyday speech so that their work with other teachers and parents will not be handicapped by difficulty in communication. In discussing the psychodynamics of a case, for instance, the members of the team first use a psychiatric term and then try to convey the implication of the term to the teachers in common parlance; then the two parties work out an appropriate common term for the psychiatric term. Toward the end of the first year of training, a glossary of this kind was drafted for trial use.

Establishment of Counselor's Office and Its Functions

After a year of training at the clinic, the first two teachers returned to the East-Gate school in September, 1963, and set up a counselor's office, the first of its sort in the country. It has six offices for individual interviewing and testing, two large group activity rooms, and a spacious playground. The mental health team consults with and supervises the counselors and also participates in a bi-weekly conference at the counselor's office which is chaired by the principal and attended by the heads of the offices of curriculum and discipline. The counselor's office thus functions as a co-ordination center for the different offices of the school which are concerned with children's progress in learning and behavior.

When the counselor's office was established in 1963, the mental health seminar became one of its most important activities. During the academic years of 1963 and 1964, the seminar was conducted by the mental health team, with the two counselors sitting in as resource persons. They had been involved actively from the beginning in the preparation of the whole year's program and also in planning, conducting, and evaluating each session. For the 1965–66 academic year, the seminar was conducted by the counselors themselves, with the mental health team receding into the background as consultants. School policy providing for in-service mental health training for every teacher implies that the seminar will be continued regularly, since every year approximately ten new teachers are assigned to the East-Gate school while some are transferred to other schools.

INDIVIDUAL COUNSELING

The basic policy in setting up the counselor's office was to encourage and assist the teachers of the school to manage as many children with behavior problems as possible. A counselor, however, often finds it useful to have personal contact with a child and his parents to formulate his own view on the case before attempting to help the teacher responsible for the child. Moreover, certain cases require special examinations or intensive counseling which ordinary class teachers cannot handle.

Every teacher who wishes to refer a child to the counselor's office first discusses the nature of the problems and the purpose of referral with a counselor. As a rule, the referring teacher is encouraged to make a systematic study of the case under question. This process frequently requires more than one meeting between the teacher and the counselor. Certain cases then have been taken over by the counselors for further assessment or intensive

Table 2: Disposition and Present Status of Children Referred to Counselor's Office, 1963–1965

	Number of Cases		
Item	Boys	Girls	Total
Year Referred			
1963	28	4	32
1964	61	11	72
1965	59	26	85
Total	148	41	189
Initial Disposition			
Carried by teachers	104	21	125
Carried by counselors	18	7	25
Group therapy	9	8	17
Referred to Taipei Children's Mental Health Center	17	5	22
Total	148	41	189
Present Status			
Graduated	7	3	10
School change	10	2	12
Under class teacher's observation after improvement	38	8	46
Carried by class teachers	59	13	72
In group therapy	9	8	17
Carried by counselors	29	6	29
In treatment at Taipei Children's Mental Health Center	2	1	3
Total	148	41	189

counseling, and some have been referred to the clinic of the Taipei Children's Mental Health Center for professional investigation or treatment, but a majority have continued to be handled by class teachers, in close contact with a counselor. As the situation permits and as each party involved feels comfortable, some cases which had been referred to the clinic are transferred back to the counselor's office, and some cases which had been dealt with by a counselor are transferred back to the referring teachers for continuing help. Table 2 shows the distribution according to disposition and present status, of the cases which have been referred to the counselor's office for the academic years 1963, 1964, and 1965.

A series of questions about the effectiveness of such a school mental health program may be asked at this point: How many of the school children who have been identified by individual class teachers as showing signs of maladjustment were actually in need of counseling? How are the "problem children" who have not been brought to the attention of the counselor's office being dealt with by individual class teachers and for what reasons? What are the results for children who have been under the care of individual class teachers? Objective answers to these questions are hard to come by. In an attempt to secure some useful data on these questions, a "behavior sheet" has been attached to each child's report card at the end of each academic year, starting in 1964. The class teacher is requested to describe on the form in concrete terms the characteristics of the behavior problem, the possible underlying factors and causes, the methods used during the school year to handle the problem, the present status of the child's adjustment, and recommendations for future handling of the child. The accumulation of such information is expected to be of valuable assistance to the next class teacher the following year and also may provide clues to answering the above questions.

GROUP THERAPY

The need for exploring the usefulness of a group approach in working with children had been a major concern of the Taipei Children's Mental Health Center for some time before two groups of children with disciplinary problems were organized in 1963. They have been meeting regularly at the counselor's office with a group therapist from the clinic as the leader. The continuation of these group therapy sessions is of utmost importance both for the training of counselors and for research purposes.

WORKING WITH PARENTS

The counselors work directly and indirectly with parents. Directly, they see only the small number of parents whose children they are counseling. It is the indirect aspect of working with parents which deserves special mention. First, the counselor usually introduces a new approach to help a teacher to establish a bridge to the family. Second, the counselor helps the teacher to gain increased understanding of the nature of adjustmental problems of children in relation to their families. Third, the parents thus are brought into the picture in dealing with a particular problem of the child, and they become more aware of all aspects of the child's life than they had been.

The value of psychological testing in working with parents also deserves mention. Owing to the incredibly severe competition in entrance examinations for secondary schools in Taiwan, parents increasingly have tended to place undue emphasis on the academic achievements of their children. This emphasis has been one of the major causes of stress both for teachers and children, especially children of modest intellectual endowment who have ambitious parents. For these parents, skillful interpretation of the results of intelligence tests has proved to be effective in helping them to accept the limitations of their children's performances and thus construct reasonable future plans for the children.

WORKING WITH TEACHERS

In accordance with the objectives set for the counselor's office, work with teachers has constituted the most important and time-consuming part of the counselor's activities. The East-Gate school decided to take advantage of its regular weekly teachers' meetings, attended by an average of 20 teachers of each grade on different days of the week, for the counselors to meet with all teachers regularly. The two-hour meetings therefore were divided into two sessions: one hour for the regular meeting to exchange experiences and discuss problems of common concern and the other for free discussion on mental health problems. The meeting is chaired by a leader of the teachers for each grade with the counselors sitting in as resource persons. In contrast to the mental health seminar, no lecture is given and no definite program or agenda is arranged. Teachers are invited and encouraged to bring up problems or cases for free discussion, to exchange experiences in dealing with specific problems or cases, and to use the occasion for initial contact with counselors for case referral. Since the school has more than 120 classes, it can be understood that this meeting has been welcomed both by teachers and counselors as one of the few avenues for keeping communication open.

The teachers themselves can be grouped roughly on the basis of their attitudes toward the project as (1) co-operative, (2) indifferent, or (3) skeptical. A number of teachers have shown a positive interest in increasing their knowledge about children generally and also about effective ways to deal with children's behavior problems. These teachers have learned quickly to identify the early signs of children's maladjustment, have met frequently with the counselors, have taken an active interest in the weekly discussion group, and have co-operated in various research programs. While these co-operative teachers have been given timely encouragement and reinforcement in working with children and parents, so far as possible they also have been made to realize their limitations as teachers in such guidance work.

The experience of Miss H., a second grade teacher, is cited as illustrative of the teachers in the first group. She was one of the teachers who volunteered to participate in the first year's seminar. She dropped in at the counselor's office one day because of her concern over the problems of a boy, T. S., in her class. T. S. was one of three children who had been transferred to her class from other schools at the beginning of the academic year. On the first day of school, T. S. was accompanied by a young, well-dressed lady who left the class very soon without saying a word to the child. In marked contrast to the young lady, T. S. looked like a beggar. His clothes seemed not to have been washed for a week; his skin was covered with mosquito bites, scratches, and eruptions. The second day, T. S. came in alone and late for class. When Miss H. tried to find out the trouble, she found that T. S., a Taiwanese who spoke a local dialect at home, hardly could comprehend Mandarin. She seated him next to a friendly, bright boy who helped him to understand what was going on in class. During the recess period she managed to learn from T. S. that he had not had breakfast and that instead of taking a bus he had walked quite a distance to school, but he could not tell her why. After that day it became Miss H.'s routine to take T. S. to the snack shop for breakfast, help him wash, and give him additional tutoring. Gradually, she found out that the young lady who had brought him to the school was not his mother but his recently married eldest sister. T. S. could not say where his mother was, though he said his father had died a few months ago in their home village, and his mother had brought him to the city to live with his sister. Until his sister's marriage, his mother had taken care of the house while his sister worked. After the marriage, the young couple did not have room for the mother and T.S., and, moreover, the bridegroom did not like their all living together. The mother then found a job as a live-in cook. T. S. had been sleeping on a wooden bench without a mosquito net in the living room of his newly married sister's home. When he woke in the morning the young couple were still in bed, and he dared not ask them for breakfast or bus fare. One day he did not show up at school. The next day he came in late with tears in his eyes. The teacher learned that T. S. had gone to look for his mother in vain. That evening Miss H. made a home visit, but no one was in. She learned from neighbors that the young couple were always out dancing or at the movies and that the boy frequently was not fed. Early the next morning, Miss H. was able to see the couple. Though their manner to Miss H. was very polite, she found that neither the sister nor her husband liked to have T. S. living with them. Miss H. was very much worried that unless his living conditions changed T. S. would be unable to settle down to learn and might quite well become involved in a gang, if simply to satisfy his need for food. The counselor agreed and suggested that Miss H. locate the mother and discuss the problem with her. Miss H. finally managed to find the mother at her employer's home. The mother apparently was surprised to find that T. S. was not being well taken care of. A few days later his mother came to Miss H. depressed and complaining that her daughter had told her to take T. S. out of her home. Miss H. went to the counselor who suggested encouraging the mother to take T. S. back to her village to live with the extended family. The mother went to their former rural home where she was welcomed back by all her in-laws and found work in their fields. T. S. was happy because he could now live with his mother and no longer be troubled by mosquitos or hunger. Miss H. went to the village to discuss with T. S.'s teacher how to help T. S. catch up with his school work; she has continued to keep in touch with the boy.

Among the teachers showing eager co-operation in the project a small subgroup has been discerned whose interest in mental health stemmed partly from their own need for psychiatric help. As might be expected, in the course of their contacts with the counselors or in discussion groups they have become able to talk about themselves.

The indifferent teachers probably constitute the second sizable group of teachers. Their attitude to the mental health project is expressed in Chinese as *pa-ma-fan*, which can be translated as "couldn't care less." Though they may appreciate intellectually the seriousness of mental health problems among children in the school and recognize that sound personality development also is a goal of education, they have shown little interest in taking part in the program. Some of them have looked upon participation in the project merely as additional unpaid work. Teachers in this category have reported a considerably smaller number of maladjusted children in their classes than have the co-operative teachers. This group of teachers also have sent only seriously disturbed children to the counselor's office, with little intention of personally sharing the guidance work.

Mrs. L., a third grade teacher, typifies this group. In the initial survey of teachers, she reported that there was no "problem child" in her class. It turned out that she had been urging parents of such children to withdraw them from class, telling them that the children should be treated "radically" before they came back to class. When encouraged to identify children who were problems to her, she sent four children with intellectual handicaps to the counselor to have them taken care of for good. In the discussion groups, she often stated that she knew that children with behavior deviations were sick and needed help, but not from a busy class teacher like herself. She kept complaining about the overcrowding of her class, the poor pay of teachers, the unfair attitude of the public toward teachers, and the unreasonable pressure put upon her by overambitious parents.

How to motivate these uninterested teachers to take an active part in the project constitutes as great a problem for the counselor's office as do the skeptical teachers. From the beginning of the project, a group of teachers showed attitudes ranging from skepticism to open antagonism. Their resistance can be attributed in part to their mistaken ideas about mental health, ideas which apparently reflect the stigma that the general public attaches to mental illness. It also may stem partly from their narrow view of education—the idea that the teaching of children is the exclusive prerogative of the teacher, since only he knows how to teach. Finally, in a few cases, the cause for such negative attitudes toward mental health seemed to be rooted in their own personal problems. These teachers as a rule have claimed that the traditional method of discipline is more effective than counseling. They have shown strong reluctance to participate in the program, asserting that they would rather spend more time with "good children" than waste their time with a small number of "bad children."

Mr. C., one of the sixth grade teachers, is illustrative of this group. He had 15 years of teaching experience and enjoyed the reputation of being one of the best teachers because he always succeeded in getting a large proportion of the children in his class into good middle schools. He felt a spartan method to be the best way of educating children. He never volunteered to participate in the seminar. In the group discussions he openly expressed doubt about the effectiveness of permissive counseling in improving children's behavior. In the initial survey of teachers, he reported several "problem children" in his class for reasons of intellectual inadequacy or lack of motivation for learning, but he never brought any of these children to the attention of the counselors. A boy, K. T., in Mr. C.'s class played truant several times and one day was picked up by the head of the office of discipline, who sent him to the counselor's office. When a counselor got in touch with him, Mr. C. said that punishment would be the most effective way of "correcting" the misbehavior. He ordered the child to hold a chair aloft for 30 minutes and then urged him to apologize in front of the class for "losing face" for the entire class by being brought to the attention of the office of discipline. A few days later, K. T. again was found on the street and was sent to the principal who suggested that Mr. C. co-operate with the counselor's office in working out a way to help K. T. Mr. C. brought K. T. to the office and declared that he would not like to waste any more time on such a hopeless child. The counselor found that K. T. was another case of a victimized child—one caught between an overpressing teacher and over-ambitious parents and hard put to measure up because of his low-average intellectual endowment (an I.Q. of 92). After a few talks with K. T.'s father, the counselor was able to help him see that for K. T., with his average ability combined with a liking for mechanics, a vocational school would be a better choice than a middle school. Mr. C. also was led to agree that there would be no problem in helping K. T. to enter a vocational school. K. T. was delighted with this decision and ceased to be truant. Though Mr. C. is still far from positively favorable toward the counseling program, he has referred several cases to the counselors for assessment of their intellectual potential.

The counselors quickly learned that in addition to their two most important requirements, i.e., time and patience in winning over resistant and indifferent teachers, they ought to work out their own counter feelings aroused by such attitudes. It has been encouraging and gratifying to witness the way in which the counselors have handled the indifferent and skeptical teachers and improved their relations with them.

Influence of Pilot Project

To encourage the interest of other elementary schools in Taiwan in children's mental health and in starting their own active programs when the situation permits has been one of the goals of the East-Gate project. Already toward the end of the first year of the project, teachers attending the mental health seminar expressed a strong wish to share their experiences with teachers of their own and other schools in the city. Thus they organized a one-day conference on their own at the close of the academic year, to which the principal and two teachers from each of the 40-odd elementary schools in the city were invited. After an explanation of the overall school mental health program by the East-Gate principal, the audience was divided into several small groups for discussion. Each person at the conference was given as reference material a booklet written by the teachers and the members of the mental health team on principles of mental health work with elementary school children, including case reports on each child handled by the teachers during the past year. A couple of teachers who had attended the mental health seminar presented their experiences with cases and their reactions to the seminar. This presentation was followed by lively and wide-ranging group discussion. At the end of the day, each discussion group presented a summary report to a plenary session.

The response of the principals and teachers of other schools to the conference was encouraging, and a similar conference has been held every year. The level of the conference has improved each year, as evidenced by the content and quality of the group discussion and also by the quality of subsequent booklets written by the teachers. It should be added that the effects of such mental health conferences have been far reaching, and several schools already have asked for assistance from the Taipei Children's Mental Health Center or from the East-Gate school in initiating a similar program. Preparations are being made to meet such demands by strengthening the counselor's office at the East-Gate school to make it a basis for expanding mental health work to other schools.

SPECIAL EDUCATION FOR MENTALLY SUBNORMAL CHILDREN

As we mentioned in passing, a serious problem for all teachers was the mixing of mentally subnormal children in the ordinary classes. It was with good reason that nearly half of the cases selected for discussion by the teachers who took part in the mental health seminar were those of children in the category of "mental subnormality with behavior problems." Each participant agreed that serious effort should be given to starting special education for the mentally subnormal children in Taiwan. This feeling also was reflected strongly in the one-day conference held at the close of the academic year, and, when one of the attending principals expressed his determination to start an experimental class for subnormal children, the strongest support came from the teachers of the East-Gate school. In fact, teachers of the

East-Gate school have been contributing to the training of teachers for the experimental class through sharing their experiences in working with emotionally disturbed children and their parents (Hsu and Lin, in press).

RESEARCH

In addition to the evaluative studies touched on earlier, the mental health team, together with the counselor's office, started in 1963 to carry out one research project each year in areas concerned with basic adjustmental problems of elementary school children. The study on the prevalence of subnormal children and their adjustmental problems in 1963 has helped the Taipei Municipal Bureau of Education in its further planning, training, and assignment of teachers in special education. Studies of bed wetters and habitual absentees were carried out in 1964 and 1965, and the results seem to shed some light on the prevalence of these problems and also give some clues for working out preventive measures. A follow-up study on the fate of children who repeated grades will be the theme for the next study. All concerned share the belief that without the experience of working with schoolteachers for several years and the existence and effective functioning of the counselor's office, it would not have been possible to investigate this series of important research questions.

Concluding Remarks

Much has been going on in the field of mental health work in the elementary schools in Taiwan, in contrast to the complete lack a decade ago. The most noticeable phenomenon so far is the change in educators' attitudes toward mental health. The enlightened attitudes of the educational administration can be witnessed in the fact that in 1963, for the first time in its history, an appropriation, though small in amount, was made for school mental health work and for the training of teachers in counseling and special education. The permission granted to the East-Gate school for a certain number of teachers to work as full-time mental health counselors is another reflection of this enlightened attitude. That the principles and techniques of the mental health approach have been integrated, from the very beginning, into the training program of teachers receiving special education is still another proof of their acceptance by the educational profession (Hsu and Lin, in press).

The question whether the school mental health activities are attaining the purposes they were intended for still remains unanswered. Are there other, more effective ways than the ones being used to attain the goals? How can we assess more objectively than now the changes in attitudes and methods of the teachers in dealing with maladjusted children? What are the criteria for assigning certain cases for guidance to class teachers, and others to the teachers who have been trained in counseling? Ample time is needed for answering these important questions.

It would not be too subjective to remark, however, that the school mental health project has been a source of pleasure to the members of the Taipei Children's Mental Health Center. Through operating the program, they feel that some way has been found to meet the increasing needs that the modern world has imposed on mankind. Through working with teachers, they have become more convinced of the urgent need for a close working relation between education and mental health. Both professions have a great deal to offer each other in contributing to the welfare of children. They also have found a wealth of material for research on the better understanding of children through the East-Gate project. Finally, relations with principals and teachers, which have been characterized by warmth and mutual respect, have been most rewarding, and this result alone would have been a sufficient reason for such an undertaking. In other words, this has been a good mental health program for all parties—the children, the teachers, and the mental health team.

REFERENCES

Bower, E. M. 1960. Early identification of emotionally handicapped children in school. Springfield, Thomas.
———. 1963. Primary prevention of mental health and emotional disorders: conceptual framework and action possibilities. American Journal of Orthopsychiatry 33:832–48.
Bower, E. M., P. J. Tashnovian, and C. A. Larson. 1958. A process for early identification of emotionally disturbed children. Sacramento, California State Department of Education.
Hsu, C. C. 1966. A study on "problem children" reported by teachers. Japanese Journal of Child Psychiatry 7:91–108.
Hsu, C. C. and T. Lin. In press. Induction of special education for the mentally subnormal children in Taiwan: the role of a mental health team in the program development. *In* Proceedings of the 18th Annual Meeting of the World Federation for Mental Health, Bangkok.
Lin, T. 1953. A study of the incidence of mental disorder in Chinese and other cultures. Psychiatry 16:313–36.
———. 1960. Teaching of psychiatry at National Taiwan University. British Medical Journal 2:345–48.

12. The Structure of Rejecting Attitudes toward the Mentally Ill in Japan

SHOGO TERASHIMA, M.D.

Department of Neuropsychiatry
Kyūshū University Medical School
Fukuoka, Japan

SINCE the advent of the psychotropic drugs, it appears that a shift in emphasis has occurred in all countries both in hospital administration and in mental health policies generally. Many new patients are treated with various potent psychotropic drugs in an open-door situation, and it has become quite possible for them to be discharged within a few months. The chronic patients, particularly chronic schizophrenic patients, however, have remained in hospitals and continue to occupy the majority of the beds. In an advanced hospital these chronic patients are provided with active recreational, outside work, and psychotherapy programs in order that they too can return to the community as soon as possible. As a consequence of social prejudice and rejecting attitudes, however, there are numerous problems in returning mental patients to the community. It is of crucial importance at the practical level to know why it is so difficult to re-establish expatients in their communities. Not only have social workers told us that the reintegration of the patient with his family and community is the most difficult part of their job but also discussions with patients in mental hospitals have revealed that the patients themselves frequently are acutely sensitive to the rejection which they feel upon their return home. Furthermore, treatment programs for the mentally ill person who has stayed in his home have increased in importance. In Japan the national mental health program has urged since 1965 that each prefecture establish a mental health center in order to give professional help to expatients and the mentally ill who have remained in their homes. Many discussions among those responsible for the preventive aspects of this service have led to the belief that very little is known about the nature of preventive psychiatry or about public attitudes toward mental illness, either good or bad.

The project upon which I am reporting in this chapter was an attempt to explore the lay attitudes in Japan toward mental health and mental illness. Most studies concerned with social attitudes toward the mentally ill have revealed a wide range of attitudes extending from failure to realize that they are ill at all, combined with full acceptance of them as members of the community, to complete rejection of them because they do not conform to the norm (Gruenberg and Belline, 1957; Permins *et al.*, 1965; Star, 1957; Tershakovec, 1964). Between these extremes are attitudes of veneration, tolerance, pity, amusement, morbid curiosity, anxiety, prejudice, repulsion, and hostility. A number of studies in the United States and Canada (Bowen and Fisher, 1962; Permins *et al.*, 1965; Phillips, 1963, 1964; Pratt, Giannitrapani, and Khanna 1960; Ramsey and Seipp, 1948) have shown that public feeling about the mentally ill, in general, has been characterized by fear, anxiety, stigmatization, rejection, and misinformation. Star (1955), summarizing her study of a national sample, reported that, as both her data and other studies made clear, mental illness is something which people want to keep as far from themselves as possible. Cumming and Cumming (1957), working on a much smaller scale than Star, elaborated a theory of social response to the mentally ill comprising a sequence of "denial, isolation and rejection." In general, the essentially rejective and punitive picture of the social response to mental illness has become widely accepted. The final report of the Joint Commission on Mental Illness and Health (1961) pointed out that "several studies of public attitudes have shown a major lack of recognition of mental illness as illness and a predominant tendency toward rejection of both the mental patients and those who treat them. There is general agreement on these points." This finding may represent the status quo in the United States and Canada, although recently there appears to have been some disagreement with these findings and statements (Dohrenwend, Bernard, and Kolb, 1962; Lemkau and Crocetti, 1962). In the meantime, almost no information exists on the differences in culturally based attitudes toward the mentally ill and the mental hospital in Asian countries. Even in Japan, as far as can be determined, no previous study has been made of the important issue of public attitudes toward individuals exhibiting disturbed behavior, although most Japanese professional mental health workers have become fully aware that such attitudes are inclined to be largely rejective and negative.

The Communities Investigated

The populations of three communities were investigated. Table 1 shows the demographic characteristics of the respondents in the three communities.

The Osaka Community. Nose, an old village with an adult population of 6,549, is about 25 miles due north of Osaka city, the second largest city in Japan with a population of about three million, and is truly a representative small agrarian community (covering 38 square miles). Its setting is as completely mountainous as is that of any village in Japan: very steep, though not high, and the mountains form very narrow valleys. No railroad runs into the village; only a few buses pass through each day. There are some outpatient clinics and one modern public health center but no mental hospital in the village. There are six elementary schools and three junior high schools. Economically, the village is rather poor; most inhabitants engage in small farming and some in timbering. The Buddhist religion predominates. The community consists of a completely homogeneous population, without a single foreigner. Television has been rapidly popularized, and about 70 per cent of the homes have had TV sets for several years. Gradually the young people have left the village to work; this change is regarded as an effect of industrialization, urbanization, and the general rise in the economic level of Japan.

The Saga Community. The Saga study was carried out in a relatively wide area extending over Kanzaki-machi, Higashi-Seburi-mura, and Mitagawa-mura, all situated in the northern part of Saga Prefecture, Kyūshū. This area is a famous and typical agricultural area, and communications are good by rail and bus to Saga City, the prefectural capital. The area studied, an old, stable village with an adult population of 3,746 (dwelling units 1,156), is distinguished by the presence of a mental hospital. This is the only one of the three communities studied which has a mental hospital in or near it. Right in the middle of the region studied stands the government-operated Hizen Sanatorium, the sole national mental hospital in western Japan. Its presence has been a problem to people in the area because of the open-door policy of Hizen Sanatorium in recent years, and Saga was chosen for study purposely in order to investigate the opinions of those who live in the environs of a mental hospital.

The Okinawa Community. A part of Kunigami-mura, the village of Okuma, situated in the northwest part of the main island of Okinawa, was selected as the third community. Only a few buses pass through this small village each day. The village is located at the seaside, but relatively broad rice fields are near-by. The adult population is only 313, and most of the young people have drifted to big cities in Japan or to Naha, the capital city of Okinawa. The community consists of a completely homogeneous population in close face-to-face contact. It is a backward community; electric current is cut off by midnight, and only ten TV sets were found in the village.

Table 1: Percentage Distribution of Demographic Characteristics
of Respondents (N=1,191)

Characteristic	Osaka (N=549)	Saga (N=441)	Okinawa (N=201)
Sex			
Male	47	39	41
Female	53	61	59
Age			
18-24	7	12	10
25-34	23	19	17
35-44	17	18	26
45-54	18	21	19
55-64	19	17	15
65 and over	16	13	13
Marital Status			
Single	7	14	11
Married	83	74	73
Widowed/Divorced	10	12	16
Education			
No education	5	3	19
Elementary	28	17	19
Middle school	40	46	46
High school	23	29	15
College	4	5	1
Number in Family			
1-2	3	6	7
3	8	13	8
4	11	18	14
5	19	22	14
6	28	14	16
7	18	16	5
8	10	5	17
9 and over	3	6	19
Years of Residence			
Less than 5	4	5	5
5-10	5	8	10
10-15	4	3	2

(Continued)

Table 1: (Continued)

Characteristic	Osaka (N=549)	Saga (N=441)	Okinawa (N=201)
Years of Residence *(Continued)*			
15-19	6	9	6
19 and over	81	75	77
Prior Contact with the Mentally Ill*			
None	67	18	9
A member of the immediate family	1	4	8
A member of the relatives	7	8	20
A close friend	2	2	9
An acquaintance	18	39	46

* Multiple scoring.

There is a tiny grade school in the village but no junior high school. No physician lives in the village. Its economic situation is remarkably poor; most people are engaged in small-scale farming. This community was chosen for study mainly because of its isolation from both Japanese and Okinawan urban cultures.

Methodology

A randomly selected sample of the population in the three communities studied was interviewed by about 15 local college students, majoring in sociology, psychology, and public health and trained in the techniques of public opinion polling. The interviewer presented a preformulated questionnaire in a rather conversational and relaxed way. The final draft of the questionnaire was established after pretesting on preliminary forms. Wherever possible, the questions used were identical with those used in previous surveys of public attitudes toward the mentally ill in the United States (Nunnally, 1961; Star, 1955; Woodward, 1951). The polling was done mostly in homes, although at times interviews took place on the streets, in the fields, and in office buildings.

An experienced statistician and a sociologist collaborated in the selection of the population sample. The sample was selected by first listing all the tracts of each community and classifying them according to the number of people each contained. Within each tract, the interviewer followed a prescribed route on a map designed to cover most of the tract and interviewed all members over 18 years of age in a predetermined sample of the dwelling units. An attempt was made to obtain a representative sample for the variables of sex, age, and educational level.

The first study was carried out in the rural community in Osaka from September 2–5, 1963. Using a revised questionnaire, the second survey was carried out in the Saga community in exactly the same period of September in 1964. The last study was conducted with the same revised questionnaire in the Okinawan community in July, 1965. Responses were obtained from 78, 62, and 84 per cent, respectively, of all selected respondents in the three communities.

Something should be said about the response of the communities to the inquiry. During the survey in each village, no overt manifestations of either interest or anxiety were displayed. When an interviewer visited by accident a family who had kept a mental patient or a mentally deficient person at home, he was asked why the family was chosen for investigation. Otherwise the inquiry appears not to have aroused any reaction in the surveyed population either at the time of the survey or afterwards.

Measures of Orientation toward Problems of Mental Disorder

In a number of studies carried out in North America, respondents were asked whether they considered various descriptions, which were devised by Star (1955), to be those of mentally ill persons. Because several of these surveys used the descriptions of paranoid schizophrenia, simple schizophrenia, and alcoholism, we also used these three case vignettes in order to compare the public's responses in transcultural terms and also to study the ability of the population to identify given descriptions of behavior as indications of mental illness. The original stories were translated as closely as possible into Japanese and read by the interviewer in the following manner:

1) *Paranoid Schizophrenic.* I'd like to describe a certain kind of person and ask you questions about him. I'm thinking of a man—let's call him Saburo—who is very suspicious; he doesn't trust anyone, he's sure that everyone is against him. At times he thinks that people whom he sees on the street are talking about him or following him. A couple of times now he has beaten up men who didn't even know him, because he thought that they were plotting against him. The other night he began to curse his wife terribly; then he hit her and threatened to kill her, because, he said, she was working against him, too, just as everyone else was.

2) *Simple Schizophrenic.* Now here's a young woman in her twenties—let's call her Michiko. She has never had a job, and she doesn't seem to want to go out and look for one. She is a very quiet girl; she doesn't talk much to anyone, even in her own family, and she acts as

though she is afraid of people, especially young men her own age. She won't go out with anyone, and whenever someone comes to visit her family she stays in her own room until they leave. She just stays by herself and daydreams all the time; she shows no interest in anything or anybody.

3) *Alcoholic*. How about Masao? He never seems to be able to hold a job very long because he drinks so much. Whenever he has money in his pocket, he goes on a spree; he stays out till all hours drinking and never seems to care what happens to his wife and children. Sometimes he feels very bad about the way he treats his family; he begs his wife to forgive him and promises to stop drinking, but he always goes off again.

After each story the respondent was asked, "Would you say this person has some kind of mental illness or not?" This is the same question used by Star (1955), Cumming and Cumming (1957), Lemkau and Crocetti (1962), and Miura *et al.* (1963). Table 2 presents the results obtained in the three Japanese communities.

These findings, although they are much at variance, certainly indicate some public ignorance concerning the signs and symptoms of

Table 2: Percentage of Respondents Identifying Star's Hypothetical Cases as Mentally Ill in This and Other Studies

Case	U.S. National Study 1950 (Star, 1955) (N=3,500)	Canadian Study 1955 (Cumming & Cumming, 1957) (N=540)	Baltimore Study 1960 (Lemkau & Crocetti, 1962) (N=1,736)	New York Study 1960 (Dohrenwend et al., 1962) (N=87)
Paranoid schizophrenia	75	69	71	100
Simple schizophrenia	34	36	78	72
Alcoholism	29	25	62	63

Case	Tokyo Study 1962–1963 (Miura et al., 1963) (N=1,218)	Osaka Study 1963 (N=549)	Saga Study 1964 (N=441)	Okinawa Study 1965 (N=201)
Paranoid schizophrenia	63	61	64	84
Simple schizophrenia	30	36	42	74
Alcoholism	9	9	12	31

mental illness. Interestingly enough, each of the three populations identified the stories as depicting cases of mental illness in the same order; the highest number identified the paranoid case as mentally ill, the next highest, the case of simple schizophrenia, and the least, the alcoholic case. The proportion identifying the alcoholic case as mentally ill was markedly lower in all the Japanese studies than in Western studies. On the other hand, the general understanding by the Japanese of mental disorder seems not so different from that expressed in the less-educated North American populations surveyed (judging from the comments on Star's vignettes), for about the same percentages failed to recognize the two schizophrenic pictures as indicating illness.

Wittkower, in an unpublished discussion of our paper (Terashima and Nareta, 1964) at the annual meeting in 1964 of the American Psychiatric Association, commented as follows:

> As far as the questionnaire is concerned, the procedure
> adopted by them differs from that employed in Shirley Star's
> and other North American studies in one important respect.
> After presenting the vignette of the hypothetical patient to
> their respondents they asked them directly whether they
> thought the persons in the story had some kind of mental
> illness, i.e., invited confirmation of the implied suggestion that
> the person is mentally ill; whereas previous investigators on
> the American scene preceded this question with open-ended
> questions, such as "Would you say that there is anything
> wrong with this person or not? What do you think makes him
> act this way?" The direct and somewhat directive approach
> was apparently chosen in the study reported for the sake of
> establishing quantifiable cross-cultural differences. . . .

In consideration of Wittkower's comments, we tried to adopt the original questionnaire method in the Saga and Okinawa surveys and found a remarkable difference in both surveys between the view that there is something odd about the person and the concept of mental illness. The respondents' replies are summarized in Table 3.

Undoubtedly, confusion arises from a tendency to accept a broad definition of the concept of mental illness in theory but to narrow it to psychosis in practice. *"Seishinbyō"* in Japanese ("mental illness") seems to be thought of in terms of violence, incoherence, loss of reason, and unpredictability, much as uneducated North Americans thought of insanity until recently. The general public in Japan and in the West appears to picture mental illness in terms of extreme pathology (*see* Carstairs, 1959).

The case of paranoid schizophrenia was classified as mentally ill by more than a majority of people in all four Japanese populations which have been studied (*see* Table 2). It is conceivable therefore that persons of hostile and aggressive behavior who disturb others may more commonly be regarded as abnormal mentally than those who live a secluded life or have less aggressive behavior disorders. It is also quite plausible that an overwhelming majority of the population perceive the illlustrated cases of simple schizophrenia and alcoholism as within the range of normal Japanese behavior. As far as Michiko is concerned, the respondents appeared to find it difficult to differentiate the abnormal features, as described, from those normal to a Japanese girl in whom naiveté, quietness, modesty, and a retiring nature are considered rather high virtues. Even in the national American and Canadian studies, however, only 34 and 36 per cent, respectively, labeled the simple schizophrenic case mentally ill. The low percentage of Japanese in the Tokyo, Osaka, and Saga studies who regarded chronic alcoholism as a mental illness may be explained by socially and traditionally determined tolerant attitudes toward a drinker in Japan. These phenomena may be considered "culturally oriented overlay." It is not correct, however, to conclude that the population regards the drinker as a normal person. As shown in Table 3, about half of the respondents in Saga and Okinawa regarded him as odd, but far fewer saw him as mentally ill. In the Osaka study 28 per cent of the respondents could give a correct diagnosis of chronic alcoholism (*arukōruchūdoku*) to the vignette, although only 9 per cent regarded the case as mentally ill. Incidentally, the low admission rate of chronic alcoholics in Japanese mental hospitals results from the permissive attitude toward a drinker. This fact seems to be very important in transcultural comparisons of data regarding admission, incidence, and prevalence rates of alcoholism.

The identification rates of the paranoid schizophrenic, simple schizophrenic, and alcoholic cases were about 62, 39, and 10 per cent, respectively, in the two rural communities in Japan. Of the sample in

Table 3: Percentage of Respondents Viewing Star's
          Hypothetical Cases as Odd*

Case	Saga (N=441)		Okinawa (N=201)	
Paranoid schizophrenia	89	(64)	98	(84)
Simple schizophrenia	81	(42)	93	(74)
Alcoholism	45	(12)	67	(31)

* Figures in parentheses indicate percentages of respondents who
  also identified the cases as mentally ill.

the small rural Okinawan community, however, 84 per cent identified the paranoid as mentally ill, 74 per cent identified the simple schizophrenic, and 31 per cent identified the alcoholic. The proportion identifying all the cases as mentally ill was higher in the Okinawan sample than that in prior reports by Star (1955) and Cumming and Cumming (1957) and in other Japanese studies. The fact that the proportion identifying the simple schizophrenic and particularly the alcoholic was markedly higher than in prior Japanese studies may have been caused by some particularities of the community, such as an isolated, cohesive society, high identification with each other, high drive to work, and the existence of a great number of alcoholics. At any rate, the Okuma study indicated that the use of such a questionnaire can elicit different concepts of normalcy and abnormalcy.

The respondent was asked to assign a "diagnosis" to the hypothetical cases in the Osaka study. Only 4 per cent of the total respondents correctly diagnosed paranoid schizophrenia, and only 0.5 per cent so diagnosed simple schizophrenia. Only 28 per cent diagnosed the alcoholic correctly. It can be concluded that it is almost impossible for laymen to give a psychiatric diagnosis even when they have the ability to identify Star's vignettes as mentally ill.

In further analysis, respondents were classified into four groups. Group A included those who identified all three cases as mentally ill, and the proportions by community were: Osaka, 5 per cent; Saga, 9 per cent; and Okinawa, 25 per cent. Group B comprised those who so identified two of the cases, and the proportions by community were: Osaka, 24 per cent; Saga, 27 per cent; and Okinawa, 45 per cent. Those identifying but one case as mentally ill were in Group C, and the proportions were: Osaka, 41 per cent; Saga, 38 per cent; and Okinawa, 22 per cent. Group D included all respondents who said that none of the case stories described mentally ill people, and the proportions were Osaka, 30 per cent; Saga, 26 per cent; and Okinawa, 8 per cent. These findings indicate some difference from community to community in the respondents' tendency to identify the cases as mentally ill, with the Okinawan community the most successful.

Analyses were made to determine the association of respondents' tendency to identify the cases as mentally ill with various factors such as sex, age, education, and experience with mental illness. In general, sex of a respondent was not significantly associated with the ability to make a correct identification. On the other hand, it appears that an age factor was significantly associated with the ability to make a correct identification; the older the respondent, the greater the likelihood that the cases would be considered indicative of mental illness. Education was not significantly associated with the ability to make a correct identification in the Osaka and the Saga samples. In the Okinawa sample, however, the more educated the respondent, the less the likelihood that the cases would be considered representative of mental illness. Generally speaking, it can be concluded that educational level did not make much difference in the ability to identify mental illness. With regard to experience with the mentally ill, generally those having a mental patient among their family members, blood relatives, or close friends tended to identify more easily the cases as mentally ill than those having no relationship with a patient.

Popular Concepts of Mental Illness

In order to discover how people actually conceptualized the "mental illness" they responded to on the questionnaire, a multiple-choice association test was given to respondents in Saga and Okinawa as a pilot study. The proportions of response to each alternative appear in Table 4. The results exceeded expectations. Despite variations, the largest group in each community consisted of those who felt "fearful and vaguely uncanny." When this group is added to the group who felt that "he is not understandable," the proportions are 58 and 40 per cent, respectively. Those who indicated empathetic and sympathetic attitudes, stating that "he is lonesome and solitary" or that "he has a deep-seated mental trouble," were 27 and 43 per cent, respectively. It is surprising that only 14 per cent of the respondents in each community expressed feelings that an "insane" person is excited and violent. It should be emphasized that only a relatively small percentage in both communities saw an "insane" person as potentially dangerous, a finding which should be taken into serious consideration in planning community mental health programs.

Similarly the concept of "psychoneuroses" was tested as indicated in Table 5. It is evident that about one-third of the respondents in both communities believed that a neurotic person is one with a minor form of mental illness, and another one-third felt that he is fearful of something. The general public may understand psychoneuroses as a continuum with psychoses.

Popular Concepts of the Origin of and Stigma of Mental Illness

The concept of the origin of mental illness generally held within a community may affect profoundly attitudes toward the mentally ill. In some communities mental disorders are reputed to be mainly hereditary, and the remark is commonly heard that "It is in the family." This belief frequently leads to the assumption that mental illness has a poor prognosis and to rejection of a person who has had a mental disorder as a suitable marriage partner. Studies in the three Japanese communities included the use of a social-distance scale to show how close a relation a respondent was prepared to tolerate with someone who had been mentally ill.

The results indicate that in all three communities a strong stigma is associated with mental illness; this finding agrees with a Canadian report (Cumming and Cumming, 1957) which stated that about three-quarters of the respondents would strongly discourage their children from marrying

Table 4:

Statement: When I imagine an "insane" person, I usually feel:

	Percentage Distribution of Replies	
Choice of Reply	Saga (N=441)	Okinawa (N=201)
a) fearful and vaguely uncanny.	44	28
b) he is lonesome and solitary.	12	17
c) he is dirty.	1	3
d) he is not understandable.	14	12
e) he is excited and violent.	14	14
f) he has a deep-seated mental trouble.	15	26
Total	100	100

Table 5:

Statement: When I think of a neurotic person, I also think of:

	Percentage Distribution of Replies	
Choice of Reply	Saga (N=441)	Okinawa* (N=201)
a) selfishness.	7	10
b) physical weakness.	11	18
c) a fearful person.	31	30
d) a somewhat strange person.	13	8
e) a minor "mental illness."	34	27
f) someone who commits a crime very often.	4	3
Total	100	96

* Four per cent of the Okinawa sample could not understand the term "neurotic."

anyone who had been mentally ill. The Japanese respondents had an even stronger negative response than did the Canadian sample, and the proportions of negative responses in the sample by community were: Osaka, 87 per cent; Saga, 86 per cent; and Okinawa, 81 per cent. Above all, marriage to a blood relative of the mentally ill was rejected, and sterilization of a mental patient was advocated by a majority of respondents irrespective of sex, age, or educational level. Undoubtedly, the Japanese public shares with Japanese psychiatrists a very strong belief in the hereditary nature of mental illness. It is needless to say that this belief has exercised a deleterious influence upon the way mental hospitals and community mental health programs are viewed.

In the past Japanese regarded tuberculosis and leprosy as well as mental illness as indicating a weakness in the family line. At present almost everyone knows that tuberculosis and leprosy are infectious diseases, and accordingly these illnesses are no longer regarded as shameful. Mental illness or a mentally ill person in the family, however, is still regarded as somewhat shameful. Responses to direct and indirect questions regarding this matter are presented in Tables 6 and 7.

In reply to the direct question shown in Table 6, about one out of three respondents in the Saga sample felt that it would be shameful for a family member to be in a mental hospital, whereas only one out of five did so in the Okinawan sample. Cross tabulation also revealed that the older and the less educated a respondent, the greater the likelihood that he would consider mental illness shameful.

In reply to the indirect question shown in Table 7, attitudes of respondents differed remarkably from community to community. Sixty-one per cent of the Osaka sample and 38 per cent of the Saga sample stated that they would try to keep the mental illness of a family member as quiet as possible, whereas only 14 per cent of the Okinawan sample stated that they would do so. Thus the following hypothesis is suggested: In a small cohesive community with a well-developed extended family system and much face-to-face contact, it is almost impossible to make a secret of having a mental patient within a family.

It is also interesting to note that the better educated were the most conservative. In general, the findings in Table 7 on education and age indicate that the direction of change in the future will not necessarily be toward a rational and scientific viewpoint. Since the general public in rural Japan, as indicated by three communities studied, regards mental illness as shameful, the development of local mental health programs may be hindered.

Popular Prognoses of Mental Illness

All respondents, regardless of whether they could identify a given case as mentally ill, were asked to give a prognosis on each. Interestingly, as presented in Table 8, a great majority of the respondents felt that the cases which had the most favorable prognoses were the simple schizophrenic girl and the paranoid schizophrenic man. The case which was felt to have the poorest prognosis was the alcoholic man. About one-third of the respondents indicated that he could never be cured. These views on the prognosis of each case are similar to the results obtained by Lemkau and Crocetti in Baltimore (1962). Prognostic views did not differ significantly among the three communities.

As far as research of this kind can reveal, Japanese have a re- markably optimistic view on the prognosis of mental illness, contrary to psychiatrists' experiences and beliefs. It is not easy to determine the reasons for this lay optimism. A multiple-choice association test asking for prognoses of hospital patients gave additional evidence of the respondents' optimism. Table 9 indicates that 57 and 89 per cent, respectively, in Saga and Okinawa thought that a person who was then in a mental hospital probably would recover by means of psychiatric treatment. Only 40 and 10 per cent, respectively, had a very pessimistic view about the patient's future. It is also interesting that about 50 per cent of the respondents felt that a mental patient would recover if treated for a long time. The tendency seems to be similar to one shown in the research data obtained in Lafayette, Indiana (Nunnally, 1961).

It is evident that the general public in rural Japan has a strong belief that mental illness will unavoidably be inherited; however, unex- pectedly, the same public has highly optimistic views on the curability of mental illness. So far, this contradiction has not been explained.

Public Attitudes toward Mental Hospitals

Views on mental hospitals also comprise an important aspect of attitudes toward mental illness; accordingly, three statements on this subject were presented to respondents in the several communities. As indicated

Table 6:

Question: Is it shameful for a member of the family to be hospitalized in a mental hospital?

	Percentage Distribution of Replies			
Community	Yes	No	Don't Know	Total
Osaka (N=549)	49	40	11	100
Saga (N=441)	36	56	8	100
Okinawa (N=201)	20	80	—	100

Table 7:

"Suppose a member of your family became mentally ill. Do you think you would tell your friends and acquaintances about it just as though he had gastric ulcer or apopletic stroke, or would you try to keep it as quiet as possible?

Percentage Distribution of Replies

Reply	Community	Total Sample	Education			Age			
			9th Grade or Less	High School	College	18-24	25-44	45-64	65 and Over
Tell it to friends	Osaka	29	29	29	21	31	24	31	33
	Saga	41	48	27	17	14	37	48	53
	Okinawa	84	88	61	67	50	81	94	93
Keep quiet	Osaka	61	61	58	71	47	64	60	61
	Saga	38	34	46	44	55	37	35	32
	Okinawa	14	11	38	—	40	15	6	7
Don't know and no answer	Osaka	10	10	13	8	2	12	9	6
	Saga	21	18	27	39	10	4	—	—
	Okinawa	2	—	—	—	—	—	—	—

Table 8:

Question: Do you think this case can be cured or not?						
	Percentage Distribution of Replies					
	Paranoid Schizophrenia		**Simple Schizophrenia**		**Chronic Alcoholism**	
Community	**Yes**	**No**	**Yes**	**No**	**Yes**	**No**
Osaka (N=549)	69	14	74	12	56	30
Saga (N=441)	72	10	77	13	59	32
Okinawa (N=201)	79	12	80	12	70	27

Table 9:

Statement: A person who is at present in a mental hospital:			
	Percentage Distribution of Replies		
Choice of Reply	**Lafayette, Indiana* (N=101)**	**Saga (N=441)**	**Okinawa (N=201)**
a) has very little chance of ever coming home.	4	7	1
b) may get out for a while, but will probably have to return.	10	15	5
c) may come home but will never be normal.	6	18	4
d) will probably recover by himself if he is left alone.	2	3	1
e) will probably recover if treated for a long time.	41	50	63
f) will usually recover after being treated for about a year.	37	7	26
Total	100	100	100

* Nunnally, 1961.

in Table 10, a great majority of the respondents in the Saga and Okinawan communities had a favorable attitude toward treatment in a mental hospital. It is not known to what degree this response represents primarily a negative attitude toward treatment or care at home.

As shown in Table 11, a significant majority of the sample in the Saga and Okinawan communities considered that a mental hospital functions more for treatment than for seclusion from the community, while there was no meaningful difference in the Osaka sample. Generally speaking, it is conceivable that few people in Japan now regard seclusion as the primary function of a mental institution.

Attitudes toward an open-door mental hospital policy are given in Table 12. The responses show that in both the Saga and Okinawan communities the proportion of respondents with permissive, accepting attitudes was low. Even in Saga, which had been accustomed to such a policy for some years, less than one-third favored the open-door policy.

The general public in rural Japan thus tends to view a mental hospital as an institution for treatment but simultaneously objects to the open-door system. There can be no doubt that attitudes toward the mental patient and the mental hospital are ambivalent. Under these circumstances, any abrupt enforcement of an open-door mental hospital policy could be expected to encounter public resistance.

Summary and Conclusion

The ability of the population to identify given descriptions of behavior as indicative of mental illness has been explored in three rural communities, two in Japan and one in Okinawa. The most striking contrast between the results of this study and those carried out in Western countries is in the ability to identify chronic alcoholics as mentally ill; about 86 per cent of the respondents in the three Japanese communities considered collectively failed to recognize the alcoholic case as representing mental illness. In terms of community differences, the sample in the Okinawan village identified mental illness in each case markedly more frequently than did the Japanese samples in the other two communities.

A semantic difference between the terms "oddity" and "mental illness" was revealed. What the Japanese and Okinawans think of in terms of *"seishinbyō"* ("mental illness") appears to include violence, incoherence, loss of reason, and unpredictability. The mentally ill person is seen as a lost soul who lives in another world; in other words, he is imagined as an extremely pathologic entity. The Japanese and the Okinawan rural populations thus have a much broader concept of what constitutes "odd but not mentally ill" behavior than do psychiatrists or mental health workers.

Another finding is relevant to cross-cultural differences in general behavior norms in studies of this kind. What may be abnormal for the hypothetical Betty Smith in Star's study in the United States, possibly is

Table 10:

Statement: People who have some kind of mental illness are better off being
taken care of at home than being hospitalized in a mental hospital.

| Community | Percentage Distribution of Replies | | | |
	Yes	No	Don't Know	Total
Saga (N=441)	8	78	14	100
Okinawa (N=201)	9	89	2	100

Table 11:

Statement: I think that the function of the mental hospital is more for
seclusion from the community rather than for treatment.

| Community | Percentage Distribution of Replies | | | |
	Yes	No	Don't Know	Total
Osaka (N=549)	41	37	22	100
Saga (N=441)	30	58	12	100
Okinawa (N=201)	5	92	3	100

Table 12:

Statement: Suppose you were living in the neighborhood of a mental hospital;
how would you feel about mental patients coming and going freely in
your neighborhood?

| Choice of Reply | Percentage Distribution of Replies | |
	Saga (N=441)	Okinawa (N=201)
a) I wouldn't care.	29	15
b) I would object because:		
I would feel uncomfortable.	6	4
I would feel fearful.	27	11
they would bother me.	5	3
they might inflict injury on women and children.	22	36
educationally, their odd behavior might be a bad influence on children.	11	31
Total	100	100

not abnormal for her Japanese counterpart Michiko Ikeda, since her naiveté, quietness, modesty, and retiring nature may be considered high virtues in a Japanese woman. Although this study did not show any particular effect of this stereotype of the Japanese woman on case identification when compared with American studies, a cultural factor of this kind, even though it is not supported by contrasts in the particular cross-cultural material that is available, may still be important and may explain partially the difference between the percentages of rural Japanese who identified the simple schizophrenic and the paranoid schizophrenic cases. This matter needs further investigation.

It was expected that the public's response to the label "mentally ill" would tend in general to be negative and that mental illness would be felt to be incomprehensible and productive of fear and uneasiness. More than one out of three respondents, however, felt that the mentally ill are lonesome and that they have deep-seated, painful mental trouble. The evidence of sympathetic attitudes toward the mentally ill is important for those planning future community mental health programs.

It also was disclosed that there is a strong popular belief that mental illness in a family is regarded as shameful. Beyond doubt, this attitude is based on the belief that mental illness is an inherited and transmissible disease. As to the general rejecting attitudes toward the mentally ill, they are stronger in the older, the less educated, and those unrelated to a patient. Surprisingly, less than one-third of the sample regarded the mentally ill as dangerous, and a majority regarded the mental hospital as an institution for treatment. It is clear that the general public wishes the mentally ill to be treated in a mental hospital.

Differences between the various communities are to be explored in future studies. The present findings, however, indicate that the rural population has a rather complicated attitude toward the mentally ill. The following dual structure is hypothesized: The general rural public tends to assume a favorable and permissive attitude in such superficial relations as having an expatient as a neighbor and working with one, although there are slight variations from community to community. On the other hand, in close relations, such as friendship, inviting people to the house (a sign of great intimacy in Japan), and accepting a mentally ill person as a marriage partner, the attitudes are strongly negative. In these respects, the respondents were less ready to accept the mentally ill than were respondents in North American studies. It should be noted, however, that there are in general strong differences in ingroup-outgroup concepts in Japan and North America; these differences have to be grasped for a full comprehension of the meaning of the rejection of the mentally ill in intimate relations.

Finally, the data collected in this study inevitably suffer from the limitations inherent in surveys conducted by questionnaire. The development of more adequate transcultural measures of attitudes relating to mental health and ill-health would be of great value.

ACKNOWLEDGMENT
The author expresses appreciation to Dr. Toshiaki Nareta, Dr. Matsuo Araki, Dr. Junichi Oyabu, Dr. Genbu Aragaki, Dr. Seisuke Matsuo, and Dr. Kenichi Mikajiri for their co-operation during this study. Acknowledgment is also made to Dr. Tonao Sakurai, Dr. Masao Ito, and the Okinawa Mental Health Association for partial financial support of this research project.

REFERENCES
Bowen, W. T., and G. J. Fisher. 1962. Community attitudes toward family care. Mental Hygiene 46:400–407.
Carstairs, G. M. 1959. The social limits of eccentricity: an English study. *In* Culture and mental health. M. K. Opler, ed. New York, Macmillan.
Cumming, E., and J. Cumming. 1957. Closed ranks: an experiment in mental health education. Cambridge, Harvard University Press.
_____. 1959. Two views of public attitudes toward mental illness. Mental Hygiene 43:211–21.
Dohrenwend, B. P., V. W. Bernard, and L. C. Kolb. 1962. The orientations of leaders in an urban area toward problems of mental illness. American Journal of Psychiatry 118:683–91.
Gruenberg, E. M., and S. S. Belline. 1957. The impact of mental disease on society. *In* Explorations in social psychiatry. A. H. Leighton, J. A. Clausen, and R. H. Wilson, eds. New York, Basic Books.
Joint Commission on Mental Illness and Health. 1961. Action for mental health. New York, Basic Books.
Lemkau, P. V., and G. M. Crocetti. 1962. An urban population's opinion and knowledge about mental illness. American Journal of Psychiatry 118: 692–700.
Miura, T., et al. 1963. Study on the reco-therapeutic attitude toward mental health and illness. Seishinigaku 5:967–73. [In Japanese.]
Nunnally, J. C., Jr. 1961. Popular conceptions of mental health. New York, Holt, Rinehart and Winston.
Permins, M. E., et al. 1965. Public images of psychiatry: challenges in planning community mental health care. American Journal of Psychiatry 121: 746–51.
Phillips, D. L. 1963. Rejection: a possible consequence of seeking help for mental disorders. American Sociological Review 28:963–72.
_____. 1964. Rejection of the mentally ill: the influence of behavior and sex. American Sociological Review 29:679–87.
Pratt, S., D. Giannitrapani, and P. Khanna. 1960. Attitudes toward the mental hospital and selected population characteristics. Journal of Clinical Psychology 16:214–18.
Ramsey, G. V., and M. Seipp. 1948. Public opinions and information concerning mental health. Journal of Clinical Psychology 4:397–406.
Star, S. 1955. The public's ideas about mental illness. Paper presented at the Annual Meeting of the National Association for Mental Health, Indianapolis. Mimeographed.

————. 1957. The place of psychiatry in popular thinking. Paper presented at the Meeting of the American Association for Public Opinion Research, Washington.

Terashima, S., and T. Nareta. 1964. A rural community's opinion and knowledge about mental illness in Japan. Transcultural Psychiatric Research 1:97–100 (abstract). (Paper presented at the Annual Meeting of the American Psychiatric Association, Los Angeles.)

Tershakovec, A. 1964. An observation concerning changing attitudes toward mental illness. American Journal of Psychiatry 121:353–57.

Woodward, J. L. 1951. Changing ideas on mental illness and its treatment. American Sociological Review 16:443–54.

13.　Shaman and Client in Okinawa

WILLIAM P. LEBRA, Ph.D.

Social Science Research Institute
University of Hawaii
Honolulu, Hawaii

PREVIOUSLY I have described the general characteristics of Okinawan religion (Lebra, 1966) and the role of the shaman in Okinawan culture (Lebra, 1964). In this chapter I should like to consider certain aspects of the shaman-client relation, in particular: (1) the client's expectation of the shaman's character and role performance; and (2) the shaman's resolution of possible conflict and dissonance engendered by these expectations which may be at variance with her (the overwhelming majority are female) actual experience.

　　　The principal functions of the shaman in contemporary Okinawa (*circa* 1960–61) relate to the diagnosis, explanation, and suggestion of remedial action for illness, disease, and all other forms of major misfortune which defy ready, rational explanation. The absence of any concept of impersonal causation in traditional Okinawan thinking leads to the ultimate ascription of all misfortune to supernatural causes. Although there are a variety of shaman types, they alone are credited with the preternatural powers of seeing, hearing, and reterocognition which permit understanding of the nature of supernatural involvement in any specific instance of misfortune. Their numbers are large, estimated at 1:600 of population, in contrast to modern medical practitioners who are in a ratio of approximately 1:3,000. Despite recent and steady increases in the numbers of medical doctors, apparently shamans are not dwindling; rather, the trend has been toward simultaneous employment of doctor and shaman, for, as one informant put it, "Even if there is cure [by an M.D.] it doesn't explain why."

Public expressions of the shaman's validity do not provide an accurate index to involvement. Women constitute the overwhelming bulk of the shaman's clients. Taping of 67 shaman-client sessions (with the same shaman) on ten separate occasions during the period of May to November of 1960 revealed only three males involved as principal clients (men sometimes accompanied their wives or mothers but did not participate actively in the interchange). This proportion is not unusual, since in traditional Okinawan religion and society women were ritually superior to men, and to this date they tend to predominate in spiritual matters. Moreover, unlike Western society, where the basic unit of reference in society is the individual, the Okinawans think of the family as the lowest common denominator. Within the family (or household), the senior female member usually has charge of ritual matters, and hence it is she who visits the shaman on behalf of her family. Educated people, males in particular, frequently scoff at or make light of the shaman, but not uncommonly as acquaintance lengthens even these will relate accounts of unusual or "strange" insights evidenced by a particular shaman. When real misfortune strikes, their rather ready compliance with the shaman's prescription is rationalized in terms of humoring a wife or an old mother since "It will do no harm." Newspapers and schoolteachers particularly have been vocal in their public pronouncements against the shaman, but familiarity with shamans reveals schoolteachers and journalists among their clientele. Suffice it to say that their influence is pervasive in Okinawan society, and on a household basis their utilization is close to universal. I also have been impressed by accounts of reliance upon shamans among first- and second-generation Okinawan-Americans residing in Hawaii.

To their clientele, shamans are viewed as possessing significant attributes which qualify them for their role. First of all, they are acknowledged to have been born with *kami*-spirit and are said to be possessed (or "carried") by the *kami* (*kami nkai mutariing*), which distinguishes them from *musang* ("ordinary people, normal people, laymen"). According to Okinawan thinking, the capacity to become a shaman is inherent; therefore it is not something which can be learned or acquired by study or application. It is recognized, however, that this capacity is not implicitly recognized by those born with it; consequently, the *kami* is forced to send notifications (*shirashi*), usually not until the individual is old enough to understand. These notifications may commence with strange or unusual occurrences or experiences; hallucinatory experience (*imi-gukuchi*, "dream-like sensation or experience") is a certain sign of supernatural notification. It is recognized further that most potential shamans not only do not aspire to their pre-destined role but also will attempt to ignore these signs, even though no escape is possible. As a result, the *kami* becomes angered, and the potential shaman falls victim to divine retribution (*kami-daari, kami* curse, or more commonly *taari*). *Taari* is commonly described as a type of sickness which cannot be diagnosed or cured by any doctor, modern or traditional, and which is accompanied by seeing and hearing strange things, usually of the spirit world. The only cure for a *taari* victim is to seek her *chiji* ("guardian spirit"), a particular *kami* spirit whom she must serve and who functions as her mainstay. In a sense the *chiji* is a guardian spirit. The *chiji*-quest requires an intensification of ritual efforts, especially prayers for guidance and visits to many major ritual sites. Ultimately, the identity of the *chiji* and its abode are revealed in the course of *imi-gukuchi*—the dream-like sensation or experience which I equate with hallucination or waking vision. Once the *chiji* has been properly identified and a regular ritual relation established, it is incumbent upon the individual to use the powers and abilities conferred by the *chiji* to help others. Thereafter, the new shaman has a lifelong obligation to serve her personal *kami* and to help others; any slackening of effort in either direction supposedly will result in a recurrence of *taari*.

In terms of Okinawan ethnopsychology, shamans are not regarded as normal persons, a point previously noted. They are believed to be selected by *kami* and marked for *kami* service from the time of birth, which sets them apart from ordinary people. They are regarded as endowed with the capacity for spirit possession and the ability to see and hear events of the past as well as the future. They are decidedly not regarded as mental cases after establishment in office, although it is recognized that temporary behavior disorders can be inflicted upon them by the *kami* when they reject the call to office or slight their ritual duties after assumption of the shaman role. Essentially, the shaman is viewed by Okinawans as different—deviant, we would say—not pathological. Claimants to the title of shaman who persistently resort to manifestly extravagant behavior readily are termed "crazy" and quickly lose their clients. The performance of the shaman in Okinawa is mild in comparison to that reported from other cultural areas, especially the Siberian area. In this respect, established shamans do not diverge too widely from the Okinawan ideals of moderation and mildness in overt behavior.

From the Okinawan point of view, hopeless mental pathologies are evident at birth and can be detected at an early date. Such conditions are regarded as punishment inflicted by the supernatural (the *kami* spirits in nature and the ancestral spirits) for sins of omission or commission by ancestors. These conditions are regarded as beyond cure, although desperate efforts, nonetheless, may be resorted to by the family with the minimal hope of forestalling recurrence. Behavior disorders occurring later in life also are symptomatic of impaired relations with the supernatural, either through the action or inaction of living relatives of ancestors or of self. These disorders need not be regarded as hopeless, especially when the behavior can be interpreted as simulating the action of other people, living or dead. Such behavior is viewed as an indication of supernatural notification and requires that intensive efforts be undertaken to determine the cause of supernatural displeasure and to initiate remedial action. The type of behavior which the disturbed person simulates provides clues to the causal agent. A potential shaman emerges in Okinawan society by virtue of asserting that insight into, and remedy of, her condition was achieved by special birth and supernatural assistance. In brief, emphasis is given to self-discovery and self-enlightenment through supernatural assistance.

Paying clients do not accept unreservedly all self-proclaimed shamans. Claim to the role must be validated by surmounting a series of tests. The important first test is recovery or at least a large measure of recovery from *taari*. Failure to recover is synonymous with failure to identify correctly or to establish a relation with the proper *chiji*. A recurrence of *taari* after entering office implies a slackening or inattention to ritual efforts or false identification of the *chiji* in the first place. A second necessary test which, in effect, is continually being met throughout the remainder of the shaman's life is validation through performance. In other words, the shaman must establish a fairly consistent record of success in providing explanation or in prescribing remedy for misfortune in others or both. A critical ingredient here is the client's belief that the shaman experiences possession in communicating with the spirit world. In the Okinawan language a number of words express possession—to be possessed, to be held, to be carried, to be ridden, to be leaned on, and so forth. All these imply that a spirit takes over full or partial control of the shaman's body and faculties. The insight, explanation, and advice obtained from the shaman therefore issue from the supernatural. Such is the stereotype of the shaman in Okinawa.

How well does this cultural stereotype of the shaman accord with the evidence obtained from observing, interviewing, and testing? The life histories of shamans revealed long records of discord in interpersonal relations. Early life was characterized by frail health and recollections of playing alone, doing unusual things, and being slighted by parents. Relations with siblings tended to be strained and distant, if not actually unfriendly. Marital life was marked by sexual incompatibility, frequent divorces, and bickering with spouses and in-laws. Performance in terms of work and meeting responsibilities was consistently poor. If I were to use a single word to describe their lives prior to becoming a shaman, "failure" would be most apt. They have met with failure in home, school, occupation, sex, marriage, and life in general, but essentially theirs has been a failure in interpersonal relations and achievement.

My shaman informants readily asserted that their childhood, adolescent, and adult life experiences were decidedly different from those of ordinary people; in particular, they emphasized the *taari* experience as setting them off from others, and years afterwards they spoke of it as a period of extreme anxiety, misery, and helplessness. Some of the commonly described somatic disorders accompanying *taari* included generalized stomach disorders, prolonged and intense headaches, pounding noises, difficulties in breathing (asthmatic conditions), pains or stiffness in the limbs (especially the legs), skin disorders, and sometimes impairment of vision. Along with these disorders, hallucinatory experiences (seeing or hearing or both) occurred and sometimes spells of complete dissociation. The total effect was one of debilitation precluding performance of normal routine work and role relations. By this point, the individual (or family in her behalf) simultaneously was consulting several or more specialists, medical practioners as well as shamans. It is my impression that commitment to the *chiji*-quest usually came as the last resort, when all other means of cure were thought to have been exhausted.

What the Okinawans describe as identification of *chiji* and the clearing of *taari* (i.e., recovery), I would equate with conversion experience. We have long recognized the psychotherapeutic effect of religious conversion, and I am convinced that for the Okinawan shaman the greatest intensity of overt pathology occurs prior to taking office, especially during what is termed the *taari* period. Thus, after taking office, the skin affliction covering the hands, arms, and breasts disappears; the seemingly hopeless asthmatic breathes easily; the stiffness, pain, or partial paralysis in the leg is gone; pounding headaches and roaring noises become infrequent; and so on. Moreover, the whole lifetime experience to date—failure, inadequacy, pain, and misfortune—at last makes sense as supernaturally imposed.

So far, what I have related concerning the potential shaman's experience does not differ appreciably from the public image of them. Even the consistent record of failure and maladjustment can be explained away as positive proof that only one role was open to them. After their somatic ills have diminished, some dissonance arises. My shaman informants were insistent that it was not their intention, after identifying the *chiji* and the clearing of *taari,* to establish a professional following. Rather, it was their hope to pray regularly to their *chiji* and to attempt to realize a normal life. Instead, they contended, neighbors, kinsmen, and others who had heard of their experience pressured them into using their *chiji's* power on behalf of others who had met misfortune. There is a strong tendency toward fadism in the Okinawan use of shaman, and when a new one appears the word quickly spreads and potential clients begin to seek her out. This practice is reinforced by the belief that a shaman who refuses help to others will suffer a recurrence of *taari* and ultimately will die or become hopelessly insane. Consequently, a clientele may build up rapidly, and a somewhat reluctant shaman soon finds herself in business, receiving fees and gifts.

It was noted before that clients believe that the shaman experiences possession in contacting the spirit world and that the Okinawan language has a rich range of terms to express possession. The language also very clearly distinguishes "hallucination," "possession," and "dream." I am convinced that all of my shaman informants repeatedly have experienced hallucinations, especially during the *taari* period prior to taking office. Vivid descriptive accounts of hallucinatory experiences were rendered with little hesitancy or reserve. In respect to possession, however, I found that older, well-established shamans referred to it far more frequently than did the younger, newly established shamans. Moreover, the younger ones with whom I had closest contact frequently expressed doubt about the validity of their role performance, making statements such as: "Am I doing the right thing?" or "Is what I am doing real?" In brief, I submit that new shamans consciously recognize that they are resorting to acting and showmanship in satisfying the public expectation of possession and that the matter is a source of considerable anxiety to them. Even assuming a capacity for self-induced trance, it would be nearly impossible in terms of time and energy expenditure to give a valid performance for each and every client when their numbers run as high as 15 to 30 per day. In any event, whether the answer is inability or energy conservation, stagecraft and showmanship are used to simulate possession.

This inconsistency between public expectation and the shaman's knowledge of the situation can be and is obviously rationalized by the shaman in terms of helping people and thereby preserving her own health through aiding others. Not to be overlooked is the material gain derived from being a shaman and, most important of all, the fact that this heretofore failure, this inadequate person, now has recognition as an important and useful member of society.

At this point, it may seem quite appropriate to apply such labels as showman, fake, phony, imposter, and the like to the shaman. This labeling would be inaccurate, however, for it overlooks the daily life experiences of the shamans throughout the whole of their professional careers. The continuing demands of clients for performance and the need to meet these demands in order to preserve their health force the shamans into expending most of their time and energy on communion with the spirit world. Increasingly, I suspect, the distinction between reality and nonreality diminishes and conscious acknowledgement of deception recedes.

Observation, interviewing, and analysis of projective tests give ample indication of pathological thinking and acting among Okinawan shaman, and I feel quite sure that, in terms of general personality configuration, deviants are recruited for this role. Although no clear single pattern of overt pathology has emerged, I have suggested (Lebra, 1964) that intelligence, verbal fluency, and perhaps any one of a number of pathologies which can be implemented or adjusted to this role are some of the necessary traits for a successful shaman in Okinawa. That the shaman has achieved social adjustment is incontestable from any point of view. While the question of the shaman's mental health best can be left to the psychiatrist, the interesting and presently unanswerable question for the anthropologist is the sort of culture which requires one deviant personality to tend to the needs of each 600 population.

ACKNOWLEDGMENT

The support of Grant M-3084 from the National Institute of Mental Health is gratefully acknowledged.

REFERENCES

Lebra, William P. 1964. The Okinawan shaman. *In* Ryukyuan culture and society. A. H. Smith, ed. Honolulu, University of Hawaii Press.
————. 1966. Okinawan religion. Honolulu, University of Hawaii Press.

14. Psychiatric Study of the Shaman in Japan

YUJI SASAKI, M.D.

Department of Neuro-psychiatry
School of Medicine
University of Tokyo
Tokyo, Japan

SHAMANISM is a form of primitive belief which developed mainly among the Ural-Altaic tribes; the key persons of the belief rituals are called shamans. The most widely accepted definition of shaman (Iwai, 1938: *see also* Harada, 1949) is:

> the medium between the human and the supernatural worlds, he who communicates freely as a human medium with the "heavenly world" where gods and good spirits reside, and with the "under-world" where the devils reside . . . , through offering sacrifices or doing prayers to the supernatural spirits and bringing himself to the state of trance and thus makes prophecy or even cures the illness of the clients.

Shamanistic practices can be seen not only in their supposed place of origin among the Tungus tribe but also in many other cultures in the East and West, although with certain differences in their appearance, rituals, and contents. In fact, the phenomenon is said to be rare only among the Africans (Eliade, 1951, 1961).

Another psychological phenomenon called fox possession contrasts with shamanism in being a nonvolitional psychopathological condition, while shamanism is a trance state induced at will. In Japanese the words *kitsunetsuki* ("fox possession") and *miko* (a type of shaman) are used to differentiate the two; a similar verbal differentiation is found between *imu* and *tsusu* for the Ainu tribes, *shie-pin* and *fu-i* among the Manchurian tribes, *yumu-oloshiona* and *bo* for the Mongols, *fu-pin* and *mudan* for the Koreans, and so on. Both possessed patient and shaman can be regarded as examples of the possession syndrome, which, together with *amok* or *latah*, can be considered culture-bound syndromes (Yap, 1960). As a brief review of the literature demonstrates, however, these phenomena have attracted little attention from psychiatrists (apart from a few among the French) in either the East or the West. Such studies as there are have mainly been of the possessed patient. Among distinguished psychiatric studies of this sort are those of Oesterreich (1930) published in France; Morita (1915) in Japan, who after reporting such cases proposed for them the term *kitōsei-seishinbyō* ("invocation psychosis"); Uchimura, Akimoto, and Ishibashi (1938), which is a frequently cited study on *imu;* Tamura (1940) and Ko (1943) on the Mongol possession syndromes; Murakami (1950) and Ogino (1950) on the psychopathological interpretation of possessed states; and Shinpuku and Miyashita (1958) on fox possession.

Of the shaman there has been very little study from the psychiatric point of view. In 1961 Boyer and Klopfer stated, "There has been no detailed study of shaman by well trained psychiatrists." Only recently has the shaman become the focus of psychiatric study, and the emphasis in recent studies seems not to have been on the personality or psychopathology of the individual shaman but rather on client-shaman relations within the context of a specific culture (Jahoda, 1961; Murphy, 1964; Kiev, 1964) or on the possession process, such as in religious dance (Field, 1960). In North America Boyer tried to investigate the public acceptance of shamanism by use of Rorschach responses (1964). In Japan, Uchimura, Akimoto, and Ishibashi (1938) and Tamura (1940) touched on the issue of shamanism in their study of *tsusu* and *fu-i*. More recently there was a social psychiatric study of shamanism in Aomori prefecture (Kakeda *et al.*, 1959; Nakamura, 1961), and Nakagawa (1964) has started a rather extensive study on *tsusu* of the Ainu.

In contrast to the paucity of psychiatric studies on shamanism, there have been many studies on shamanism from the points of view of ethnology, folklore, cultural anthropology, sociology of religion, and sociology, among others. Typical examples are those on shamanism among the Tungus tribe in Siberia by Shirokogorov (1933), Czaplicka (1914), and Michael (1963) and many similar studies on North American and Mexican Indians and in Tibet, China, Malaysia, Norway, and other cultures. Eliade's extensive comparative historical review of shamanism (1951, 1961) is an excellent contribution to the field. May (1956) surveyed the phenomenon of glossolalia. In Japan studies of the shaman from the folklore point of view started with Yanagida (1913). Studies by Nakayama (1930), Wakamori (1943), and Hori (1953) focused upon religious history. Fairchild (1962) and Eder

(1958) based their accounts of shamanism in Japan upon the many papers which have been published by Japanese investigators.

In ancient times in Japan shamanistic beliefs and customs centering around the shamans, commonly known as *miko*, prevailed in the administrative, military, and religious affairs of the state; from the Middle Ages onward, these became the main current of folk beliefs and even nowadays are found in every part of Japan, although religious functions and ceremonial patterns have undergone various changes.

Shamanistic trends are found, moreover, in most of the numerous new religions which have been prospering since World War II, and, in spite of the enormous growth of modern medicine, a large number of patients, especially psychiatric patients, still flock to various magico-religious sects for cure (Akimoto *et al.*, 1964, 1966). Thus the abnormal psychological phenomena of possessed states remain the legitimate object of psychopathological study, and the sociocultural background of the particular society which accepts and allows the continued existence of such conditions is also an important area for social psychiatric studies. Comparative studies of the individual psychopathology of the shamans as well as the social psychiatric aspects of shamanism would open a fruitful avenue for future cross-cultural study and should shed light on problems arising from religious phenomena which thus far have been rather hard to approach through psychiatry.

This chapter gives an account of 56 shamans studied in four districts of Japan. My research was focused mainly upon the following areas of interest:

1) In a given community with its traditional sociocultural heritage and current psychological needs, what kind of person would become a shaman and through what sorts of processes.

2) The historical vicissitudes of the religious function of the shaman within a community and the classification, if possible, of certain types of shamans on the basis of the evolution of their religious functions.

3) Clarification of the specifically religious phenomena experienced by the shamans during their professional activities. In other words, special attention was paid to the psychosocial motivation which led persons to become shamans, to the psychopathological process of their professional practice as shamans, and to the specific subcultural needs of each district which accepts the existence of and determines the modes of social function of the shamans. It is hoped that such a study will stimulate similar researches in other cultures and eventually lead to comprehensive comparative cross-cultural studies on shamanism from the mental health point of view.

Methodology

The 56 shamans studied are from four districts of Japan, as indicated in Table 1. All these persons have been living and functioning professionally or semiprofessionally within their communities. Many other persons perform similar activities within the society, such as professional prayers or beadsmen, priests, fortune tellers, witches, and so forth. The present study, however, is concerned only with shamanistic activities characterized by communication with gods or souls to reveal the "divine will" through glossolalia, although within the sample are a few cases who are no longer engaged in conveying the "divine will" through glossolalia as they had done in the past.

Techniques used for communicating with religious groups and for obtaining information from them have been controversial. In the present study I avoided the technique of pretending to be a client or a believer in shamanism. Instead, from the very beginning, I presented myself as a psychiatrist who was interested in religious relief and cure phenomena and in understanding the relation between the shamanistic approach and psychotherapy. I explicitly expressed a desire for the shaman's co-operation. My observations were made by making as many visits as possible to the homes of the shamans, to the places for their *shugyō* ("self-training"), and to other sites where they practiced. I was interested especially in obtaining information relevant to the shaman-client relation. Sometimes I even was able to discuss their practices with the shamans, from a psychiatrist's viewpoint, and to offer comments or suggestions upon request. All but two shamans were quite co-operative. Though psychological tests were not available, all the 56 cases presented here were interviewed personally and frequently, and their shamanistic rituals were observed carefully. Several cases for whom data were insufficient are excluded from the report.

As mentioned before, the sample was drawn from several districts, each with its specific subcultural background and needs, thus providing interesting material for comparative studies of shamanism from the socio-religious standpoint. Only the samples from four districts in Japan with which I am fairly familiar were studied in depth. In addition, I studied some ten shamans from other districts in Japan by means of psychological tests,

Table 1: Place of Residence of Shamans Studied

District	Male	Female	Total
Hirosaki and vicinity			
(Tsugaru District)	4	21	25
Tōgane and vicinity	0	4	4
Hachijō Island	1	11	12
Aogashima Island	5	10	15
Total	10	46	56

EEG studies, or treatment as inpatients, but since they were from communities with which I was insufficiently familiar, they are excluded from the presentation.

The Communities Surveyed

The city of Hirosaki and Its Vicinity, Aomori Prefecture (Tsugaru District). This district was surveyed during the summers of 1958 and 1959 for a total of about six months while I was working in the mental hospital of Hirosaki City. Since the establishment of a castle by the second feudal lord of Tsugaru in 1611, the city of Hirosaki has been the center of politics, economy, business, communication, culture, and education for the district of Tsugaru. After the city annexed several villages in the vicinity in 1955, the population increased from 70,000 to the present 150,000. The villages within the vicinity are situated on the Tsugaru plain, famous for its apple and rice production. The economic gap between the rich and the poor, who constitute the majority of the farming population, is enormous, presumably in consequence of the frequent floods. The long, cold winter season is gray both economically and emotionally. This particular district is characterized by a contradiction: despite the city's having been the center of culture and education for centuries, it still maintains many traditional, rather superstitious annual ceremonies, though they have been becoming more or less folk recreational activities. The two kinds of shaman groups in the district are called *itako* and *gomiso*; compared with *gomiso*, *itako* have slightly more believers in villages than in towns.

The City of Tōgane and Its Vicinity, Chiba Prefecture. This district was surveyed for about a month in the summer of 1960 when I was a member of a research team for an epidemiological survey of mental illness (Arai *et al.*, 1961). This district is situated in the northeastern part of Chiba Prefecture and includes two farming and fishing towns, together with the chief city of the locality, Tōgane. The economy is mainly agricultural. The total population is approximately 52,500. This district has maintained few local traditions, and even in the fishing villages there is very little local color, presumably because they are very near Tokyo.

Hachijō Island. This island was surveyed for six months starting in August, 1960, and again for ten days in the summer of 1961 while I was a member of a research team for an epidemiological study of mental disorders on the island (Akimoto *et al.*, 1964). Hachijō Island is situated about 290 kilometers south of Tokyo. Its land area is approximately 70 square kilometers, and it accommodates 3,000 households with a population of approximately 12,000. There were ten medical doctors on the island but no psychiatrists at the time of the study. The main means of communication with the Tokyo area is by a ship which comes to the island every five days and also by a recently introduced tourist aircraft which arrives at the island at least once a day. Since the development of a tourist industry, Hachijō has lost its isolated characteristics, and the pace of acculturation now is rapid, though the island still relies principally on fishery and farming as its sources of income. The traditional Hachijō Island still is there, however, in terms of its many local traditional annual ceremonies.

Aogashima Island. This small island, which is situated 70 kilometers south of Hachijō Island, was surveyed in the summer of 1961 for 20 days when I was once again an investigator in an epidemiological study of mental disorders on the island (Sasaki, Takano, and Ozawa, 1964). The size of Aogashima is only 5 square kilometers; it is a volcanic island accommodating only 100 households with a population of 380. It is literally an isolated island since it does not have even a good harbor for the monthly ship. At the time of the study, there was no medical doctor on the island. The main food is imported rationed rice from the mainland and fish, which is not abundant. As a whole, the life is very poor and remains at a rather primitive level. Rainwater is the only source of drinking water, and, of course, there is no electricity. Very naturally, the young people have had to choose their marital partners within the island, and, consequently, the family tree of each household is related to others in very complicated ways. A marriage, death, or other crisis in any household becomes an island-wide community affair. This community closeness has been responsible, in part, for the maintenance of the traditional village ceremonies.

Functions of Shamans within Their Local Settings

The professional activities of shamans within the communities studied can be grouped roughly accordingly to the needs of the clients into the following three categories: (1) Prophesying (called *uranai*), typically by means of *kamioroshi* (*kami-kuchi*), that is, the shaman brings himself to a trance state, communicates with the "god," and then conveys the "divine will." (2) Following the prophecy and against or in support of it, the magical ritual (called *majinai*); the performance of *majinai* sometimes is unrelated to the prophecy, and then it is called *katarimono*, in which the shaman tells folk tales in a rather amusing way. (3) Mediumship (called *hotokeoroshi* or *shini-kuchi*), which is a shamanistic performance called upon the request of a client (an individual or a group) to communicate with particular dead persons. Since each shaman performs all three activities to a certain degree, it is futile to attempt precisely to classify the shamans by these means. I follow here the line of functionalism in the sociology of religion, and I have tried to understand the functions of shamans of different districts in terms of their public functions on behalf of the community (such as the public *uranai* and *majinai* on the occasion of village ceremonies) and their private functions to deal with the emotional needs of individual clients. This functional approach is believed to lead to a more comprehensive understanding than others of the social background of a given community in which shamanism continues to persist.

The aspect of service to individuals, that is, the private function, is practiced by all shamans. Service to the public, the public function, however, is another matter. The public function is strongest among the shamans of Aogashima and diminishes in the movement to larger communities—from Hachijō Island to the Tōgane district to the area of Hirosaki.

Shamans in Japan have been under the influence of religious forces including Shintoism, Buddhism, Taoism, and the mountain religions; in a way, the groups of shamans which I studied denote the various states of historical change of shamanism in the country. The extent of the public functions performed by different groups of shamans indicates historical background. For example, the Aogashima shaman is historically the oldest of the existent shaman, and, along with the *noro* of Okinawa, functions as an officiating priest of the community, while the Hachijō Island shaman retains only a fragmentary function as a village ceremonial leader, and the public function is even less in evidence in Tōgane and Hirosaki.

Social Characteristics of Shamans

Although there was some variation within the four communities studied, the general characteristics of the group of 56 shaman were similar. They were fairly old: only 16 per cent were less than 40 years of age; 46 per cent were between 40 and 59 years of age; and 38 per cent were 60 or more years of age. They were rather poorly educated; 19 per cent had no formal schooling; 47 per cent had six years or less of schooling; and 34 per cent had more than six years. There were 10 males, and 46 females. All the males were currently married. Of the 46 females, only 29 (63 per cent) were currently married; 16 (35 per cent) were widowed or divorced; and 1 (2 per cent) was single. In comparison with other residents in their communities, the bulk of the 56 shamans was in the middle economic range: 49 (88 per cent) were middle or working class, while only 4 (7 per cent) could be called upper class and only 3 (5 per cent) really lower class.

Glossolalia and Revelation:
Two Basic Religious Experiences of Shamans

The following is a case illustration of a typical shaman, which serves to clarify some of the terminology associated with shamanism.

> *Case Number 12.* S. Y. is a 56-year-old man, a resident of the city of Hirosaki. He is known as a *gomiso*. He is assertive, aggressive, argumentative, stubborn, and occasionally explosive in his emotionality, and yet, on the other hand, he is simple-minded and easily trusts in others. He is the eldest son of a cook in the city of Hirosaki. His

childhood was characterized by emotional and financial hardship because of the habitual heavy drinking of his father. After completing the eighth grade, he lived in a shop as an apprentice. After army service, he married at the age of 22 and started a small shop of his own, selling fish. The drinking of his father became more and more serious a problem, and because the father behaved sometimes in such an undisciplined way the son even contemplated killing his own father. Starting at the age of 23, S. Y. was taken by one of his friends to Mt. Iwaki, which is a "sacred" mountain, where he started his *shugyō* ("self-training"). Since then, his only source of emotional tranquility has been to go up to the mountains for a few days to engage in meditation, standing under a waterfall, praying in a special posture, climbing up and down the hill repeatedly, and so on. In the third year, during the last night of the last day of his two-week meditation and fasting, he suddenly heard a "voice" telling him in his ecstatic state, "Your father is like a devil; yet he still is your father." A feeling of such religious happiness continued even after he had awakened from the ecstasy that he extended his stay. One night, during his meditation, both his praying hands were pulled up and at the same time he felt something rushing up from his bosom to his throat as he also became chilled; his throat muscles became tight, and he was unable to talk. After experiencing this paresthetic sensation and these involuntary motor activities, he gradually started to murmur fragmentary words and later sentences of some relevance, but he confided that he cannot remember what he was made to speak. One day, at the age of 30, he finally heard the "voice" of the "god" telling him to "save the people," and so he gave up his business of selling fish and took up the career of a shaman. Currently, upon the request of a client, he will do *uranai*, that is, give meanings and interpretation to those ideas which emerge at random out of his mind as the "god's will," but he rarely brings himself to the state of trance. He confided also that sometimes even though he is in a state of trance he still is alert enough to be able to guess the emotional reaction of his client and adjust the content of the "god's will" accordingly.

This case illustrates clearly how the initial spirit-possessed state developed and how it degenerated as time elapsed. In other words, the quality of the "divine will" the shaman communicates to his clients changes or degenerates as the shaman becomes more "professionalized."

It seems that the shaman perceives the "god's will" by means of two different religious avenues. The first is through glossolalia; being possessed by either a god or a soul, he talks or acts as a medium of that which possesses him. The second is through receiving certain revelations or inspirations. Both of these two means of access are preceded by getting into the state of trance or ecstasy. The state of trance, as shown in this case, is usually achieved through the so-called *shugyō* ("self-training"), which consists of repetition of simple bodily movements and sensory stimulations which bring about the gradual dimming of consciousness both physiologically and psychologically, leading to diminution of ego activities. This state also presumably may be facilitated by extreme exhaustion caused by hypoglycemia. Under such physiological conditions, it is probable that anyone would become highly suggestible, a condition which favors the creation of a special religious state. This is the state of trance as I understand it, though thus far there has not been a commonly acceptable definition of it. The transformation of personality which is brought about under such a state through autosuggestion is the "glossolalia," and the vivid sensory experience brought about is the "revelation or inspiration," and I wish to use "spirit possession" as a general term to include both these experiences. As has been shown, however, both the glossolalia and revelation gradually degenerate so that the glossolalia becomes an act and the revelation becomes attaching meanings to or interpreting ideas emerging out of his own mind at random. As the shaman becomes more experienced and businesslike, it becomes hard to differentiate the real trance state from what is only an act. The difficulty of differentiating the two can be the same as that of differentiating a real hysterical reaction from simulation. There seem to be many quantitatively different levels of consciousness during real trance. It is quite rare to have a state of complete loss of consciousness or what Jaspers (1948) called the "alternate consciousness"; rather, in the majority of cases there is a partial dimming of consciousness, a condition called by Oesterreich (1930) "continuous consciousness."

At this point a re-examination of the definition of shaman is pertinent. It appears that both Eliade and Shirokogorov consider ecstasy as the essential part of shamanism. Eliade (1961) stated: "The shaman knows how to employ ecstasy for the benefit of community." Shirokogorov (1933) said: "The shaman knows the method of falling into ecstatic states." My case material suggests, however, that trance states precede the states of ecstasy in shamanistic experience and therefore should be considered primary in explaining the origin of the shaman's experiences. Moreover, many religious experiences are not accompanied by ecstasy.

For operationally screening the shaman from other religious practitioners, such as seers, magicians, diviners, saints, prophets, and priests, glossolalia should be considered the differential, since in many cases it is practically impossible to determine the existence of states of trance or ecstasy and since some individuals can get "possessed" without the accompaniment of the abnormal sensory experiences that are supposed to be the basis of revelation.

Psychodynamic Studies of Shamans

Intensive analysis of the histories of individual shamans indicates that the process by which a shaman first achieves spirit possession varies. Grossly, there are two types of processes, the *shugyō* type and the spontaneous type. The spontaneous type, in turn, can be divided into two subtypes.

I. Shugyō Type. These are the shamans whose first spirit possession took place after *shugyō* ("self-training"). Forty of the 56 shamans studied belong to this category, and Case Number 12 cited above is typical. Disappointed, hostile to his ill-disciplined father, and tortured by real life, S. Y. found an escape in *shugyō* on Mt. Iwaki. The "voice" he heard in his first trance state saying "Your father is a devil, but he still is your father" can be understood psychodynamically as self-blame over having negative and even homicidal impulses toward one's father. As Kishimoto (1958, 1961) put it so pertinently, "*Shugyō* is a device to get to one's deep mind through a strenuous bodily maneuver." *Shugyō* is a most effective way to facilitate the state of trance.

II. Spontaneuos Type. These are the shamans whose first spirit possession happened not through *shugyō* but spontaneously, and 16 of the 56 cases pertain to this category. Typical cases fall into two subgroups (IIa and IIb).

IIa. Shamans in the first subgroup of the spontaneous type experienced their initial possessed states without any other psychopathological syndrome. Five of the 16 cases belong to this type. The following is a typical case.

> *Case Number 43.* K. T. is a 33-year-old housewife living in the suburbs of Hirosaki City. She is one of the *gomiso*. She is serious-minded, fanatic, and tenacious. At the age of 25, after a love affair with him, she married her present husband (Case Number 18), who was two years older than she and a schoolteacher. Three years after the marriage, the husband lost his job, became a *gomiso*, and secluded himself in a mountain for *shugyō*, leaving the two children and her at home. She suffered from the desertion and financial difficulty, and was pushed to the brink of divorce. At the age of 32, she was forced by her husband to participate in the annual festival of a shrine which her husband believed in fanatically. On coming home, she suddenly fell into a state of possession and shouted, "You devil, I have found out what you are. Now the right god is with me. You devil, follow my god." This was apparently spoken to her husband, who was stunned by it.

Psychodynamically this case can be interpreted as a hysterical reaction through which defense K. T. became possessed and thus reversed her status in marital life so that in the field of belief she became dominant over her husband: hers is the right god and his is a devil.

Other shamans have their spontaneous first religious experience not through glossolalia but through revelation. The following case is illustrative.

Case Number 42. K. N., a 51-year-old female, is a *gomiso* in the city of Hirosaki. She was the fifth of ten children in a poor farmer's family. Since her mother also was a *gomiso*, K. N. had liked to play "god" since early childhood. She recalled that one day at the age of 10, she was afraid of being scolded by her mother for coming home late. On her way home in the dark, shivering with the fear of being punished by her mother, she saw a tall man with a white coat, high nose, and red face who stared at her. Frightened by this, she rushed home crying. Her mother prayed for her and told her that the tall man she saw was her tutelary divinity. She was shown the picture of the tutelary divinity next day and was surprised to find that it looked exactly the same as the being she had seen the day before. Though she did excellently in elementary school, she had to quit school to work and thus had a hard time. Since then, she often had "dreamed" of the tutelary divinity appearing to her and encouraging her by saying that every hardship she had been experiencing was for her *shugyō* and therefore should be endured. She married at the age of 16. Her marital life also was a hard one because of poverty and excessive demands of her mother-in-law. Her physical health was not good. Around that time, the tutelary divinity not only "appeared" to her for encouragement but also in her dream would give her an injection in the arm and even soothe her by stroking her bosom while she was pregnant. About ten years ago, after all of her eight children were grown, she went up to Mt. Iwaki for *shugyō*, obeying the "voice" of her tutelary divinity. She now is one of the most popular *gomiso* of the district. Twice every year she performs to big audiences, during which sessions she walks through burning charcoal. She says that while she is praying sincerely to her tutelary divinity before a performance he appears in the sky and encourages her, so that she will not get burned, and thus have the courage and emotional ease to walk through the fire. At present she uses both glossolalia and revelation according to the nature of the clients. As for glossolalia, she has said: "The god somehow jumps into my chest and causes me to speak. I am aware of this but just cannot keep myself from expressing the god's will." In the case of revelation, she has said that she only interprets the figures which appear to her mind symbolically. She is rather simple-minded and gets excited easily; yet sometimes she appears to be stubborn and quick-tempered.

In this case also the initial religious experience was related to the wish for escape from hard reality, that is to say, to wish fulfillment. Interestingly, this shaman prefers to employ visual revelation in making prophesies. This preference, coupled with the fact that her first religious experience was in the form of visual revelation, strongly suggests the type of personality described by Schneider (1927), who easily experiences visual hallucination under powerful emotion. Moreover, this case is interesting because her mother, aunt (Case Number 27), younger brother (Case Number 11), and niece are also *gomiso*. No signs of personality disintegration, discrepancy of thought processes, or other symptoms of paranoid schizophrenia were noted in her.

The following case is rather similar to the foregoing one (Number 42) in the experience of the first revelation, but differs from it in showing the presence of a paranoid schizophrenic tendency.

> *Case Number 45.* N. K. is a 54-year-old female *gomiso* in Hirosaki City. She was born into a rather well-to-do farming family as the fourth of six sibs. She had an elementary education and appears to be equipped with average intelligence. Her father was a sincere believer in the gods, and thus she started to worship the sun and moon in early childhood. At 17, she married a candy peddler. They have three children, and except for the fact that her husband has lost one leg, no financial or emotional difficulty is apparent in her marital life. Since the age of 30, she has been experiencing a shivering feeling all over her body at midnight and thus has been awakened to see the souls of famous people standing by and talking to her. She writes down their sayings, but most of them consist of fragmentary words and do not form sentences. Her facial expression is rather loose and lacks emotional expression. She is overtalkative with anybody, and her speech content is grandiose and stereotyped, with loose associations. The "divine will" she communicates comes from famous figures, such as Emperor Meiji, Empress Shōken, Buddha, Christ, Confucius, and Emperor Jimmu. Her glossolalia very often starts with speech in the first person and suddenly shifts to the third person. Its content is irrelevant most of the time. Though superficially she still is orderly in her daily routine life, her speech content and thought processes strongly suggest the presence of paranoid schizophrenic pathology.

The characteristics of the initiation into spirit possession for this group of shaman, Type IIa (except Case Number 45), are its involuntariness and its association with some emotional need, which explains it psychodynamically.

IIb. Eleven of the 16 cases of the spontaneous group belong to this subtype. For them, the initial spirit possession was associated with other psychopathological symptoms, such as fox possession, which persisted and sometimes led to hospitalization of the possessed. They resemble the cases described by Morita (1915) as *kitōsei-seishinbyō* (so-called invocation psychosis) in that hallucination, delusion, confusion, stuporous states, and so on accompany the initial religious spirit possession and that the symptom complex lasts for a perceptible length of time. Except for 1 case (Number 56, from Aogashima) who manifested catatonic excitement, the remaining 10 cases in this group raised problems of diagnostic categorization. It was possible, however, to formulate the psychodynamics of 6 of these 10 cases from the information obtained. The following is an illustration of such a case.

> *Case Number 47.* K. H. is a 52-year-old female. She
> was born and raised on the island of Aogashima. She is
> a conscientious, serious-minded, hard-working woman with a
> strong sense of duty. Since her youth she has been worshipping
> *Kompirasama* as her *oboshina* ("tutelary divinity"). At the
> age of 44, as the climacterium approached, she started to
> suffer from numbness of her extremities and loss of appetite
> and consulted a shaman of the island. By mistake, the prayer
> was carried out at the wrong shrine, not that for *Kompirasama*
> who had been her tutelary divinity. She had strong feelings of
> guilt, especially toward her divine god and her dead mother-
> in-law who had been a famous shaman. After she underwent
> a few days of torture from guilt feelings, the numbness
> of her extremities reappeared in exaggerated form and was
> associated with uneasiness and agitation. For three weeks she
> suffered the delusion of being possessed, personality dis-
> integration, and severe feelings of guilt and mental confusion.

Psychodynamically, this case can be interpreted as an acute psychotic reaction to overwhelming guilt feelings that had been culturally instilled in K. H. since childhood.

The other four cases are differentiated from the first six in that the situational and emotional factors which are supposed to have precipitated the psychotic conditions appear to have been minimal, although the clinical psychiatric pictures manifested were more severe. For each case, after one or two acute psychotic episodes, recovery seemed to come without sign of personality disintegration or deterioration. Psychodynamically it is hard therefore to understand the onset of the psychotic condition with its possession symptoms and also to find an appropriate diagnostic category within the established psychiatric nomenclature. These cases may be, as stressed by Yap (Chapter 3), classified under the "culture-bound syndromes of psychogenic or reactive psychosis." The following is an example of one such case.

Case Number 52. K. S. is a 55-year-old female on Hachijō Island. She was born as the second of nine siblings in a farmer's home. Her older brother has hebephrenic schizophrenia. She is tenacious, responsible, conscientious, and apprehensive. After finishing elementary education with excellent achievement, she went to Tokyo in the hope of getting a higher education, but because of financial difficulty she had to work as a laborer in a factory and thus had no further schooling. She felt disappointed and was anxious. Under such conditions, at the age of 20, she started to suffer from insomnia, swaying sensations of the body, and a decline in work efficiency. She had to return to the island. Then she suddenly refused to eat any cooked foods, and ate only seeds and plants which were considered inedible on the island. She became confused, tore off her clothes, shouted out words of the dead, prayed loudly and irrelevantly. She was taken to a shaman (Case Number 55) for treatment, and the psychotic condition improved rather dramatically. After the psychotic episode, she lived in the shaman's house for three years for training in shamanship, and at the age of 23 became a shaman upon the *kamisode* ceremony. She married at the age of 28 and her husband was a heavy drinker, as her god had "told" her he would be. When she was 32, her newborn baby suffered from high fever. Again, she became confused and psychotic. She became irritable and aggressive, stripped the clothing off the baby and precipitated the child's death by exposure to cold. The psychotic condition cleared up rather quickly soon afterwards.

At present she has inherited the profession of her teacher and is a leader of the shamans in the island. Her daily life is characterized by energetic activities, politeness, sociableness, with natural facial expression and emotional expression. There is no evidence suggesting the presence of personality disintegration or emotional deterioration.

For reference, Table 2 gives the most probable clinical psychiatric diagnoses of the 56 shamans at the time of this study.

Personality Factors in Spirit Possession

Although it is obvious that sociocultural factors play a very important part both pathoplastically and pathogenetically in spirit-possession, many investigators have failed to stress the role of individual personality factors, particularly for the shamans of the spontaneous type.

The mechanism of the initial possession state common to the spontaneous type (Type II) can be summed up as a psychodynamically understandable defense mechanism manifesting itself unconsciously. This mechanism is quite in contrast to the mechanism of the initial possession state of the *shugyō* type (Type I), who, at a conscious level, try to deal with their anxieties through faith and *shugyō*. In other words shamans of the *shugyō* group initially bring about trance states by conscious effort, while trance states of shamans of the spontaneous group take place altogether unconsciously. Logically, one can infer that the shaman of the spontaneous type would enter easily into trance states by minor autosuggestion. In practice these shaman, in fact, do bring about trance states rather easily and thus enjoy more clients than do shamans of the *shugyō* type. Two-sidedness of personality is certainly more marked among the spontaneous group of shamans than it is among the *shugyō* type. They are simple-minded, highly suggestible, and naive, while also stubborn, serious, tenacious, argumentative, and easily involved in conflicts with others in social life. These findings may suggest that a shaman of Type II is better fitted to become a successful shaman than one of Type I.

It also has been reported that many of the *fu-i* in Manchuria (Tamura, 1940; Ko, 1943), the *mudan* in Korea (Watanabe, 1943; Akiba, 1949), and the *yuta* of Amami Islands and Okinawa (Oguchi, 1959; Takagi, 1957; Yamashita, 1964) have episodes of psychiatric illness and that the *tsusu* shamans of the Ainu all were in a state of *imu* (an acute psychotic condition) in the past (Uchimura, Akimoto, and Ishibashi, 1938). Many other investigators (e.g., Eliade, 1951, 1961; Friedrich and Buddruss, 1955; Kiev, 1961, 1964; Murphy, 1964) have pointed out that most shamans have a history of psychiatric episodes, but these investigators have failed to associate the personality predisposition leading to psychosis with the capacity

Table 2: Diagnostic Classification of Shamans at Time of Study

Diagnosis	I. Shugyō Type	II. Spontaneous Type		Total
		IIa	IIb	
Hebephrenic schizophrenia	4	0	0	4
Catatonic schizophrenia	0	0	1	1
Paranoid schizophrenia	0	1	0	1
Alcoholic psychosis	1	0	0	1
General paresis	1	0	0	1
Personality deviation	4	4	2*	10
Without evident signs of psychiatric symptoms	30	0	8*	38
Total	40	5	11	56

* These had a history of transient psychotic episodes.

for being a successful shaman. All these findings, however, seem to indicate that the basic underlying disposition to spontaneous spirit possession is the essential factor in shamanism.

Although clinical observation has not been substantiated by psychological testing, most of the present cases seemed articulate (as were those described by Lebra, 1964) and shrewd (as noted by Murphy, 1964). Most of them were assessed to be of average intelligence, 8 of the 56 belonging to the upper level and 5 to the borderline level.

Sociocultural Factors and the Initiation Process through *Shugyō*

While for the spontaneous type of shaman, preshaman personality factors play an important role in the initial possessed state, it appears that for the *shugyō* type sociocultural factors play the key role. Also, the degree of acculturation and modernization of the community in which the shaman exists seems to have an important effect.

In the most primitive and isolated area, Aogashima, the inhabitants as a whole still believe strongly in tutelary divinities such as *oboshina* or *mikoke,* and a prospective shaman who has had a history of psychotic episodes is considered to have a better potentiality for becoming a shaman. The community as a whole can be said to live in a shamanistic atmosphere, and the inhabitants are quite ready to accept shamanism. These islanders even voluntarily practice shaman *shugyō* for recreation. Here therefore the shaman applicant can be led very easily into a state of possession without any strenuous *shugyō* in the collective ecstatic atmosphere of the *kamisode* (a ceremony held by a group of shaman).

In the more modern Tsugaru District, on the other hand, a good many of the shaman applicants are blind or physically crippled women. Their motivation for becoming shamans is no more than a vocational choice. In this particular district a blind girl can choose only between becoming a shaman or a masseuse. It has been a centuries-old social custom in this district for a blind girl to apprentice herself to a noted shaman (an *itako*) in order to become a professional. After an approximately two-year preparatory training, the apprentice finally is brought to a state of readiness in which she is able to become possessed through the ceremony of *kamisode* (which requires a seven days' starvation). To become an *itako* therefore requires a very strenuous *shugyō*, but the training follows a clearly prescribed ritual course, as automatic as travel on a conveyor belt.

In contrast, for *gomiso* in Tsugaru, the *shugyō* required for spirit possession is (as shown by Case Number 12 cited earlier) even more strenuous, without any tutoring, and initiated completely by the prospective shaman's personal emotional needs.

These findings suggest that the more shamanistic the community, the wider and easier in every sense is the way to spirit possession. In Table 3 *shugyō* type shamans in the four districts surveyed are classified according to their motives for becoming shamans.

Conclusion

In conclusion, I would like first to stress the danger of lumping all the shamans in one collective category. The analysis even of 56 cases has shown that the shamans in different districts of Japan differ from each other according to: (*a*) the mechanism of their experiencing the first possession state, (*b*) the different sociocultural situations, (*c*) the motives of shaman applicants, and (*d*) the types of *shugyō*, they underwent.

In summary, in a primitive or shamanistic community, an individual without specific psychopathological needs can become a shaman relatively easily. In other communities which are less primitive and less shamanistic, where shamanism has been considered, for example, as a career for the blind, strenuous self-training under well-arranged tutoring is required. In

Table 3: Motives for Becoming *Shugyō* Type Shaman (40 cases)

Motive	Tsugaru District	Tōgane and Vicinity	Hachijō Island	Aogashima Island	Total
To provide a vocation for blind or crippled female	8	0	0	0	8
Because of poverty and family trouble	5	0	0	0	5
Because of a sick family	3	0	0	0	3
Because of a question over God's existence	2	0	0	0	2
For consolation	0	0	2	5	7
Because of own sickness:					
Physical illness	3	1	0	2	6
Neuroses	1	1	1	0	3
Schizophrenia (hebephrenia)	0	0	2	2	4
Other psychoses	0	0	0	2	2

still other, rather modernized communities, in which an individual tries to escape into shamanism as a defense against his own psychopathological needs, even more strenuous self-training and self-discipline are required. Shamanistic status also may be reached spontaneously without *shugyō* by some people because of their shamanistic predisposition; in practice, these persons seem to be better able to meet the realistic needs of their clients. It is also among this latter type of shaman, however, that one encounters the most psychopathological symptoms in association with the possessed state.

REFERENCES

Akiba, T. 1949. Fu to hi. Minzokugaku Kenkyū 14:13–16.
Akimoto, H., N. Arai, J. Sugamata, Y. Sasaki, *et al.* 1964. Hachijō-jima ni okeru seishin-shōgai no ekigaku-idengaku-teki oyobi shakai seishinigaku-teki kenkyū. Psychiatria et Neurologia Japonica 66:951–86.
Akimoto, H., J. Sugamata, Y. Sasaki, T. Fujisawa, and Y. Ono. 1966. Socio-psychiatric study on religious group. Seishinigaku 8:928–32.
Arai, N., Y. Shibata, O. Mori, J. Murata, *et al.* 1961. Chiba-ken ka ni-ka-chōson no issei-chōsa ni okeru seishinigaku-teki kenkyū. Minzoku-Eisei 27:1–10.
Boyer, L. B. 1964. Folk psychiatry of the Apaches of the Mescalero Indian Reservation. *In* Magic, faith and healing. A. Kiev, ed. New York, Free Press.
Boyer, L. B., and B. Klopfer. 1961. Notes on the personality structure of a North American Indian shaman. Journal of Projective Techniques 25:170–78.
Czaplicka, M. A. 1914. Aboriginal Siberia. London, Oxford University Press.
Eder, M. 1958. Schamanismus in Japan. Paideuma 7:367–80.
Eliade, M. 1951. Le Chamanisme et les techniques de l'extase. Paris, Payot.
———. 1961. Recent works on shamanism. History of Religions 1:152–86.
Fairchild, W. P. 1962. Shamanism in Japan. Folklore Studies 21:1–122.
Field, M. J. 1960. Search for security: an ethno-psychiatric study of rural Ghana. Evanston, Northwestern University Press.
Friedrich, A., and G. Buddruss. 1955. Schamanengeschichten aus Sibirien. München, Barth.
Harada, T. 1949. Buraku-saishi ni okeru shamanism no keikō. Minzokugaku Kenkyū 14:7–12.
Hori, I. 1953. Wagukuni minkan-shinkō-shi no kenkyū. Tokyo, Sōgensha.
Iwai, T. 1938. Shaman-kyō (Tōyō-bunka-shi taikei). Tokyo, Seibundō-shinkōsha.
Jahoda, G. 1961. Traditional healers and other institutions concerned with mental illness in Ghana. International Journal of Social Psychiatry 7:245–68.
Jaspers, K. 1948. Allgemeine Psychopathologie. Berlin, Springer.
Kakeda, K., T. Nakamura, Y. Shibuya, T. Tajima, *et al.* 1959. Tōhoku-chihō ni okeru shamanism no seishinigaku-teki kenkyū. Medical Journal of Juntendō 5:199–210.
Kiev, A. 1961. Spirit possession in Haiti. American Journal of Psychiatry 118:133–38.
Kiev, A., ed. 1964. Magic, faith and healing. New York, Free Press.

Kishimoto, H. 1958. Shūkyō-shinpi-shugi. Tokyo, Taimeidō.
————. 1961. Shūkyōgaku. Tokyo, Taimeidō.
Ko, R. (Chia Lien Yuen). 1943. Manshū-koku zaikan-minzoku ni okeru Wuji narabi ni Hsieh-Bing ni kansuru kenkyū. Psychiatria et Neurologia Japonica 47:569–98.
Lebra, W. P. 1964. The Okinawa shaman. *In* Ryukyuan culture and society. A. H. Smith, ed. Honolulu, University of Hawaii.
May, L. C. 1956. A survey of glossolalia and related phenomena in non-Christian religions. American Anthropologist 58:75–96.
Michael, H. N., ed. 1963. Studies in Siberian shamanism. Toronto, Toronto University Press.
Morita, S. 1915. Yo no iwayuru kitōsei-seishinbyō ni tsuite. Psychiatria et Neurologia Japonica 14:286–87.
Murakami, H. 1950. Geijutsu to kyōki. Tokyo, Misuzu.
Murphy, J. M. 1964. Psychotherapeutic aspects of shamanism on St. Lawrence Island, Alaska. *In* Magic, faith and healing. A. Kiev, ed. New York, Free Press.
Nakagawa, S. 1964. Ainu-minzoku no tsusu ni tsuite. Psychiatria et Neurologia Japonica 66:233–34.
Nakamura, T. 1961. Aomori-ken ni okeru shamanism no shakai- seishinigaku-teki kenkyū. Medical Journal of Juntendō 7:872–900.
Nakayama, T. 1930. Nihon miko-shi. Tokyo, Ōuokayama Shoten.
Oesterreich, T. K. 1930. The possessed (Translated into English from French by D. Ibberson). New York, Smith.
Ogino, K. 1950. Hyōi-jotai no seishinbyōrigaku-teki kōsatsu. Nō Kenkyū 6:115–34.
Oguchi, I. 1959. Noro to yuta. Jinrui kagaku 11:120–24.
Sasaki, Y., R. Takano, and M. Ozawa. 1964. Tokyo-toka Aogashima-jūmin no seishinigaku-teki kenkyū. Psychiatria et Neurologia Japonica 66:252 (abstract).
Schneider, K. 1927. Zur einfuhrung in die religionspsychopathologie. Tubingen, Mohr.
Shinpuku, N., and N. Miyashita. 1958. San'in-chihō no kitsunetsuki ni tsuite. Medical Journal of Yonago 9:212–21.
Shirokogorov, S. M. 1933. Social organization of the Northern Tungus. Shanghai, Commercial Press.
Takagi, H. 1957. Yuta ni tsuite. Jinrui kagaku 9:188–93.
Tamura, Y. 1940. Manshū-koku ni okeru Hsieh-Bing, Kuei-Bing, Wui oyobi Kuoyinche, narab ni Mōko no Bironch. Psychiatria et Neurologia Japonica 44:40–54.
Uchimura, Y., H. Akimoto, and T. Ishibashi. 1938. Ainu no imu ni tsuite. Psychiatria et Neurologia Japonica 42:1–69.
Wakamori, T. 1943. Shugendō-shi kenkyū. Tokyo, Kawade.
Watanabe, M. 1943. Chōsen ni okeru seishinbyō. Psychiatria et Neurologia Japonica 47:747–48.
Yamashita, K. 1964. Amami ni okeru yuta ni tsuite. Minzoku Kenkyū 1:151–230.
Yanagida, K. 1913. Miko no kenkyū. Kyōdo Kenkyū 1:13–24.
Yap, P. M. 1960. The possession syndrome. Journal of Mental Science 106:114–37.

EFFECTS OF SOCIAL STRUCTURE
AND CULTURE ON HUMAN BEHAVIOR

15.   The Psychological Function of Witchcraft Belief:
The Burmese Case

MELFORD E. SPIRO, Ph.D.
Department of Anthropology
University of California, San Diego
La Jolla, California

The Burmese Perceptual Set: The Hostile World

The Burmese—like most of the peoples of South and Southeast Asia—inhabit a world which is believed to be populated not only by benevolent and kindly beings but by hostile and dangerous ones. Evil ghosts, lurking at the outskirts of villages, may attack without warning. Irrascible spirits, both petty and powerful (both of whom are termed *nats*), are to be found in forests and fields as well as in villages and even in one's dwelling. These spirits, although not intrinsically evil, are easily offended when slighted or ignored, and they respond with punitive actions ranging from petty annoyances to serious harm such as illness and even death. Frightening demons and ogres—cannibalistic and noncannibalistic—also abound. In addition to all these harmful beings, every village is believed to contain witches (the Burmese folk saying has it that one out of seven Burmans is a witch) malevolent human beings who innately or through learning possess harmful magical power capable of causing illness and even death.

Hostility is not confined to the supernatural world of spirits, ghosts, and witches. (Although witches are human, they are included in the "supernatural" category because their power is supernatural.) It is a characteristic of the ordinary human world as well. One of the striking characteristics of the Burmese is the frequency with which they allege that they are disliked, even hated, by their fellows. In conversation with Burmese friends and informants alike, one is almost invariably told that "everybody hates" (the speaker) because he "dares" to tell "them" the truth, or because he is "afraid" of no one, or because he has the "courage" to say what is on his mind, or for numerous other ostensible reasons.

It is this perceptual stance—"everyone hates me"—that gives special poignancy to Burmese beliefs concerning harmful supernaturals, for it is this stance that, in consistency with witch beliefs, renders everyone suspect and, in consistency with all other supernatural beliefs, interprets all harm as the result of punitive or malevolent intention. Thus the suspicion of the Burmese villagers with whom I lived that because of my spitting habits, I might be a witch tells us more about the characterological basis for the belief in witchcraft than it does about witches. To have observed and noted that I did not spit on the ground—a fact of which I had been unaware until it was pointed out—implies a cautious, watchful attitude, constantly alert to cues which might identify an apparently harmless person as being other than he appears (or claims) to be. If it be argued that there is insufficient evidence for my conclusion—I was, after all, a strange and mysterious foreigner, from whom anything might have been expected—I hasten to add that the Burmese approach each other with the same wary attitude. Suspicion of others, fear of their putative, hostile designs, accusations of deceit and duplicity—these traits are recurrent features of Burmese interpersonal relations. The Burmese say that *no one* can be trusted because, in the expression that became for me a constant refrain, "How can anyone know what is in the mind of another human being?" Since, clearly, one cannot know what is in another's mind, one can only watch for cues. In foreign anthropologists, one can watch for—or, at least, be struck by—blatant cues. In fellow villagers, the signs are more subtle: "We must watch their mood and manner, their facial expressions, and then maybe we can know what kind of people they are." This is why witches are believed to turn their faces away from the speaker—a somewhat silly tactic, however, for any witch to adopt because, of course, that action is a sure sign that he is a witch.

The true measure of the Burmese perception of others as hostile may be gauged by the fact that, although malevolence can be identified in another, benevolence never can be established with certainty. No one can be taken at face value. The most vicious witch may appear to be the most pious Buddhist; the bitterest enemy may appear to be the warmest friend. Hence, the more affectionate a man's smile, the more pious his devotions, the more cautious one must be.

It is my assumption, then, that the Burmese perceptual set—"everybody hates me"—is reflected in their beliefs concerning harmful supernaturals; it both reinforces these beliefs and, given Burmese psychological reality, is an obvious conclusion that someone intended harm. When the harm cannot be traced to some natural agency, it is an equally obvious conclusion, given their culturally constituted reality, that it was caused by some super-natural agency. Hence when I asked Ma Hlain, an attractive woman in her thirties, to describe the congestion in her chest, of which she com-plained, she told me, instead, that her pain had been caused either by a witch or a ghost. When I asked how she knew this to be so, she said, "I always feel that a witch or a ghost is about to do me some harm."

Although the Burmese perceptual set—"the world is hostile"—is an important feature of Burmese character, and although this orientation to the world may properly be characterized as paranoid-like, I strongly dis-agree (for reasons to be adduced below) with those who therefore conclude that the Burmese are paranoid. That their paranoid-like orientation does not erupt into genuine paranoia is related, at least in part, to their belief in malevolent supernaturals, especially witches, to which I shall confine this discussion. If this personal orientation is the important perceptual basis for the Burmese belief in the existence of witches—conferring credibility on these cultural beliefs, these beliefs also serve to mute the pathological con-sequence (paranoia) of this potentially pathogenic perceptual set. This latter thesis can be defended only after examining the possible bases for this set.

The first clue to an explanation for the Burmese perception of others as hostile is provided by their belief in witches and other malevolent supernaturals, for, on the assumption that supernatural beings do not exist, their putative character traits, such as a desire to harm, must be attributed to them by those who believe in them. If this reasoning is so, it is at least plausible that the Burmese perception of their fellows as hostile also may result from the attribution of hostility to them. The basis for this attribution can consist in one or both of two types of psychological processes. First, it can be based on the *generalization* of perception, the process by which an attribute—such as hostility—perceived to characterize one segment of one's social field is believed to characterize other segments of the field as well. Second, it can be based on the *projection* of drive, the process by which one of one's own drives—such as hostility—is imputed to others. Among Burmans, I submit, both processes are at work.

I suggest, first, that the Burmese perception of their fellows as hos-tile is a generalization from their childhood perception of their parents. Since this is not the place to describe Burmese socialization, I can only record, without documentation, two findings that suggest that this explana-tion may be so. Following a period of warm nurturing and free indulgence, Burmese children are often subjected—especially by parents, more espe-cially by mothers—to the withdrawal of affection and other kinds of emo-tional support which they had formerly experienced. In addition, Burmese children often perceive their parents as rejecting and sometimes as brutal. It is my assumption that these findings are not unrelated, but that, on the contrary, the parental behavior is the cause of the child's perception of his parents as rejecting. I further assume that perceptions and cognitions deriving from primary-group experience are generalized by the child to apply to his entire social field, a process by which everyone is perceived to be hostile and potentially rejecting.

Generalization is not the only possible basis for the Burmese hostility-oriented set. A second, theoretically possible, basis for such a set is the process of projection. Typically, projection may be taken to be a defense mechanism which, like all defense mechanisms, is motivated by an attempt to reduce, if not to resolve, psychological conflict. If, for example, one is hostile to others, and if, according to one's own values, such hostility is deemed immoral or wrong, the consequent conflict between one's drive and one's value can be very painful. One of the ways to reduce this conflict is to project the drive, to locate it in agents other than the self. The paradigm for this process is a simple one: "I am not hostile; they are hostile." Sometimes, this process not only localizes the drive in some *alter* (or group of *alters*) but it inverts the agent-object relation such that the perception "I am hostile to you" is transformed into the new perception "You are hostile to me." The Burmese perception of others as hostile does, in fact, exhibit such a quality; they believe that their fellows are hostile and, as shown above, this hostility is directed toward them. This perception is partly formed, so I believe, by the projective process. Threatened by his perception of the hostility of others, the child responds in a typically threatened manner: he becomes hostile to them. Then, feeling threatened by moral anxiety, the child projects his hostility onto others.

If this argument is correct, the Burmese hostility-oriented set is deep-seated. It conjoins the child's belief in the hostility of others, based on perceptual generalization, with his belief in their hostility, based on drive projection. Perceptual sets formed in early childhood are notoriously difficult to destroy and form the basis for later motivational and cognitive styles. Hence given their childhood-based belief in the hostility of their fellows, the Burmese continue, in later life as well, to project their hostility on them. The evidence of this twin thesis—that the Burmese are hostile, and that they project their hostility—can only be summarized briefly here.

That the Burmese can be, and often are, a kindly, generous, and gay people is easily documented and frequently recorded; that they are also a hostile people is as easily documented and as frequently recorded. The Burmese have a long history of violence and aggression—cruel warfare, massacre of populations, dacoity, insurgency, factionalism of all kinds—that have been, and continue to be, endemic features of their life. Whatever else these aggressive acts reflect, they surely express deep-seated hostility. (As I am using these terms, "aggression" refers to overt acts of harm, and "hostility" refers to the motivational disposition to cause harm.)

Hostility is observed individually as well. In the course of field work among the Burmese, one is struck by their almost compulsive denigration of their fellows: everyone else—in the village, or in the monastic order, or in the party—is uneducated, or ignorant, or impious, or evil, or self-seeking, or dishonest. It is because of these faults in others, one is frequently told, that some impending disaster is the inevitable fate of Burma. Now, I submit, this denigration of others is as much an expression of hostility as is the overt aggression on the group level. Although the speaker may view his criticisms as objective descriptions of his fellows, the observer cannot help but view them as the speaker's barely disguised expressions of hostility.

Whatever the adult sources of Burmese hostility, it is hard to escape the conclusion that, as in childhood, their own hostility to their fellows is one of the bases for their perception of their fellows as hostile to themselves. Although this conclusion is admittedly inferential, suggested more by theoretical expectation than by firm evidence, some indirect evidence, derived from the structure of witchcraft accusation, nevertheless supports this inference. That the victim's prior aggression to the alleged witch is the basis for his belief that the latter has worked magical harm against him is all but acknowledged by the Burmese themselves.

Let us, then, examine a typical case of witchcraft accusation. This case exemplifies one type of witchcraft accusation in which a patient suffering from a physical illness attributes it to witchcraft. A second, more dangerous type, is one in which the belief that one is being bewitched is the cause of psychological illness. In the first type—exemplified in the first case presented—witchcraft accusation is the response to illness; in the second—exemplified in the case presented next—illness, explained as witch possession, is the response to the belief that one is the victim of witchcraft.

Because of appetite loss, Do Han Yi, a married woman in her middle fifties, became progressively weaker and weaker, until, quite ill, she sought help from an exorcist, claiming that she was bewitched by Do Θan Nu. How did Do Han Yi know that she was bewitched by Do Θan Nu? Immediately prior to her loss of appetite, she had quarreled with and, in the heat of anger, insulted Do Θan Nu. Offended, Do Θan Nu, so she believed, had retaliated by making her ill.

Notice, the projective—specifically, the paranoid—process. In Burma the first question a patient asks when he falls ill is, "Who would wish me harm?" The automatic assumption is that if he is suffering some harm, it is because someone, either human or supernatural, intended that he be harmed. In order to answer, the patient asks himself a second question, "Whom have I harmed or wished to harm?" The assumption here is that if someone wishes him harm, it is in retaliation. Hence, since Do Han Yi had insulted Do Θan Nu, she concluded that the latter, injured by the offense, wished to harm her. Then, given her culturally constituted behavioral environment, it was obvious to Do Han Yi that her illness was caused by witchcraft, for, unless Do Θan Nu were a witch, how could she have executed her harmful intentions?

We can observe here the process of paranoid projection with only minimum disguise. Do Han Yi, to be sure, did not say that she had been hostile to Do Θan Nu, let alone that she had wished to harm her. She merely said that Do Θan Nu had injured her in consequence of her having been injured (insulted). I think it fair to assume, however, that the insult was an expression of Do Han Yi's hostility and her inference that an angry Do Ɵan Nu had injured her in retaliation supports this assumption. Since, however, projection is an unconscious process, Do Han Yi remained unaware of her own hostility to Do Ɵan Nu.

Lest I be misunderstood, I emphasize the point I made previously. Although I cite witchcraft accusation as an expression of paranoid projection, I do not characterize as paranoid the typical Burmese perception of others as hostile. I merely have used witchcraft accusation as evidence for the thesis that the latter perception is based on the projection of hostility, for, since this process in its paranoid form can be observed in Burmese witchcraft accusation, it is not far-fetched to assume (especially since the assumption is consistent with theoretical expectations) that the same process in a non-paranoid form is one of the bases for the Burmese perceptual orientation to others. The latter perception, although projective, is not paranoid, however, because unlike the case of witchcraft accusation, it is not persecutory. Although the Burman believes that "everyone hates me," he does not believe that some one person or group of persons is intent on harming him. Since they do not intend to harm him, he does not fear them; they are hostile, but they are not dangerous. Granted that he is cautious in his dealings with others, his caution stems not so much from his belief that they will harm him as from his difficulty in identifying who, among them, is a witch. Since any one may be a witch, it is best to offend no one lest the offended person be a witch and turn his evil power against his offender.

I stress, then, that although believing that he must be cautious in his dealings with his fellows because he can never be sure that one of them is not a witch, the typical Burman does not believe that his fellows *are* witches. Moreover, even when he believes that one of them is a witch and therefore harmful, he does not believe that the putative witch is hostile toward *him* or wishes to harm *him*. From the point of view of the typical Burman, those who are hostile to him (his fellows) do not wish to harm him, and those who are harmful (witches) are not hostile to him. In short, neither his belief that some humans are witches nor his belief that most humans are hostile to him reflects a true paranoid attitude. Only if he believed that his hostile fellows were intent on harming him or that the harmful witches were hostile to him (and therefore were intent on harming him) would his attitude properly be characterized as paranoid. One has only to compare a typical Burman, who subscribes to the two generalized beliefs that *everyone* hates him and that witches exist, with an atypical Burman who believes that one of his fellows hates him and is attempting to bewitch him (i.e., is both harmful and hostile to him) to discern the difference between a paranoid and a paranoid-like personality and between paranoid and paranoid-like behavior. It is only when the two generalized beliefs are conjoined in the particularized perception—"U khin (a particular individual) is bewitching me"—that one observes Burmese paranoia. One only has to observe one such case to realize that if the Burmese were truly para-noid, i.e., if they generally behaved as putative victims of witchcraft, Burmese society would not be a viable society. I shall illustrate this point with an example of a man who believed that his wife was bewitching him.

I first encountered this case when the friends of Maung Oun Yi, the victim, were attempting to obtain an exorcist to treat what to them was an obvious case of "madness" caused by witch possession. That morning Maung Oun Yi, in a trance (from our point of view) or possessed by a witch (from their point of view), had been extremely violent, using abusive and obscene language and indiscriminately attacking everyone with a dagger. At the same time he (or, as his friends put it, the witch who had possessed him) challenged them to bring in any exorcist they desired, pro-claiming that "none can defeat me." This episode, however, was merely the last of a recurrent series that had started nine months earlier. In the first episode Maung Oun Yi was neither abusive nor violent but, in a trance-like state, had wandered into the fields after experiencing what he described as a choking feeling which did not permit him to breathe. The exorcist, who was called in to treat him ten days after the onset, diagnosed the illness as witch possession. His second attack came four months later while working in the fields. Shouldering his tiffin-bowl, he wandered about the paddy fields, disorganized and confused, in a state of great emotional turmoil. Some time after this episode, an exorcist was called in, who seemed to cure him, but three months later, again in the paddy field, he had a third similar attack. The same exorcist treated him, again with apparent success. Seven days prior to my encounter with him, Maung Oun Yi had his fourth attack; his be-havior was almost the opposite of what it had been in the previous episodes. Seated in his house in a catatonic-like state, both motionless and emotion-less, he was stimulated to action only when the healer arrived. He (or, if you will, the witch who possessed him) challenged any exorcist to treat him; he would have "revenge" on all of them. "All exorcists," he shouted, "are powerless," and he had no "fear" of any of them. For seven days he alternated between catatonic-like withdrawal and violent acting out against anyone he encountered. On the second day of this episode, another exorcist, who happened to be in the village, attempted to treat him, but on the fol-lowing day the patient again became violent. On the sixth day, the local exorcist attempted to treat him, encountering only abuse, as the patient threatened to smear him with vaginal discharge—a deadly insult in Burmese culture—should he come near him. It was at this point that I was requested to bring his former exorcist to the village.

Belief in Witchcraft as a Culturally Constituted Defense Mechanism

Let me recapitulate my argument thus far. The Burmese percep-tion of their fellows as hostile to them is not in itself a paranoid perception because it is not accompanied by the belief that their fellows wish to harm them. It is only when these two perceptions are conjoined, as they are in cases of witchcraft accusation, that one can observe a true paranoid perception and characteristic paranoid behavior. In witchcraft accusation a fellow human being is transformed into a witch when the alleged victim of witchcraft projects onto him his own hostility to, and desire to harm, him. This projection for the most part can occur only in a society whose culture postulates the existence of witchcraft and for whom witches therefore are an accepted element of the behavioral environment. On the assumption, however, that witches do not exist, the generalized belief in their existence also must be projected in character. If this reasoning is so, then the same cultural belief which provides the cognitive basis for the (typical) personal belief that one is bewitched can also constitute the cognitive basis for the (more general) personal belief that one's fellows, although hostile, are not harmful. Indeed, only on the assumption that the Burmese project their harmful impulses onto their culturally acquired witch beliefs can one explain the curious Burmese perceptual bifurcation noted above, namely, those who are hostile to ego (his fellows) do not wish to harm him, while those who are harmful (witches) are not hostile to him. In order to explicate this thesis the perceptual and motivational bases for the belief in witchcraft must first be examined.

Witches, it will be recalled, are malevolent beings who, though human, are endowed with magical (supernatural) powers of evil and destruction. I submit that the psychological driving power for the acceptance of a cultural belief in which sheer malevolence is conjoined with magical power for the execution of one's desires can derive only from the earliest fantasies of childhood. If hostility is induced by frustration, then sheer rage, which is the emotional basis for malevolent and sadistic fantasies, is the frustration-induced response of the immature ego of a child—either because its frustration tolerance is low or because its anxiety-binding processes still are undeveloped. Similarly, psychoanalysis has taught us that it is the immature ego, its reality orientation still undeveloped, for whom the omnipotence of thought—the psychological analogue to the cultural belief concerning magical power—is the basis for the execution of its desires. In short, it is in childhood that private fantasies corresponding to witchcraft beliefs develop. By means of his omnipotent thought, the child, in a fitful rage, hopes to destroy the frustrating, threatening object.

This process, there is reason to believe, is universal. All children experience frustration-induced rage; all children are characterized by the omnipotence of thought. Although the process is universal, its dimensions are culturally variable. First, the intensity and frequency of rage is a function of culturally instigated threat. Second, the persistence of the cognitive stage of infantile omnipotence is a function of culturally constituted reality. In a society, such as Burma, in which lavish nurturing is followed by abrupt rejection, the child's frustration—and, hence, his frustration-induced rage—is intense. In a prescientific culture, such as Burmese culture, in which magical beliefs play a prominent role, the child's private belief in the omnipotence of thought is reinforced by his culturally transmitted magical world view.

It is my thesis, then, that their childhood fantasies concerning their own sadistic and destructive powers constitute the perceptual basis for the Burmese belief in witches. On the assumption that witches have no objective reality, the belief in their existence must be based on psychological, or phenomenological, reality. This psychological reality, I argue, is provided by the fantasies and perceptions of the believers.

Witch-like fantasies, *internal* to the believer, are not a sufficient basis for the belief in witches independent of, and *external* to, the believer. The latter belief can only be based on the externalization of the believer's internal fantasies. This is my second thesis. By externalizing their witch-like fantasies and projecting them onto their cultural beliefs concerning witches, the Burmese not only transform their own phenomenological reality into cultural reality but thereby transmute these culturally postulated beings from mere items of belief in a cultural inventory into what is for them existential reality.

Projection, as mentioned earlier, is a defense mechanism, and like all defense mechanisms represents an attempt to cope with threat. In this case the threat, so I have postulated, consists of the Burmese rage-produced childhood drives of sadistic and malevolent destruction. Drives of powerful intensity—whatever their nature—assume traumatic proportions for the immature ego; they create internal pressures which threaten to overwhelm, even to destroy, it. One means of coping with these traumatic pressures is to externalize the drives and project them onto some other being. By this process, they are no longer part of the ego; they have become ego-alien. Projected onto others, they no longer arouse traumatic anxiety in the self. In short, by using traditional witch beliefs as a vehicle for the projection of its own witch-like fantasies, the immature Burmese ego is protected from the potentially traumatic consequences of powerful forces with which it could not otherwise cope.

It is not only in childhood that traditional witch beliefs can serve as the basis for a culturally constituted defense. They also may serve defensive functions for adults. If, as I argued above, hostile impulses arouse for the Burmese painful self-perceptions, harmful impulses must be doubly threatening. Especially in the context of Buddhist culture, with its emphasis on compassion and loving kindness, the wish to harm others surely must arouse an intense degree of moral anxiety. Given the belief in witches— evil beings intent on harming others—the Burmese, so I think, can reduce their moral anxiety, as they reduced their childhood traumatic anxiety, by externalizing their harmful impulses and projecting them onto these culturally acquired witch beliefs.

To be sure, these perceptual and motivational explanations for the Burmese belief in witches are speculative, but how else can one explain the set of data which requires explanation? If the projection of witch-like fantasies of childhood does not constitute the psychological basis for the conviction that the cultural belief concerning witches is true and on the assumption that culturally constituted fantasy (like any other form of cultural behavior) is motivated, how else can the persistence of the Burmese belief in witches be explained? By the same token, if the harmful impulses of adults are not projected onto witch beliefs, how else can one explain the curious Burmese perceptual bifurcation earlier alluded to, namely, that those who are hostile to ego (his fellows) do not wish to harm him, while those who are harmful (witches) are not hostile to him? These speculations can explain this bifurcation, and this bifurcation, as discussed in the next section, points to one of the important psychological functions of the Burmese belief in witches—its contribution to Burmese mental health.

Witch Beliefs and Burmese Mental Health

Burmese childhood experience, I have argued, provides the experiential basis both for the Burman's personally acquired belief that his fellows are hostile to him and for his culturally acquired belief in the existence of witches. The former belief is a generalization from the child's realistic perception of his parents as rejecting. Rage, aroused by the latter perception, produces witch-like impulses in the child which are defended against by their externalization and projection onto the culturally postulated belief in the existence of witches. Since the latter belief, however, does not have a vectorial dimension—it merely asserts that "malevolent people, with magical power to harm, exist"—the projection of witch-like impulses onto this belief is similarly nonvectorial and, specifically, non-paranoid. Although the externalization of their childhood witch-like impulses allows the Burmese to defend themselves against the traumatic anxiety attendant upon them and although the projection of these impulses onto the cultural belief in witches strengthens their conviction concerning the truth of this belief, neither process produces the perception that "malevolent people, with magical power to harm, are intent on harming me." In short, this projection makes the Burmese cautious about witches, but it does not lead them to believe that they are bewitched or are about to be bewitched.

The projection of their own witch-like impulses onto the cultural belief in witches not only does not create the paranoid fear of bewitchment but also serves to protect the Burmese from the paranoid consequences of converting their fellows into witches. If their witch-like impulses were not projected onto the cultural belief in witches, these impulses conceivably would be projected onto their fellows. Given their personally acquired belief that their fellows are hostile to them, the latter would then be viewed as witches, who, hostile to *them,* would be intent on bewitching *them.* Having, however, projected their witch-like impulses onto the cultural belief in witches, they disconnect their belief in the hostility of their fellows from the possibility of their being witches.

This childhood-rooted disjunction between the personally acquired belief in the hostility of others and the culturally acquired belief in witchcraft, and, hence, between the perception of hostility and the perception of harm, continues throughout life. Given the cultural belief in witches, the Burmese learn very early to bifurcate the projection of their own aggressive drive into its two dimensions of hostility and harm. Hence when in post-childhood, they feel aggressive to their fellows, they project its harmful dimension onto their belief in witches and its hostile dimension onto their fellows. In short, given their differential beliefs concerning witches and people, the aggressive impulse, "I hate you," is bifurcated and projected into the two beliefs: "They (their fellows) are hostile to me," and "Witches are harmful." This disjunction between harm and hostility protects the Burmese from the fear both of witches and their fellows. A Burman therefore can feel that, although witches are deadly harmful, he need not fear them because their hostility is not directed toward him and that, although his fellows are hostile, he need not fear them because they intend him no harm.

According to this argument, it is the culturally acquired belief in witches that, paradoxically, protects the Burman from paranoid fear of his fellows, and it is his personally acquired belief in the hostility of his fellows that protects him from paranoid fear of being bewitched. If the harmful dimension of his aggressive drive, now projected onto witches, were to be projected onto his fellows, the latter would be perceived not only as hostile toward him but also as wishing him harm. By projecting this fear onto witches instead, his fellows are perceived as hostile to him but not as harmful. Similarly, if the vectorial dimension of his aggressive drive were not projected onto witches, the Burman would be in constant fear of being bewitched. If the vectorial and harmful dimensions of this drive were conjoined in one projection, witches would be perceived not merely as harmful but as wishing to harm him. It is the splitting of the aggressive drive into separate projections that protects the Burmese from delusions of persecution.

That this is not wild speculation can be seen in cases of witchcraft accusation—clear instances of paranoid projection—in which, by cognitive distortion, a fellow human being is transformed into an evil, attacking witch. It is only when the culturally constituted (normal) defense—"witches exist" —breaks down that the pathological (paranoid) defense—"a witch is trying to harm me"—occurs. This latter projection, it is noted, is constituted by an idiosyncratic conjunction of what is typically a perceptual disjunction; that is, the belief that one is the victim of witchcraft occurs when the culturally acquired belief in the existence of witches, conjoined with the personally acquired belief in the hostility of one's fellows, is focused on one person. This produces the paranoid delusion that *he* is an evil witch and *I* am the victim of his witchcraft.

The latter analysis provides a possible explanation, though not necessarily the one intended, for the curious Burmese belief that "without witches we cannot build our villages." Without the projective disjunction of their aggressive fantasies, made possible by the belief in witches, social solidarity would be effectively undermined. The belief that one is an imminent victim, either of the plotting schemes of one's fellows or of the harmful designs of witches, would, if generalized, render an orderly village life all but impossible.

As in most parts of this essentially speculative discussion, one can only speculate here, too, about the conditions that lead to the conjunction of these two otherwise bifurcated projections. Data suggest that the conjunction occurs, i.e., the culturally constituted defenses break down, when the aggression-arousing frustration is one that reactivates the childhood trauma of rejection. The aggressive response then becomes one of sheer rage, with all the magically destructive fantasies characteristic of this emotion. For reasons which I do not understand, the combined moral and traumatic anxiety produced by this rage does not instigate the typical (non-paranoid) bifurcated projections but does instigate, instead, a unified (paranoid) projection which transforms the frustrater into an attacking witch. The witchcraft case already described may help to elucidate this process. Although many facets of the case remain obscure, data obtained from the exorcistic seance and from interviews conducted with the patient and his relatives provide an explanation in which one may be reasonably confident.

At the age of 22 Maung Oun Yi was married to a 16-year-old girl. As he and his friends tell the story, his wife, after four years of marriage, committed adultery. Maung Oun Yi, although knowing of her infidelity, was ashamed to discuss it with anyone. His relatives, incensed by the wife's behavior, however, told him in her presence that she did not really wish to live with him, and they accused her of having two lovers whom they named. To this, Maung Oun Yi replied that nevertheless he would not leave his wife, for he had faith that she would abandon her immoral ways. The wife persistently denied that she had been unfaithful to him.

Shortly after, before leaving for an extended period of work in the jungle, Maung Oun Yi sent his wife to live with his parents so that they could watch her during his absence. Despite their surveillance, she entered into still a third affair. Returning from the jungle and being informed of her infidelity, Maung Oun Yi, ashamed that others would learn of it, told his wife that although he would not divorce her he would kill her if he discovered her in an adulterous act. It was almost immediately after this warning that Maung Oun Yi had his first attack; it was because she showed no concern for him that most people assumed that his wife—wishing finally to be rid of him—had bewitched him.

After an exorcistic seance Maung Oun Yi was cured, but four months later—shortly after his discovery that his wife had again been unfaithful—he had his second attack. Again, his wife showed no concern for him either during the attack or during the seance. His third attack occurred a few months later, and the fourth attack occurred after his wife eloped with one of her lovers and after he, therefore, had become engaged to another woman.

When I questioned him, Maung Oun Yi said that he and his wife had no sexual relations between the first and second attacks, because he had felt no sexual desire for her during that period. Upon further inquiry, I learned that because of his weak sexual interest they had never had an active sexual life. (It is not improbable that it was his weak sexuality, among other reasons, that had driven his wife, a highly sexed girl, into her adulterous affairs.) When I asked Maung Oun Yi why he thought that his wife was attempting to harm (bewitch) him, he said it was because she hated him. Only, however, at the end of a lengthy interview, did he concede that her hatred might have been provoked, at least in part, by his behavior toward her. It seems that even before his first attack—and despite the earlier picture which he and his relatives had painted of a long-suffering husband—he had, when learning of his wife's infidelity, beaten her severely and threatened to kill her. One can only assume since his first attack occurred shortly after this threat that his mounting violence, becoming too much to handle, was projected onto his wife by the paranoid process. This projection of his own rage together with his fear of her retaliation for his beating combined to transform her into an especially virulent witch. He then defended himself against his fear of the witch by identifying with her—in Burmese terms, she possessed him—in his trance aggression, a maneuver, moreover, which permitted him to act out his aggressive impulses with impunity, for since he was possessed it was not he, but the witch, who—so it was believed—was in control of his body. Since in a trance Maung Oun Yi attacked especially his parents and other close relatives, his earliest important frustraters, it appears that his trance-aggression was overdetermined, stemming not only from his defensive identification with his wife, the agent of his current rejection, but also from his repressed hostility to his childhood rejecters. The threat signified by his wife's rejection served to reactivate the threat experienced as a consequence of early childhood rejection.

Conclusions

In a recent perceptive analysis, U Sein Tu, a Burmese psychologist, pointed to four salient "syndromes," as he called them, of Burmese character; orality, aggressiveness, other-oriented self-esteem, and cynicism (Sein Tu, 1964). Except for aggressiveness, the other "syndromes," though not always functional, are at least not dysfunctional with respect to the maintenance of a viable social system. Aggressiveness, at least in the intensity in which it is often found in Burma, is and always has been a potentially disruptive force in Burmese society. The coming of the British greatly diminished the possibilities for the displacement of aggression onto out-groups in the form of bloody and highly destructive wars and subsequent sadistic cruelty expressed toward captured enemies. Opportunities for the expression of aggression in various forms of competitive athletic and gambling contests also were lessened because of British prohibitions, still in force in postcolonial Burma. Thus the Burmese have been left with few socially sanctioned, institutionalized means for the overt expression of hostility. The projection and displacement of hostility onto supernatural beings, and its displacement in preindependence political behavior (agitation against the British and riots against the Indians domiciled in Burma) and in postindependence political machinations, have been the main vehicles in modern times for culturally sanctioned expressions of aggression. I am disregarding the nonsanctioned, highly disruptive aggression expressed in continuing insurgency and dacoity—manifestations which are often difficult to tell apart.

This chapter has concentrated exclusively on the way Burmans use supernatural beliefs for the expression of hostility, specifically on their use of witchcraft beliefs as a means for its projection. That the belief in witchcraft has dysfunctional consequences which contribute to the Burmese attitudes of wariness and suspicion toward their fellows is obvious. If the argument of this paper is valid, however, the functions of this belief seem to outweigh its dysfunctions. Without the opportunity for the projection of their hostility which this belief affords, it is not unlikely that Burmese hostility would be turned either inward, with serious psychopathological consequences, or outward, with serious sociopathological consequences. In either case, given the characteristically high incidence of noninstitutionalized aggression found in Burma, the dysfunctions for Burmese society would assume serious proportions. The use of culturally acquired witch beliefs as a culturally constituted defense contributes therefore to the viability of Burmese society and to the maintenance of Burmese mental health.

ACKNOWLEDGMENT

A grant from the National Science Foundation supported field work in Burma in 1961–62, during which time the data on which this paper are based were collected. This chapter stems from a general comparative study of religion, supported by the National Institute of Mental Health.

REFERENCE

Sein Tu, U. 1964. The psychodynamics of Burmese personality. Journal of the Burma Research Society 47(Part 2):263–86.

16.   Cultural Values, Concept of Self, and Projection:
The Burmese Case

HAZEL HITSON WEIDMAN, Ph.D.
Department of Psychiatry
School of Medicine
University of Miami
Miami, Florida

IN THIS CHAPTER a hypothesis is set forth about systematic relations between cultural values, concept of self, and reliance upon projective mechanisms in ego defense. Relevant literature on projection is reviewed, and in the course of discussion the logic involved in formulating the major hypothesis is outlined. Briefly, relations between cultural values and concept of self are examined, utilizing material from field research in Burma. Relations of possible theoretical importance between concept of self and reliance upon projective mechanisms in ego defense are suggested. Finally, the implications are discussed of such a formulation for future research.

This chapter rests upon three major assumptions about the occurrence of mental illness: First, that characteristic features of the major illness categories utilized in the West occur universally; second, that different cultural systems allow or encourage different specific patternings of mental disorder; and third, that in large areas of the world projective mechanisms frequently prevail in the symptomatology of mental disorders. If it is true, for example, that "Paranoid schizophrenia appears to be fairly frequent everywhere, . . ." (Wittkower *et al.*, 1960) then it should follow that processes of denial and projection have a prominent place in such disorders. It also should follow that there is a heavy reliance, generally, upon projective mechanisms in many normal individuals in a variety of cultural systems.

The above conclusion rests upon the assumption that various cultural systems encourage certain basic personality dispositions in individual members. If ego functioning fails under stress, mental illness will develop in accordance with the culturally influenced set of the personality. If these assumptions are valid, then, despite great differences in the cultural detail and symptomatology of mental disorder, some rather fundamental similarities must be accounted for in the reliance upon projective mechanisms in widely scattered areas of the world. This chapter, by focusing upon projective processes in normal personality functioning, may, by extension, contribute to the understanding of the pathological use of projection in ego defense.

Review of Relevant Literature on Projection

It should be made clear at the outset that this chapter is not intended to be a definitive work on projection. There is perhaps no vaguer concept than that of projection in all the literature dealing with personality processes. In relation to experimental psychology, Murstein and Pryer (1959) said: "One would be hard pressed to find a concept so capable of multiple interpretation and so varied in meaning as the concept of projection." Salzman (1960) referred to the same lack of precision in the concept in relation to psychiatry: "I shall speak about a process that will be immediately recognizable as the mechanism of defense which we call projection, externalization, transfer of blame, or anything else in which the individual assumes or accuses someone else of something that is designed to protect his own, omnipotent self."

One of the major criticisms made by Murstein and Pryer is that in experimental psychology definitions of the concept of projection have not been related specifically to clinical meaning and that such definitions imply nothing about the unconscious or a self-concept. They argued that "Projection should not be a function of cognition, but of emotional involvement." They concluded: "If projection is to be a phenomenon involving emotional values with regard to the self, it is the task of the experimenter to indicate in what manner the judgements of the perceiver are indicative of these values rather than of relatively extraneous cognitive-response habits."

Although I am not undertaking such an experimental task, I suggest a theoretical approach which may clarify the relations between specific cultural values, concept of self, and reliance upon projective mechanisms. "Projective mechanisms" is used in this paper to stand for categories of symptoms such as those outlined by Chakraborty (1964) in his study of paranoid symptomatology in Indian schizophrenics, namely, delusions of persecution; delusions of grandeur; ideas of reference; ideas of influence; suspicious-evasive behavior; aggressive, hostile, attacking behavior; shifting the blame; intellectualization; and psychotic thinking presented in a logical, systematic, pervasive manner.[1]

One assumption made here, in contrast to the position of Murstein and Pryer, is that projection cannot be a function of emotional involvement without also being a function of cognitive and perceptual processes. In fact, the defensive use of projection may represent one type of cognitive and perceptual orientation based upon particular cultural values, concept of self, and therefore emotional involvement. It is increasingly evident in the literature of anthropology and psychiatry that others are beginning to make similar assumptions.

This concept inevitably is linked, in the psychiatric literature on projection, to discussions of the etiology, dynamics, and therapy of paranoidal disorders, whether they fall within the diagnostic categories of paranoia, paranoid state, or paranoid schizophrenia.

Freud saw projection as a defense against repressed homosexual impulses and also as a certain kind of distortion or misinterpretation of reality based upon the displacement of energy or affects from within the individual onto external objects. A growing body of recent literature, however, points to the inadequacy of this theory. Bindelglas (1965), for example, argued that the classical Freudian theory of projection sometimes leads to incorrect diagnoses and results in the therapist's overlooking the real pathology. He reported that some cases of projection may respond to therapeutic approaches differing considerably from the classical approach, and he indicated that new awarenesses at the cognitive and perceptual levels can sometimes bring about changes in the emotional structure of the patient. Salzman (1960) too, emphasized cognition, mentation, and rational thought processes in the etiological, dynamic, and therapeutic aspects of paranoidal disorder even while recognizing the unconscious elements. He wrote, for example, that "conscious and rational conclusions . . . can be derived from the false premises that initiate the pathological process." He added that "the awareness that the paranoid delusion often flows logically from false premises involved in the patient's grandiosity would allow us to pursue the meaning and significance of the delusion as a logical consequence of conscious mentation."

Among those writing in a different vein, Carr (1963) pointed out that Freud's theory of paranoid delusions as a defense against unconscious homosexuality has been challenged by evidence of two general types: (1) no homosexual problem is reflected in many cases, and (2) the paranoid delusion often co-exists with overt homosexuality. Ovesey (1955), one of the major theorists in the group concerned especially with the problem of homosexuality in Freud's theory of paranoia, argued that "the paranoid phenomena can stem from nonsexual adaptations to societal stimuli, and motivationally need have nothing to do with homosexuality whatsoever." He stated (1954) that:

> The great majority of so-called homosexual anxieties are
> motivated by strivings for dependency and power. These
> anxieties, . . . stem from pseudohomosexual fantasies that are

misinterpreted by the patient as being evidences of frank
homosexuality. In reality, the sexual component, if present at
all, is very much in abeyance. More often it appears to be
entirely absent. In these cases it would perhaps be better to
drop the term "latent homosexuality" altogether and refer
instead to "the pseudohomosexual conflict."

Schwartz (1963, 1964) argued that it is the need for meaningful-
ness which motivates projection in a paranoid person. He stated (1964):

> Projection, the defensive maneuver of choice in the
> paranoid person, has often been described in terms of such a
> person's need to deny his own unacceptable feelings. However,
> the projection of benign and laudatory feelings seen in
> grandiose or benign delusional systems can hardly be explained
> in this way. Projection makes most sense if it is conceived of
> as a placement of thoughts which establish the meaningfulness
> and significance of the individual, into a locus where they are
> themselves meaningful: i.e., into other people.

Schwartz (1963) wrote:

> the paranoid person is uncomfortably confronted by feelings
> of inadequacy, insignificance, and unimportance. Paranoid
> illness, in an oversimplified way, may be conceived of as an
> elaborate denial of this confrontation, by means of various
> devices which add up to a counter proposal: "I am important,
> if not to the people in my immediate interpersonal world, then
> to vast and countless others." . . . The particular nature of
> the paranoid defense is that it represents an explanation . . . .
> the paranoid defends by explanation, in an intellectualizing
> way.

Schwartz (1963) has made an important theoretical contribution
by stressing the importance of a particular self-concept which may underlie
all paranoidal processes and therefore, by definition, the major projective
mechanisms in ego-defense. He suggested that the denial of such a self-
concept takes the form of *"centrality,* . . . the assertion of overwhelming
and pervasive importance to others."

Schwartz is not alone in pointing out the importance of the self-
concept in the etiology of paranoidal processes. Others have noted a deep
sense of inadequacy, inferiority, worthlessness, meaninglessness, insignificance, and similar feelings. While this observation is implicit in the writings
of many clinicians, it has been made explicit by Sullivan (1956), Fleischl
(1958), Cameron (1959), Bullard (1960), Salzman (1960), and Coleman
(1964), among others.

Of those who have attempted synthesis of the major views on

paranoidal forms of illness, only Schwartz has looked closely at the concept of self. Waelder (1951) went so far as to point out that denial underlies the whole paranoidal structuring of reality and even to suggest that projective mechanisms represent various forms of denial, but he specifically left open the question of what it is that is denied. Salzman (1960), among others, specified that "the paranoid development ... is an attempt to deal with extreme feelings of worthlessness through a process of denial and reaction formation." It is Schwartz, however, who has tried to describe the particular way in which the self is inadequate and to examine the implications of such a self-concept for the operation of projective process generally.

Schwartz (1963) postulated a paranoid mode of adaptation lying at one extreme of a "paranoid-depressive existential continuum" which is based upon the tendency to refer responsibilities to others or to the self. He described the self-concept underlying the paranoid mode of adaptation as that of meaninglessness and insignificance. He linked such a self-concept to an incapacity for self-referral of responsibility, an incapacity for ambivalence in the self-concept, and a need for the recognition of others. This set of factors he referred to as "the essential paranoid constellation." Although using different words, Schwartz seems to have said that because of an inability to refer responsibility to the self, the self is defined as a "nothing," a "zero." If the self is so defined, any meaningful definition of the self must come from others. Because a concept of self as a "nothing" is unacceptable, an acceptable definition which comes from others may not include the slightest suggestion of worthlessness or insignificance. He suggested that under these conditions the preferential use of projection in ego-defense follows naturally: "when one lacks any reasonable capacity for self-reference, then projection must become part of the major defensive maintenance of ego-integrity." For Schwartz, the paranoid mode of adaptation underlies all paranoidal disorders. It is his thesis that all the symptoms of paranoid illness are derived from the essential constellation of factors set forth above.

Schwartz (a psychiatrist), working primarily from personality functioning to family patternings, seems to have arrived independently at a position very similar to that of Hitson (an anthropologist) and Funkenstein (a psychiatrist) working primarily from family patterns to personality. The latter authors (1959) also postulated a depressive-paranoidal continuum, and in their study of families of depressed and paranoidal patients they described very different patternings for the two groups. The nearly identical conclusions of these authors suggest that their work may be the beginning of a more adequate theory of paranoidal disorder and a better understanding of the use of projective mechanisms in ego defense than now exist.[2]

Utilization of a broader conceptual approach than that heretofore employed in either the anthropological or the psychiatric literature may make it possible to state which specific features of social systems are related to particular conceptions of the self. It also may permit a better understanding of the individual's reliance upon projective mechanisms generally as well as upon particular projective techniques. Finally, it may permit a better understanding of paranoidal disorder in different cultural contexts, at different points in time, and as part of a dynamic process capable of evolution and change toward increased or decreased pathology.

Cultural Values and Concept of Self

Hitson and Funkenstein (1959) and Schwartz (1963, 1964) have suggested that there may be a depressive-paranoidal continuum which reflects basic dispositions transcending the clinical picture of depressive and paranoidal illness. In different ways these authors have hypothesized that the ego-defensive mechanisms of projection which define the paranoidal process can be derived from a generic type of self-concept. Consequently, the more general patterning must be accounted for if projective mechanisms are found to predominate in the symptomatology of mental disorder: (1) in a particular culture or widespread in certain cultural areas; (2) associated with different social strata or with particular types of social structure; and (3) in migrant situations or in certain situations of acculturation. Presumably, a generic paranoidal type of self-concept should be found underlying such phenomena and functioning in psychodynamically equivalent ways under varying situations of stress.

Exactly what is the relation between cultural process and the particular type of inadequacy of the self-concept which gives rise to the preferential use of projective devices, and, with failure in ego-functioning, to the paranoidal structuring of "reality"? Must such a self-concept be "acted upon," as Hitson and Funkenstein have suggested? Must it be "meaningless and insignificant," as Schwartz has hypothesized? Or are these, perhaps, functional equivalents at one level of generality of a more basic conception of self as "inadequate," i.e., "powerless" or "without control"? Or, following a particular *definition* of the self, should one go further and think of a particular *experiencing* of the self?

Assuming that a generic concept of "self as inadequate" underlies a reliance upon projective devices in the maintenance of ego-integrity, one may ask, inadequate in what way?—inadequate-"acted upon"? inadequate-"meaningless"? inadequate-"incapable"? inadequate-"insignificant"? inadequate-"nothing"? inadequate-"worthless"? inadequate-"unimportant"? Regardless of the specific way in which inadequacy is defined for a particular individual, such a self-concept apparently must be denied. In Schwartz's (1963) words, "the self is tautologically meaningful and significant to the self." When culture, family, and socialization processes therefore define the self as inadequate in any of these ways, does it indeed follow that such a definition is inevitably denied?

The answers to such questions must wait. The theoretical task now is as follows: On the personality side, a self-concept which gives rise to the preferential use of projective processes must be explained—a self-concept which allows for cultural differences in preferred type of projection, symptom, or content of full-blown pathology when breakdown occurs. On the cultural side, the occurrence of such a self-concept despite great differences in cultural minutiae and regardless of differences in broad social-structural features, value orientations, or institutional emphases must be explained.

Based on the assumption that emotionally motivated cognitive processes are inevitably linked to some sort of basic premises which influence perception, the contribution of cultural values in the formation of such a self-concept must be considered. It is my thesis that such a self-concept derives from implicit cultural values which act as basic premises underlying the social structure. When these values are internalized by the individual, they enter into the formation of the self-concept, they influence perception, and they help to explain the particular cognitive structuring which is inherent in projective processes. Specifically, I hypothesize that such a self-concept derives from the way in which human nature, man's relation to man, and man's relation to nature and supernature are defined culturally.[3]

The remainder of this chapter is devoted to setting forth this central hypothesis by focusing upon the relation between values, concept of self, and projection in Burma. The supporting data are from field research in a village in lower Burma during 1957–59.[4]

The operation of almost every projective process discussed in the literature could be illustrated in Burma, falling into place as part of the overall culture pattern, which, I feel, could not indicate anything other than a concept of self as inadequate. Since it is impossible in the space available to present a total view of Burmese culture, several facets of Burmese culture are presented to indicate the basis for this belief. Following a brief sketch of structural features and specific values which may influence the self-concept is a quick review of certain parental attitudes, socialization techniques, and verbalizations which seem especially meaningful for the formation of a concept of self as inadequate, generally, and as acted upon, specifically. Thereafter, the relation between cultural values and projective mechanisms in Burma is examined.

STRUCTURAL FEATURES AND CULTURAL VALUES

The concept of self in Burma is a self which is acted upon by the environment, and, furthermore, acted upon in potentially harmful ways. The two major social structural features which help to form this concept are founded upon the tacit premise that human nature is, if not basically evil, at least unpredictable and potentially harmful.

The first major structural feature is vertical. Burma is an age-graded society—respect obtains between an individual and anyone older than himself. Wealth, government position, personal power, and education are further criteria for positions of authority. These criteria also are tied to the status hierarchy and evoke respect relations which provide the basic guidelines for behavior in every interpersonal situation. Social stratification does not stop with human beings; it extends into the supernatural world of spirits as well. Increased potentiality for harm attaches to each ascending position.

There is genuine reason for one to fear the power of another who has greater socially sanctioned authority than he. Anyone in a legitimate position of authority has the power to give or to withhold rewards. He has the power to treat kindly or to punish, to bring harm to those lower in the hierarchy, and, in Burmese opinion, even to cause death. From the point of view of those of lower status, all things both good and bad come from above. In consequence, one carefully shows the appropriate degree of respect and attempts in every way possible to avoid harm by not rousing the anger of a person of high status.

At the same time, it is the better part of wisdom to insure the greatest number of rewards from above by unobtrusive, ingratiating behavior or by becoming a follower of a person of high position. Such a dependency relation holds as long as it is sufficiently gratifying. When it is no longer so, the ties are broken, the leader repudiated, and a new protector adopted.

Because it is hierarchically ordered by means of several major criteria, the very structure of Burmese society seems to produce exquisite sensitivities to status in every interpersonal relation. Self-esteem is continually at stake in the balance of power inherent in the dynamics of relations. Until some indication of status shows the way, there is no basis upon which to act. Inevitably, the relative ranking of individuals in a group determines the amount of respect and deference to be shown—to whom—by whom. Only when people are roughly equivalent in age and status may they speak and act without restraint and without fear of offending by somehow calling positions of authority into question.

The second major structural feature is horizontal. Burmese society is organized in terms of oppositions. The environment consists of areas of relatively greater danger the more removed they are from the family and all that is familiar.[5]

At the same time that a child in Burma begins to learn the intricacies of the status hierarchy, he also begins to realize that the world is a very dangerous place. He begins to realize that he is safe only within his own family. He is dependent upon it for survival. He must rely upon it for sustenance, co-operation, freedom of movement, and protection. He learns that each family member therefore must be concerned with the welfare of the family group for the family to flourish and the individual to survive.

The whole socialization process in Burma conveys to the child the belief that all safety, all privilege, all righteousness, and all loyalties lie within the family. His family is always presented in the best light. His is superior;

others are inferior. His is good; others are evil. It steps in to defend the child who quarrels with unrelated children by denying his responsibility and attacking all who accuse him. It protects the family member who commits a crime by proclaiming his innocence and bargaining for his freedom with bribes. The family expects something in return, of course. It expects children to be *lain-mah-deh*. *Lain-mah-deh* children are good, dutiful, respectful, and obedient. They involve the family in no trouble with others and bring to the family every possible advantage in the way of food, money, protection, and the like. Along this horizontal dimension, man's relation to man is such that interpersonal relations are fraught with danger. For example, people are reluctant to visit or trade in villages in which they have no relatives. Without relatives there is no house to which they can go with the assurance of being greeted and welcomed. Without relatives there is no place to stop for a rest or a visit. Most importantly, without relatives there is no one to legitimize their presence in a village in which they do not live— or to protect them in case of trouble.

Such views are clearly reflected in the following comments regarding the events leading to marriage. A young man was asked whether he visited his fiancée in her village after the agreement by their respective families for their marriage. As presented by Weidman (MS), he said:

> No, it isn't the custom; parents don't like it, and I might have enemies in that village, so I didn't go. I didn't know anyone in that village, didn't have relatives there, and they wouldn't like my coming frequently. Even if the parents approved, other villagers would talk and not like it. I didn't know how many others wanted this girl, too. They might have been jealous and might have beat me up. They might even have killed me. I would be one against the whole village; so it is best not to go.

Certainty, or at least degree of predictability, in any situation outside village routine is linked directly to kinship, friendship, and acquaintanceship in that order—thus the reluctance of young men to seek employment where they have no contacts; thus the reluctance of villagers to enter the hospital for treatment when they know no one there.

Such are the implications of the tacit premise that man's nature is unpredictable, potentially harmful, and therefore possibly even basically evil. In Burma similar assumptions are made about the potentiality for harm from the natural and supernatural. With such perceptual approaches in the social, the natural, and the supernatural realms, the experiencing of the self cannot be one of mastery over the total environment. Instead the experiencing of the self in situations of stress must be of lack of control, i.e., powerlessness in varying degree depending upon ritual forms of control offered by the culture and upon its traditional ways of coping.

Should not, then, the kind of reaction formation reported in the psychiatric literature be expected as an attempt to deny such a self-image and to overcome such feelings of helplessness? Of course, and there is a great deal of supporting evidence, particularly clear in the changing work situation in Burma.

Burmans are very sensitive to any implication of low status, especially low status or servility in the work situation. Any menial task is avoided which might be viewed as something someone in authority would not do himself. Laborers quit their jobs to maintain self-esteem when it appears to them that they are being pushed too hard or asked to do more heavy work than someone else of otherwise equal status. When workmen perceive themselves to be oppressed by their supervisors, they engage in whatever unco-operative, undermining behavior is at their disposal. In certain situations the Burmese laborer tries to do as little as he can to show that he does not really have to work or that he is slave to no man. To do otherwise would in fact be equivalent to the admission of a degree of subservience that in an earlier period of Burmese history would actually have constituted slavery.

Why such sensitivity when dominance and submission enter into every respect relation in this hierarchically ordered society? Perhaps for the following reasons: Submission to the socially sanctioned authority of another is, indeed, culturally prescribed. Also, voluntary submission to another in a leader-follower relation is perfectly acceptable. Anyone is viewed as completely evil, however, who by word or deed implies that he has placed himself in a position of authority over another without adequate social sanction, prior consent, or voluntary submission of the individual to his authority. He is considered a potentially harmful enemy. Such an implication of dominance and submission must be rejected; this rejection almost always takes the form of silent, indirect aggression but sometimes takes the form of direct violence.

This sort of concern with status enters into any work situation— but something more is involved, namely, Burmese conceptions of poverty and guilt as well as attitudes which place a premium upon slyness and cunning to avoid hard work. Poverty supposedly represents punishment for sins committed in a previous existence, and it is the sly, cunning person, who, through his cleverness, will have first place in everything without having to work for his rewards.

Thus self-esteem is continually at stake in the balance of power inherent in the dynamics of status relations. When the emotionally charged concepts regarding poverty, subservience, and punishment for past sins are injected into the work situation along with normal considerations of status, the overriding concern must be protection of the self. Such a convergence of emotional elements in the work situation constitutes so great a threat to the self that ego-defensive measures must take precedence over economic security and other important matters.

I submit that such patterened behavior provides fundamental insight into the basic nature of the self, particularly among males, in Burma. In situations of stress, however defined, the self is helpless, defenseless, and powerless to much greater extent than it is meaningless or insignificant. That the problem seems to be one of control, of course, is congruent with a perceptual set which reflects the self as being acted upon by a potentially destructive environment.

My sketch of Burmese culture should begin to show how basic assumptions which underlie and support the social system come to be built into the personalities of the participants of the system and how cultural values are related directly to the formation of a self-concept.

PARENTAL ATTITUDES TOWARD CHILDREN

In Burma parents make a number of major assumptions about the nature of children, the logical implications of which ramify in specific ways throughout the socialization process. Children are assumed to be incompletely formed human beings, something less than full-fledged members of society, and therefore are treated as less important and less dangerous than adults. Parents assume that children are to be treated as objects of teasing for adult enjoyment, as objects of blame, as useful in running errands, as caretakers for aging parents, and (if girls) as household help, or (if boys) as a means of gaining merit for parents through special religious ceremonies.

It is assumed that children will make no internal demands upon themselves. It is thought that they cannot be relied upon and will indulge themselves in every way, by stealing, lying, taking things by force, arguing, fighting with others, and so on. It is assumed that they cannot be trusted in the absence of parents and elders, that they will be mischievous and destructive. It is assumed that children will be difficult to control unless made to obey through the use of force or fear. Finally, it is assumed that children are helpless and defenseless in the functioning of the social system, that they do not know or understand cultural values, that they unintentionally will transgress norms, and that they do not know how to take care of themselves properly. They must, for example, be protected from outsiders who may try to punish them or who, supposedly, will try to take advantage of them in some way.

In such views, there is little which can convey to a child an awareness of his own potentialities, a sense of responsibility, or a feeling of adequacy through mastery or control.

SOCIALIZATION PRACTICES

In terms of social structure, the child is the recipient of orders from everyone higher in the hierarchy than he. Any adult throughout the system has the right to tell any child what to do. Within the family, it is the child's duty to do what he is told. Even though a child may do the same thing day after day, he is told anew each day when to carry out his tasks. Older children can tell younger ones what to do, but the younger cannot command the older. Parents make decisions for their children, buy their food and clothing, and arrange their marriages. It is the parental prerogative to sell (against a child's wishes) property given to him by other relatives. Formal weddings cannot take place without the consent and participation of elders, and elders will not arrange a marriage for a child with someone of whom they disapprove.

Teasing is very frequent in Burma (Weidman, MS). Both adults and adolescents generally direct such teasing toward young children. A mother, for example, described the way the family tease a dark-skinned, ten-year-old son:

> We say, "You're ugly. You're black." He gets very
> angry and abusive, and goes around hitting everybody. We all
> laugh. This makes him more angry. When we laugh too much,
> he sits down and cries. We still laugh. This is a form of
> amusement. . . . We tease like this when we are feeling very
> dull among ourselves. The baby is too young to tease like
> this [about three years]. When she is about seven years old, she
> will be teased this way.

Aside from the fundamental attitudes of parents toward children, there are implications in such socialization practices for a concept of self as helpless and acted upon. These implications are reflected in a wide range of impingements upon the child from above—commands, decisions, punishment, and teasing. All these factors suggest lack of control by the child, which is increased by many different kinds of inconsistency and unpredictability in the behavior of those about him.

There is, at the same time, an enormous amount of indulgence of many of the child's needs, indulgence which, in itself, hardly is designed to increase the strength of the ego structure. Adults seem to identify with the young and the helpless. They pity them and want to fulfill all their wishes. There is genuine empathy for the lowly little figure at the bottom of the social system who has the entire superstructure sitting on his head and cannot make his wishes known, but such empathy and indulgence do not add to a child's social skills. Instead, they tend to support a view of the self as helpless.

In addition to these characteristics of child rearing in Burma, a parent's particular phrasing of admonitions in many situations contributes to the formation of a concept of self as a target. Verbalizations such as the following (Weidman, MS) help to prevent a child from focusing upon his own behavior as "cause" or the consequences of his acts as "effect":

> Children who are careless in play are shouted at to
> "Be careful; the child's face will be hit." A child playing
> beside a calf is told in a rough voice, "The cow will stamp on

you." Children who are too active are told in angry voices,
"You'll fall. You'll be hurt." Children making toys and using
dahs are gruffly cautioned, "You'll be cut. You'll lose a hand."
A child waiting eagerly for mangoes to fall is told loudly that
"The branch will fall on you." A child keeping an exhausted
chick running is shouted at, "The little chick will die."
A child squeezing and hurting a kitten is told, "The kitten is
angry, it will bite you."

Diffuse sanctions are involved here. These pervasive practices in the
course of everyday life continually add weight to the concept of the self as
acted upon or as powerless, to a degree. The coupling of these patterns with
those inherent in the structural aspects of Burmese society shows how some
of the important features of social systems seem to be significantly related
to the formation of a self-concept as inadequate, and as inadequate in a
particular way.

CULTURAL VALUES AND PROJECTION

Throughout the literature on paranoidal disorders runs the theme of
disordered perception, defective reality testing, and through time the development of delusions which misrepresent "reality" as defined by others. Carr
(1963), for example, seems to me to have said that in order for a delusion
to develop (i.e., a disordered perception with an unalterable conviction
about it), a disordered relation must exist between perceptual experience
and reality testing. Such disordering is possible only when perceptual organization does not permit absolute certainty of interpretation during the early
years of the development process. He thus postulated that the pathological
process leading to delusional formation begins in early development when
others deny the validity of a perception which the child experienced as real
and true.

The reliance upon projective mechanisms is widespread in Burma.
If one assumes that delusions do, indeed, represent projective processes
developed to the extreme, then, in terms of premorbid personality structure,
one must expect as part of the Burmese cultural pattern the kind of denial
hypothesized by Carr, some form of perceptual ambiguity in the individual,
and some kind of disordered relation between perceptual experience and
reality testing. I believe these key elements of a pathological process are
present in Burma, as I will attempt to show. The second goal of this section
is to indicate the relation of cultural values to projective processes generally.

There are many elements in Burmese culture which might cause a
child to doubt his own sense perceptions; there are also suggestions that many
events of the sort postulated by Carr are experienced by the Burmese child.
For example, one of the clearest images I retain from field research is that
of very young children looking inquiringly into the faces of adults and older
children alike to see whether a threat was genuine or in fun. In situation

after situation, the Burmese child is forced to judge whether behavior is motivated by affection or hostility, love or hate. A mother's feelings, for example, may change visibly before the observer's eyes. Behavior which at one moment is a serious threat to harm a child a moment later will have turned into play. Conversely, a mother may show genuine affection for her child, but a moment later its intensity will have brought him close to tears.

One fat, cheerful infant of eight or ten months was loved by everyone; yet no one could have been more of a target for the amusement of adults. He was constantly being fed, poked, squeezed, rolled about, and made to cry through frustrations of various sorts—all because he was so appealing and was loved so much. Such behavior assumes special significance in the light of Carr's (1963) postulation regarding the experience of events at a time when perceptual organization could not permit absolute certainty of interpretation, and also as an example of behavior he has described as the expression of sadistic impulses while verbalizing a different morality.

There are other relevant patterns. For example, much behavior within the Burmese family might make a child feel that he is not wanted and is not safe in the hands of family members; yet there is every kind of verbalization to belie this perception. At times children are teased until they are helpless with rage, but they are told that they are teased because they are loved. Parents threaten to give their children to strangers, who are defined as dangerous; yet they are told that no one is better to them than their own parents. Children are threatened with being beaten to death by their parents; yet they are told that parents love their children and will not hit so hard as step-parents would. Children are told about the kind of cruel behavior they could expect from foster parents if they were orphans; then they are teased by being told that they are not really the offspring of their mothers but were found on the road.

There are more blatant forms of denial than these in Burma which could disorder the relation between perceptual experience and ordinary corrective influences, but they are not as temporally specific as Carr has suggested, because children of 10 and 12 sometimes are punished for perceiving clearly a parent's true motivations or attempts at deception. One girl, for example, was punished for "talking back" and for not wanting to do the housework her mother did not want to do. Her real transgression, however, was an awareness of her mother's laziness. A boy was switched for being "too cheeky" when he saw that his soiled shirt had simply been folded and placed for him to wear a second time instead of washed, as his grandmother, who raised him, had claimed.

An even more pervasive pattern of denial than the preceding one exists in Burma which could have much greater impact on a child's ability to test reality. It is a pattern which seems to derive, on the one hand, from the assumptions made about human nature and man's relation to man and, on the other hand, from what seems to be an associated concept of self as acted upon. I call it the "ambiguous situation."

There are many ambiguous situations in Burma; in fact, ambiguity is a characteristic of almost every interpersonal relation in which there is not fairly complete harmony and accord. People relate to each other in a double-edged way when they are not on good terms or when there are uncertain elements in a situation. People protect themselves from such uncertainties by phrasing their conversation so that no one really is positive what is intended. By the time Burmese are adults they have become experts in presenting their views in such a way that two meanings are always possible. Very genuine concern for someone is at the same time a criticism of that person; the interpretation of any single statement depends upon the people present and their ties of loyalty.

If words were presented in cube form, the Burman would never be so foolish as boldly to present an entire face of the cube to another person in any group outside the family. He would present a corner instead, so that two sides could be present at once. Then, as situations later required it, he would emphasize one side or the other, without conscious awareness. In one situation he would believe that he really had shown one side of the block only. He would believe equally strongly in another situation that he really had shown the other side only. Thus he would protect himself in any eventuality. Denial in the face of accusations comes naturally under such circumstances and has the virtue of being expressed as truth.

Just as the words of villagers generally permit two possible interpretations by themselves and by others, so, too, does their behavior. It is largely an unconscious process, and people themselves are unaware of the two-sidedness of their own motivations and their own behavior. Consequently, everyone must always watch to see what others actually mean. Generally, the context and several particular factors in a situation will make one possible meaning more probable than another, but one is never really sure.

A consequence of the ubiquitous use of ambiguity in social settings is that people are reluctant to accuse others openly. Not only is the appropriate side of the "corner" of ambiguity presented as an expedient, but any direct accusations are met with denial. Such denial and the righteous indignation accompanying it are so convincing that the person who believes himself to have been mistreated in some way comes to doubt the validity of his own feelings. An accused individual very adeptly turns the situation so that the person challenging him appears to be the aggressor. He lets it be known that punishment awaits the challenger for even thinking such obviously untrue thoughts, let alone being so foolish as to speak them openly.

Because of the ambiguity inherent in so many situations, people are unwilling to act upon their convictions. They begin to doubt. An individual *may* actually be innocent of a transgression. He *may* actually have meant no offense. No one can know for sure, and to accuse unjustly is a sin that is punishable in the next existence. Furthermore, if someone acts upon his convictions and charges another with a transgression, his behavior generally is considered to be most inappropriate. An example of this is the case of a stolen *aingyi* ("blouse"). A village elder commented about the open accusations (Weidman, MS) as follows: "They're just trying to outdo each other. The owner is only loud-mouthed. At once she suspected K.K.A.'s wife and at once accused her. The thing to do is to keep quiet and watch. If they *see* her wearing it, or washing it, or keeping it, *then* they can go and accuse her. As it is, they're just being loud-mouthed and tactless."

As long as a person is not seen in an act of transgression he is safe. When faced with open confrontation he can always make his accuser look foolish, and no one will ever really know the truth of the matter.

These patterns are widespread in Burmese life. It is by means of such processes that Burmans come to doubt their own sense perceptions. They can be absolutely sure of some particular motivation or harmful intent on the part of another, and they will be made to believe that they have thought or seen or heard incorrectly. They will be made to feel guilty for having perceived a situation as they have. "What is said becomes truer than what is seen."[6] The sense of reality is thus disturbed. I submit that the need for such ambiguity and defensive procedures can be premised only upon some sort of assumption about a hostile world and a concept of self as inadequate in some particular way. It is my belief that this premise is of crucial importance in the use of projection in ego-defense.

The relation between cultural values and a reliance upon projective mechanisms in ego-defense can be examined best through use of a dyadic scheme. What, for example, are the respective stances of persons A and B when A is confronted by B with an accusation of a transgression?

Hypothetically, A assumes the nature of man to be unpredictable and potentially harmful. He perceives his environment as a hostile, dangerous place. His concept of self is that he is acted upon by such an environment. Consequently, he experiences himself as powerless in a potentially destructive world. The self in such a threatening environment must always be "good" and "right" and "blameless." Otherwise, "destruction," "abandonment," or "annihilation" would be the consequence. It is important, therefore, to deny any behavior which in the eyes of others might reflect unfavorably upon the self. There is need for ambiguity in interpersonal relations as a means of protecting the self. In the face of confrontation (accusations) by B, denial is relied upon. It carries the elements of "truth," however, for it represents only one side of a two-sided "corner" of ambiguity. Ambiguity in the social situation may, in fact, function through the mechanism of denial to prevent ambiguity in the self-concept.

So far as B is concerned, sense perceptions are initially believed to be true, to represent "reality." B believes that A has transgressed against him, but, in the face of a pervasive pattern of ambiguity coupled with the frequent use of denial, he begins to doubt. There is need but little basis for confirmation. This need may lead to open confrontation, which results in vociferous denial instead of confirmation. Furthermore, denial is coupled with transfer of blame by A to B. B is "punished" for thinking that he has seen what he has seen. He is made to doubt his own sense perceptions to the point that what A says becomes truer than what B believes he has seen. This paradox is unacceptable to the self. In the interest of a sense of reality, confirmation is essential. There is heightened awareness of the motives of A. Since human nature is defined as unpredictable and potentially harmful, such sensitivity, in all probability, will focus upon the hostile intent of A.

Frustration and great anger must be part and parcel of such a process. First, there is a denial by A of the validity of a perception experienced by B to be real and true. Second, A "punishes" B for believing his perception to be real and true and for acting upon that belief. Third, B experiences negative social sanctions from significant others for acting upon his belief. Since B's concept of self is similar to A's, i.e., a self acted upon by a potentially harmful environment, such a response may represent as much of a threat of abandonment, destruction, or annihilation for B as his own accusation did for A.

It becomes vitally important to B's experiencing of reality to substantiate the claim of the senses through further reality testing. This is difficult in a culture which defines human beings as unpredictable and potentially harmful, which views open confrontations as tactless and inappropriate, and which maintains that, unless one sees with his own eyes behavior which reveals the actual intent of others, there can never be certainty about what people really do mean or intend. One can only watch and try to establish a measure of certainty. When one sees with one's own eyes, one can act.

The patterns of interaction described above are common for adults in Burma, and children learn fairly early in life to relate in similar ways. Such patterns combined with those described earlier seem to include the essential features hypothesized by Carr as providing a basis for the eventual development of delusions in mental illness in instances in which the ego fails to maintain a sufficient degree of integrity. There may not be the disordered perception, per se, or the unalterable conviction about it which define the delusional process. There is, however, widespread denial of the validity of perceptions experienced to be true. There is perceptual ambiguity, and there is the beginning of a disordered relation between perceptual experience and reality testing. In accordance with the theory presented in this chapter, in these interpersonal and psychological processes lie the bases for a reliance upon projective mechanisms in ego-defense.

In the process described above B's experiencing of reality is at stake. As Weisman (1958) pointed out, more than sense perception is required for the feeling of reality: "the reality of an object depends not only on its emotional ties, but upon verification. In order to compel lasting belief, the processes that we call reality sense and reality testing must fuse in vivid, uncontradicted sensory experience." According to Weisman, reality sense is emotional, intuitive, and perceptual; while reality tests are intellectual, rational, and conceptual. The final truth of an intuitive proposition about experience depends upon reality tests. The first requirement of reality testing is the repetition of experience, and its essential function is "to determine to what extent our definitions are faulty, our meanings vague, and our knowledge thereby incomplete" (Weisman, 1958). The important corroborative element of reality testing, however, is that the common ordering principles of experience be shared by others.

Reality in interpersonal relations in Burma is built upon shifting sands. Attempts at corroboration frequently are thwarted. If reality testing fails to establish the true nature of an experience, how does one arrive at conviction? This is important, for, as Weisman (1958) stated: "It is in the fact of belief—the confidence we have in our own acceptances (propositions) and the willingness to take action on our ideas—that reality sense and reality testing are ultimately fused."

It seems that for B the "ambiguous situation" in Burma tends to create discrepancies between the beliefs derived from the sense of reality and the knowledge obtained from reality testing, so that he does not have the confidence and willingness to act. Is this not the kind of disordered relation between perceptual experience and the ordinary corrective influences of which Carr has spoken?

While I, at present, cannot demonstrate that such a process underlies a reliance upon projective mechanisms in ego-defense, it is possible to speculate about reasons why this may be so. Presumably, the co-ordinated interaction of reality sense and reality testing in the complete reality experience represents the individual's mastery and control. It signifies belief and willingness to take action on one's ideas. It should follow, then, that the greater the discrepancy between reality sense and reality testing, the greater the feeling of unreality, helplessness, and lack of control. In this context the concept of self is relevant, as is the experiencing of self. As Weisman (1958) said:

> Part of the intangible "boundary of the self" is marked off by what we can control. When we can control, there self is; when we are controlled, there the world is. Control and countercontrol are transfigurations of the self and the world.
>
> Action and volition . . . are two aspects of control. What cannot be controlled, even if perceptually recognized as part of ourselves, is still experienced as something alien which opposes the effective operation of the self. . . .
>
> Control is the capacity to alter objects and to determine experience. Control does not imply absolute authority freely to manipulate human experience, but refers to the *conviction* that the sources of experience are within us and are directly related to ourselves. . . . What can be controlled falls within the libidinal field of the ego and thus carries a strong sense of

> reality. Where libido extends, there is an extension of the
> self. . . . Analogously, any extension of the self used to control
> the environment is included to the libidinal field of the ego.

What Weisman was talking about here is the *experiencing* of the self, which in my view, is best considered in the light of a *concept* of self. Both aspects of the self need to be taken into consideration in the present context when thinking about a reliance upon projective mechanisms.

I have argued, for example, that the concept of self in Burma is that of being acted upon by a total environment (social, natural, and supernatural) in potentially harmful ways. I also have suggested that the actual experiencing of a self so defined would be as "powerless" to a degree. By returning now to the dyadic interchange used to analyze the structure of the "ambiguous situation," the significance of such a distinction for the defensive reliance upon projection in the maintenance of ego-integrity may be shown.

For person A, the only way a powerless self can avoid the threat of abandonment or annihilation by a powerful, destructive environment is to define the self constantly as "good" and "right" and "blameless." Whenever the environment encroaches upon a powerless self in the form of accusations of evil or error or blame, the very experience of self is threatened. For A the main problem is to escape "destruction." Denial, with outwardly expressed aggression, transfer of blame, or rationalization represents the projective measures relied upon. Presumably, a degree of increased "control" comes through counter measures aimed at destroying the immediate threat to the "existence" of the self.

B presumably encounters the same kind of threat to the experience of self when A denies so convincingly the perception B feels is true. For B two additional problems arise: Both stem from the disturbed relation between perceptual experience and reality testing; both give rise to attempts toward control through the mastery which accompanies the total, integrated experience of reality.

The first additional problem is related to the need to confirm a vivid perceptual experience believed by the individual to be true. This need seems to give rise to a heightened awareness of the hostile intentions of others. Such awareness represents at once a denial of powerlessness and an attempt to bring knowledge obtained from reality testing into better alignment with a belief arising from reality sense. It is an attempt at confirmation, a bid for certainty which serves as the guide to action. Does not this process also describe typical projective patterns—such as ideas of reference, which may lead ultimately, in the event of failure in ego-functioning, to the delusions of persecution so pronounced in paranoidal disorders?

The second additional problem is related to the need to extend the experience of the self through explanation. A self experienced as powerless and threatened with annihilation is explained by focusing less upon confirmation of the hostile intentions of others than upon the logical connections between events which "account" for the feelings of helplessness, e.g., simple themes or complicated plots as contexts for this particular type of feeling of inadequacy. Since "Reality sense is most vividly appreciated in self-perception" (Weisman, 1958), cannot an intellectual process of this sort be viewed as a similar attempt to bring reality tests in line with reality sense? By so doing, is mastery not therefore achieved? When one "knows" why one feels helpless, one feels some relief. Is it possible that explanation is the functional equivalent of control and that in a more elaborate way the self as powerless therefore is denied? Does this possibility not also describe projective mechanisms, such as ideas of reference or ideas of influence which may enter into delusional processes with persecutory or grandiose elements?[7]

In the one instance, the sense of powerlessness is denied by bringing reality tests into line with reality sense to increase the feeling of control. In the other, the sense of powerlessness is recognized but made meaningful through a logical system which connects isolated events in such a way that they explain the experiencing of the self as powerless. In the achievement of logical consistency comes conviction and something close to a complete reality experience. Does this achievement in itself not represent a different form of control and attempt at mastery?

It would seem, on the basis of the Burmese data, that the reliance upon projective mechanisms in ego-defense involves at least the three major configurations described above. It is my thesis that they are systematically linked to a concept of self as inadequate and the experience of self as powerless. Furthermore, it is postulated that such a concept of self has its ultimate genesis in cultural definitions of human nature, of man's relations to man, and to the social, natural, and supernatural environments.

In order to be experienced as powerless, must the concept of self be inadequate in a specific way, or do different conceptions of self as acted upon, meaningless, insignificant, and so on, act as functional equivalents to the degree that they all eventuate in the experiencing of the self as powerless?

On the other hand, are there other cultural definitions of man which are functionally equivalent to the degree that they also give rise to similar types of inadequacy in the self-concept and to the experiencing of self as powerless? How many possible variations in social structural features can be supported by similar definitions of man? Is the experience of self as powerless to a degree inherent in *any* hierarchically ordered society?

Implications for Future Research

Up to this point, I have focused upon systematic relations between specific features of cultural systems and certain facets of personality. While the assumption has been that these are fairly enduring linkages, it may be well to pose this as a question to be examined further. Just how closely or loosely linked are they? To what degree are there elements of lag in their interrelations? Additional questions along these lines might profitably be considered in further inquiry into the major hypothesis itself.

Earlier I suggested that the utilization of a broad conceptual approach of the sort employed in this chapter might lead to better understanding of the general reliance of the individual upon projective mechanisms in ego-defense and of the reliance of the individual upon particular projective techniques in different cultural contexts at different points in time and as part of a dynamic process capable of evolution and change toward increased or decreased pathology. Limited space permits here only the briefest indication of what I have in mind.

SOCIAL CONTEXT AND PARTICULAR PROJECTIVE DEVICES

Since denial is viewed as underyling defensive processes of projection, is denial of a particular self-concept associated with a particular type of projective mechanism? If so, in what ways do social context and cultural factors enter into such a relation?

Bhaskaran (1965) in India, who studied hospitalized Bengali Hindu paranoid schizophrenics of middle to upper socioeconomic status, suggested that: "Rarity of grandiose delusions in women is attributed to culture-imposed restrictions on women's aspirations." Similar suggestions have come from Chakraborty (1964), who looked into paranoidal symptomatology in Bengali Hindu schizophrenic outpatients. He reported that women of low educational level and men of middle to high educational level "shared self-confidence, were grandiose in their ideas and felt persecuted by magic, whereas men and women in reverse positions (i.e., women of middle to high educational level and men of low educational level) were unsure of their role and had fear of being ridiculed." Such findings seem particularly significant in a male-dominated society undergoing changes which allow women increasing degrees of freedom and recognition. I believe that the theoretical approach which has been outlined provides a useful framework for further inquiry along these lines.

Another question is whether the great use of projection in childhood is related not only to the emergence of a concept of self as a maturational stage of development but also to *de facto* degrees of "powerlessness" as a consequence of physical immaturity or social inadequacy (i.e., a peripheral position in the ongoing social system)? Is this kind of powerlessness also involved in the increased use of projection in old age?

DISEASE AND PROJECTION

Will the theoretical formulation advanced in this chapter help in understanding relations between certain crises and reliance upon projective mechanisms? For example, is the amount of denial and projection often seen in cases of progressive disease, such as cancer, or in cases of lost function through accident or stroke related to a redefinition of the self as "helpless" in the face of disease, or as "incapacitated" by accident and stroke? If projective mechanisms do not become more pronounced in situations such as these, is there a definition of self as something other than "helpless" or "incapacitated"? Are the significant areas of mastery in the experiencing of the self revised to exclude the damaged portion of the self? Does the patterning of reliance upon projective mechanisms differ according to whether such catastrophic situations affect the total body ("one's life") or are partially destructive?

MIGRANCY AND PROJECTION

If, as a great deal of literature suggests, paranoidal features play a prominent role in breakdowns of migrants—whether from one cultural system to another, or from rural to urban settings, or from one social class to another—is not some degree of "loss of control" always involved?

Take, for example, migrancy from one social system to another very different one. What could be more threatening to the feeling of mastery than to find suddenly that one's past cultural modes of communication, conformity, acceptance, achieving, regard by others, and self-esteem no longer fit the new cultural situation? Regardless of initial basic value orientations regarding man, nature, and supernature, is the experiencing of self as "powerless" sufficient to channel defensive maneuvers toward increased reliance upon projection? Pederson (1949) stated emphatically that this is true of refugees. While many have speculated about the frequent association of paranoidal disorder with migrancy and displacement, Tyhurst (1951) made explicit his view that "The uncertainty about self and the environment is responsible for the feeling of general helplessness of the individual at this time."

At the present information is insufficient to establish a fixed relation between migrant or refugee status and reliance upon projection in ego-defense, but it is my hope that this chapter offers a theoretical basis for inquiry.

HOMOSEXUALITY AND PROJECTION

Finally, since projection in psychoanalytic theory has been so tied to problems of homosexuality, a word must be said about this. It is apparent that I do not hold to the central Freudian hypothesis that projection is the result of repressed homosexual tendencies. My entire effort has been to set forth a very different hypothesis about projection.

I feel, however, that problems of homosexuality may be perfectly consistent with a hypothesis which relates reliance upon projective mechanisms to particular types of cultural values, perception of environment, concept of self, and experiencing of self as powerless. It is my feeling that the same factors which seem to be related to a reliance upon projective mechanisms in ego-defense also may be related to problems of identity which, genuine or spurious, may be phrased in homosexual terms.

Taking into consideration horizontal, relational factors, such as a feeling of inadequacy in interpersonal situations, ambivalence about others, impaired interpersonal relations, poor performance in social roles, and so on, and by applying them to a vertical dimension involving power and authority, control or lack of control, dominance and submission, we have a meaningful theoretical context for examining problems of overt or latent homosexuality or pseudo-homosexual problems of the sort discussed by Ovesey (1954, 1955). I suggest, in brief, that the most recent revisions of psychoanalytic theory regarding homosexuality and paranoia may be encompassed by a broader theoretical approach such as that presented here.

Summary

This chapter is a theoretical exploration of possible relations between cultural values, concept of self, and projection. Data from field research in Burma are utilized as a springboard and, in this respect, this chapter is to be viewed as a questioning, probing, first attempt to bring anthropological and psychiatric views on projection into close alignment.

Based on examination of some of the theoretical issues of psychology and psychiatry, it is proposed that there is a basically paranoidal structuring of personality which transcends the clinical picture of paranoidal disorder. It is hypothesized that a generic type of self-concept is linked to a reliance upon the ego-defensive mechanisms of projection which define the paranoidal process and that this concept of self, in turn, is related to cultural values.

It is my thesis that a generic concept of self as inadequate derives from implicit cultural values underlying the structure of the social system. When these values are internalized by the individual, they enter into the formation of the self-concept, influence perception, and help to explain the particular cognitive structuring which is inherent in projective processes. Specifically, it is hypothesized that such a self-concept derives from the way in which human nature is defined culturally and the way in which man's relations to man and to nature and supernature are defined culturally. This central hypothesis is examined in detail in separate discussions of cultural values and concept of self, and cultural values and projection.

On the basis of the Burmese data, it is concluded that in the Burmese culture human nature is defined as unpredictable and potentially harmful, as is also man's relation to social, physical, and supernatural environments. The particular type of inadequacy of self-concept is described as that of being "acted upon." The experience of self is seen as being "powerless" to a degree. These factors are thought to enter into at least three major cognitive and perceptual configurations involving a reliance upon projective mechanisms.

While the proposed relations are presented as fairly enduring for individuals within a single cultural system, at another level of analysis they also may be viewed profitably as dynamically linked to specific social contexts within various cultural systems and therefore as changing with social setting through time. A number of questions are raised for future inquiry about relations between social context and particular projective devices, disease and projection, and migrancy and projection.

Finally, because homosexuality is inextricably bound to the Freudian theory of projection, it is noted briefly that the same factors which seem to be associated with a reliance upon projective mechanisms also may be associated with difficulties in identity which might involve problems of overt or latent homosexuality or pseudo-homosexuality. The general theory advanced here seems to offer a more acceptable approach than do others to both projection and relations between homosexuality and paranoia.

ACKNOWLEDGMENT

Funds for this research were provided in part by the Supreme Council, 33rd Degree, Scottish Rite, Northern Masonic Jurisdiction, U.S., and in part by Research Grant M-945 from the National Institute of Mental Health. The major part of the field research was supported by a United States Public Health Service Pre-Doctoral Training grant. A grant-in-aid was also provided by the Asia Foundation through its Burma office.

NOTES

1.   Chakraborty (1964) included denial in the symptom category "intellectualization"; however, my view, in accord with that of Waelder (1951) and others, sees denial as underlying the ego-defensive processes of projection. He also included "persistent use of projection" as a symptom category; however, I see the persistent use of projection as defining paranoidal symptomatology, generally. While I have not attempted to extend Chakraborty's classification, I suspect that other categories could be included.

2.   The reader is urged to compare Schwartz (1964) with an earlier article by Hitson and Funkenstein (1959). Hitson and Funkenstein stressed the assumption of responsibility to initiate action in social situations, while Schwartz spoke of self-referral of responsibility. Hitson and Funkenstein spoke of directionality in the perception of environment, but Schwartz wrote of causation. Hitson and Funkenstein described the self as "acted upon"; Schwartz spoke of centrality arising from a feeling of meaninglessness and insignificance. Hitson and Funkenstein focussed to a degree upon guilt, and Schwartz, too, considered guilt. Schwartz speculated about conditions in the family which may be important in the genesis of a basically paranoidal outlook, and Hitson and Funkenstein presented evidence which bears directly upon this problem. While their study antedates Schwartz's speculations, it tends to support his hypotheses. Interestingly, in his discussion of therapeutic goals Schwartz has come very close to my theoretical position. He specifically formulated the therapeutic problem of the depressive patient as being related to conceptions of too

much power which may be destructive. He also stated that "In the treatment of the paranoid patient one needs not to decrease the patient's sense of power but rather to increase it. One needs to help the paranoid patient to recognize that he has more power to influence his environment than he thinks he does."

3. A discussion of these basic premises in terms of the concept of *implicit culture* is contained in Weidman (1965); also, *see* Kluckhohn (1951) and Kluckhohn, and Strodtbeck (1961).

4. The description of Burmese culture included in this chapter derives from the unpublished doctoral dissertation of H. M. Hitson entitled "Family Patterns and Paranoidal Personality Structure in Boston and Burma," Radcliffe College, 1959. The study is presently under revision for publication in book form under the title *Which Way Anger?*

5. Father Jaime Bulatao suggested during the course of the East-West Center conference that the reverse may be true, that the things nearest may be more threatening and that they are made less so by increasing the social and psychological distance. Certainly, it is true that one may protect oneself from harm in the form of anything new or strange or disturbing by increasing the social distance, and I feel that this is the behavioral response to the perceptions I have described. Anything new or strange or threatening that intrudes into the area of safety and the familiar is pushed back to a greater psychological or social distance— thus making the immediate social situation safe again. The threat itself is still great. It does not become less harmful because of greater distance. It becomes less harmful simply because it has been removed from all that is safe and familiar. After reflection upon Father Bulatao's comments, I believe them to support rather than contradict my position.

6. While discussing the Burmese material upon my return to Cambridge in 1959, a colleague, Dr. Nathan Altshuler, made this comment. It was his phrase which released this insight, and I am grateful to him for seeing so clearly what is actually involved in the "ambiguous situation."

7. Many investigators have been puzzled by sets of phenomena which I think are related: (1) the reported fact that elaborate and fixed delusional systems typical of classical paranoia rarely occur in many non-Western societies; and (2) the general observation that belief in witchcraft in such countries is typically unyielding to the force of scientific logic and explanation and is not corrected by reality testing.

   I would like to suggest, in view of the theoretical position presented in this chapter, that belief in witchcraft may serve the needs of an integrative process which helps to prevent a pathological reliance upon projection in the form of markedly psychotic episodes or elaborate delusional systems. The institutionalized belief in witchcraft is a cultural "given." As such it may serve as a ready explanatory device in situations of stress or crisis for personalities in which a beginning wedge has, culturally, been driven between reality sense and reality testing. In this connection I recently wrote the following comment upon a paper by Wintrob and Wittkower (1966) to Dr. E. D. Wittkower:

   > If there is weakness in ego structure; and if denial, projection, and massive regression are the main ego defense mechanisms,

then belief in witchcraft itself might be viewed as one
mechanisms of projection. As such, it has an inherent
logic just as does the delusional system of a frankly psychotic
patient. Such "illogicality" may be seen as the consequence
of perfectly logical processes. . . . If this is so, then we can
hardly expect the same logical processes to undermine what
they have created in defense of the ego. Furthermore, we
should *expect* this kind of attempt to structure "reality"
wherever the distinctions between self and not self, inside
and outside, become blurred.

In this context, the institutionalized forms available for use in
such cognitive and perceptual processes vary from culture to culture.
Thus, witchcraft and similar belief systems may serve as the functional
equivalents of a paranoidal structuring of "reality" in the maintenance
of ego-integrity.

If the theoretical formulation presented in this chapter is correct, such a reliance upon projective processes may serve the same
purpose in each case, namely, to defend an ego organized in terms of a
particular concept of self, to deny the experiencing of self as powerless,
and, simultaneously, to explain the experiencing of self as powerless.
Presumably, the goal is constructive in each instance, e.g., to bring reality
sense and reality testing into closer alignment to achieve a better sense
of mastery. The need for such integrative measures seems to stem from
an initial disturbance between perceptual experience and reality testing,
as postulated by Carr and similar to that which I believe is operating in
Burma.

REFERENCES

Bhaskaran, K. 1965. A psychiatric study of paranoid schizophrenics in a mental
    hospital in India. Transcultural Psychiatric Research 2:110–12.
Bindelglas, P. M. 1965. Therapeutic approaches to projection. Psychiatric Quar-
    terly 39:293–302.
Bullard, D. M., Jr. 1960. Psychotherapy of paranoid patients. Archives of General
    Psychiatry 2:137–41.
Cameron, N. 1959. Paranoid conditions and paranoia. *In* American handbook of
    psychiatry. S. Arieti, ed. New York, Basic Books.
Carr, A. C. 1963. Observations on paranoia and their relationship to the Schreber
    case. International Journal of Psycho-Analysis 44:195–223.
Chakraborty, A. 1964. An analysis of paranoid symptomatology. Transcultural
    Psychiatric Research 1:103–106 (abstract).
Coleman, J. C. 1964. Abnormal psychology and modern life. Third ed. Atlanta,
    Scott, Foresman.
Fleischl, M. F. 1958. A note on the meaning of ideas of reference. American
    Journal of Psychotherapy 12:24–29.
Hitson, H. M., and D. H. Funkenstein. 1959. Family patterns and paranoidal per-
    sonality structure in Boston and Burma. International Journal of Social
    Psychiatry 5:182–90.
Kluckhohn, C. 1951. The study of culture. *In* The policy sciences, recent develop-

ments in scope and method. D. Lerner and H. D. Lasswell, eds. Stanford, Stanford University Press.

Kluckhohn, F. R., and F. L. Strodtbeck. 1961. Variations in value orientations. Evanston, Row, Peterson.

Murstein, B. I., and R. S. Pryer. 1959. The concept of projection: a review. Psychological Bulletin 56:353–74.

Ovesey, L. 1954. The homosexual conflict. Psychiatry 17:243–50.

————. 1955. Pseudohomosexuality, the paranoid mechanism, and paranoia. Psychiatry 18:163–73.

Pedersen, S. 1949. Psychopathological reactions to extreme social displacement (refuge neuroses). Psychoanalytic Review 36:244–54.

Salzman, L. 1960. Paranoid state: theory and therapy. Archives of General Psychiatry 2:679–93.

Schwartz, D. A. 1963. A re-view of the "paranoid" concept. Archives of General Psychiatry 8:349–61.

————. 1964. The paranoid-depressive existential continuum. Psychiatric Quarterly 38:690–706.

Sullivan, H. S. 1956. Clinical studies in psychiatry. New York, Norton.

Tyhurst, L. 1951. Displacement and migration: a study in social psychiatry. American Journal of Psychiatry 107:561–68.

Waelder, R. 1951. The structure of paranoid ideas. International Journal of Psycho-Analysis 32:167–77.

Weidman, H. H. 1965. Shame and guilt: a reformulation of the problem. Paper presented at the 64th Annual Meeting of the American Anthropological Association, Denver.

————. MS. Which way anger?

Weisman, A. D. 1958. Reality sense and reality testing. Behavioral Science 3:228–61.

Wintrob, R., and E. D. Wittkower. 1966. Magic and witchcraft in Liberia: its psychiatric implications. Paper presented at the Meeting of the Association for the Advancement of Psychotherapy, Atlantic City.

Wittkower, E. D., H. B. Murphy, J. Fried, and H. Ellenberger. 1960. A cross-cultural inquiry into the symptomatology of schizophrenia. Review and Newsletter, Transcultural Research in Mental Health Problems No. 9:2–17.

17. Buddhism and Some Effects on the Rearing of Children in Thailand

PHON SANGSINGKEO, M.D.
Ministry of Public Health
Bangkok, Thailand

DURING the meeting of the World Federation for Mental Health in Bangkok late in 1965, some observers remarked upon the fact that Thai children are merry and happy as well as polite, obedient, and submissive. The question arose whether these qualities in Thai children might be an effect of Buddhism, the dominant and national religion of Thailand. It is a complex question which would require long study before a full, authoritative answer could be given. This chapter represents a preliminary attempt to assess some of the effects of Buddhism upon the rearing of Thai children and is intended to encourage further research on the subject. A brief summary of the principles of Buddhist teaching in Thailand is followed by a short historical account of Buddhism in Thailand and an exposition of the part which Buddhism plays in the present-day life of the country.

The principles of Buddhism practiced in Thailand are attached mostly to doctrine supposed to have been received directly from Lord Buddha and to have been emphasized by his elder disciples. The three main principles are: (1) To do good; (2) to leave bad things behind; and (3) to purify the mind. Purification of the mind leads to the attainment of the goal of happiness, primarily by following the Middle Way. Lord Buddha's first sermon to his five disciples stated that there are "two extremes that man should avoid, over-indulgence and practicing asceticism to excess. The middle path is recommended."

Buddha was enlightened in the year 589 B.C. when he found the four truths which later became his principal Buddhist philosophy. Known as the Four Noble Truths, these are: (1) Life is suffering; (2) the cause of suffering is desire; (3) elimination of desire will remove the cause of man-made suffering; and (4) the way, called the Eightfold Path, leading to cessation of suffering has eight elements: Right views, right intentions, right speech, right conduct, right means of livelihood, right effort, right alertness, and right concentration. In order to achieve the Eightfold Path, Buddhist followers are instructed first to practice five rules of morality. These five rules of morality or Five Precepts of Buddhism are recited again and again by Buddhists: They are: (1) To refrain from taking life; (2) to refrain from taking what is not given; (3) to refrain from sexual immorality; (4) to refrain from speaking falsehood; and (5) to refrain from drinking intoxicants.

There is a code of Buddhist morality for the laity, one section of which concerns the duties of parents and children toward each other and, similarly, the relations between pupils and teachers.

Duties of parents toward their children are: (1) To prevent them from sinning (emphasis on Five Precepts); (2) to instruct them in good conduct (emphasis on politeness, obedience, and loving-kindness); (3) to teach them arts and science; (4) to provide them with a suitable husband or wife; and (5) to give what is due to them when it is time for them to inherit. Duties of children toward their parents are: (1) To support the parents in return for their kindness; (2) to help them when help is needed; (3) to uphold the honor of the family; (4) to behave in such a way as to deserve their inheritances; and (5) to perform religious rites for them after their death.

Duties of teachers toward pupils are: (1) Never to neglect giving the pupils good advice; (2) to take care to teach them what they ought to know; (3) to tell them all that is to be studied or understood; (4) to praise them to their friends; and (5) to give them protection wherever they go. Duties of pupils towards teachers are: (1) To show respect by rising in their presence; (2) to wait upon them; (3) to obey them; (4) to attend to their wants; and (5) to pay attention to what is taught by them.

It is believed that Buddhism probably came to Thailand from India in the period of King Asoka, around 269–237 B.C. The Thai sect is of the Hīnāyana or Theravāda School of Southern Buddhism, unlike the Buddhism sects of China, Japan, and Vietnam which belong to the Mahāyāna School. It is believed also that Buddhism was introduced or reintroduced to Thailand from China around A.D. 77, which belief helps to explain the close relation of some Confucian teachings and Thai Buddhism. In any case in the thirteenth century when the history of present-day Thailand began with the rise of the Sukhothai Kingdom, Buddhism had long been taught in the region.

Present-day Thailand has an area of approximately 200,000

square miles and a population (in 1965) of 30,400,000. Of this population, 95 per cent are followers of Buddhism. According to the constitution, the king must be a Buddhist. His Majesty King Phumipol, the present ruler of Thailand, spent two weeks in residence in a temple at Bangkok and was ordained a priest. Many young Thai Buddhists enter the priesthood for a period of three months in order to learn to practice Buddhist teaching and to gain maturity.

There are about 22,000 Buddhist temples in the country and around 250,000 monks and novices. The Buddhist temple is usually the most beautiful and ornate building in a village and is the social center.

In olden times schools were attached to monasteries under the guidance of the abbot. More than 500 schools for the study of Buddhism have been established with more than 20,000 students. Two monastic schools for Buddhist monks operate at the university level and give a B.A. degree in religion. More to the point of this inquiry is the fact that, when a primary school law was passed in 1921 requiring every child between 7 and 14 to attend school, many of the newly instituted schools met in temple buildings. Even today, though the Ministry of Education has erected new, large school buildings on spacious grounds, almost 40 per cent of primary and secondary schools are still on temple grounds. Buddhist priests thus have close contact with school children.

Images of Buddha, as objects of veneration and worship, appear on small tables and altars in homes, schools, and temples. They are used in police courts and courts of justice where men are required to take oaths. Servicemen and boy scouts make their pledges before them. Buddha's image appears in committee rooms and in all government buildings where officials meet.

The Thai calendar itself dates from the death of Buddha, fixed at 543 B.C., so B.E. (Buddhist era) 2509 is used in place of A.D. 1966 and so on. Various festivals and ceremonies throughout the year contribute to the support of Buddhism and have become part of Thai life. For instance, in nearly all public schools there is a ceremony held once a year which is called Veneration to Teachers. It takes the form of chants before an image of Buddha, and students present flowers to the teachers as a symbol of high respect. Many ceremonies are monastic, among them Songkran Day, Buddhist Lent, and Kathin. Buddhist families go to monasteries to perform religious ceremonies on different occasions throughout the year. Other ceremonies connected with marriage, funerals, illnesses, birthdays, and housewarmings all are conducted in accordance with Buddhist rites. Buddhist priests always are invited to be present and frequently chant, deliver sermons, or receive offerings.

Buddhist priests are supposed to have no concern for politics. Their service to the community consists in teaching the doctrine, both in and out of the temple, in exemplifying renunciation, and in enabling householders to earn merit by means of offerings and attendance at worship ceremonies.

The priests' activities are thus twofold: the monastic ideal of study to achieve detachment and contemplation and the secular impulse to further education for the sake of public instruction and service. Because of the people's sense of respect and recognition for them, Buddhist priests are considered spiritual leaders as well as community leaders.

The Buddhist Association of Thailand, aiming to encourage and foster the study and practice of Buddhism, and the Young Buddhists Association of Thailand, aiming to propagate the doctrine in various ways through young people, are established in accordance with the study and practice in the monasteries. Both are organized and run by lay people advised by Buddhist priests in certain respects.

It is, of course, not claimed that all Thai Buddhists hold to the same religious views. Highly educated adherents are attracted to the psychological and metaphysical aspects of Buddhism; they maintain that Buddhism gives first place to reason, that it anticipated modern science, and that it is the most scientific of all religions. Some view it as a philosophy rather than a religion. Other adherents are drawn to the meditative and ethical aspects of Buddhist teaching; for them this religion is a way of life. Monastic seclusion and exercises in contemplation lead to serenity and long life, an antidote for the ills and strife found in society; their emphasis is on inner peace. There also are many who are avowed but not practicing Buddhists.

We could easily find Buddhists who do not know the true principles of Buddhism. Most Buddhists, however, accept their religion as a heritage of beliefs, teachings, and customs which in time of rejoicing or death meets emotional needs and provides answers to the mysteries of life. It supplies a doctrine of man, a metaphysics, a moral law, and an ultimate goal. For daily living it provides means of earning merit for oneself or others, devotional exercises, austerities, esthetic enjoyment, and assurance of safety and good fortune by means of devotion, good conduct, and amulets.

By gradual adjustment through the centuries Buddhism has become indigenous in Thailand, and its concepts and practices are established through the personal qualities of its adherents. The followers do not formulate the teachings, but come to require of religion such answers and rites as Buddhism can provide.

I shall turn briefly to the Thai family system and consider some other ways in which the rearing of Thai children are related to Buddhism. When the Thai people migrated from southern China two thousand years ago, they brought with them an extended family system which showed the influence of modified Confucianism. In Thailand the father is the head of the family, but as a rule fathers tend to leave the task of training children at home to the mothers or to the female members of the family in general. Thai children are taught to give high respect and obedience to their fathers, mothers, and elders. When the father dies, the eldest son has to take care of the household and his younger siblings. The first son commands high respect from his younger brothers and sisters, even when the father is still living. He may have to help in the education and support of the younger ones even when the father is still alive. Grandparents and aged relatives also are paid high respect. The grandmother is considered the best person to take care of the grandchild. When young parents are away and even in their presence, the grandmother may take care of the child or give advice.

It is a tradition of the northeastern parts of Thailand that a young husband lives with his father-in-law's family. This tradition may have arisen because Thailand is an agricultural country. When a young man wishes to ask for the hand of a girl, he is apt to be asked three questions by the girl's father: namely, can he farm, can he build a house, and has he experienced the life of priesthood? The last implies good education and maturity. If he can pass the test, he can get married, build a house on his father-in-law's premises, and help him farm. Polygamy is not prohibited, but at the present time it is dying away on account of economic conditions; legally, concubines and the children of concubines are not recognized.

When the Thai people accepted Buddhism as the national religion, the rearing of Thai children and emotional interaction in the family became more or less involved with Buddhism, continuing the basic practice from the remote past. The ungrateful child is considered to have very low morals and the public condemns him. The Thai consider Buddhist priests not only spiritual leaders but also trainers of their children, especially in cases of delinquency.

The Buddhist people also believe in placing all boys under the supervision of Buddhist priests in the monasteries; they consider this a chance to learn, especially to learn moral etiquette.

In order to study the way in which the characteristics of Thai children reflect their social environment, the problems of the children must be studied both in their own culture and cross-culturally. Ideally, one of the best sources for such a study would be information secured from the parents, but, owing to the difficulty of obtaining such data, I turned to referral symptoms of children sent to mental health clinics by their classroom teachers. For this purpose, I have studied and shall summarize the findings of the survey of the East-Gate Project in Taiwan (Hsu, 1966) and the data, also drawn from schoolteachers (Bower, 1960), obtained in the United States. In addition, I have used Gilbert's (1957) data from mental health clinics. The data on Thailand were collected by Malakul (1964), also from mental health clinics. Referrals to Thailand's clinics are from various sources including class teachers, social workers, and medical practitioners.

In Taiwan it has been reported (Hsu, 1966) that elementary schoolteachers are found to be much more concerned with the acting out type of disciplinary problems than with the passive type of behavior problems among children. After analyzing the list of complaints of 291 "problem children" reported by 121 class teachers among the 8,239 school children, Hsu reported the relative frequencies of the two types of behavior problems to be 4 to 1 in favor of the acting out type of problem. The teachers in the Taiwan society also complained that problems pertaining to the category of "inadequate learning attitudes" and "intellectual inadequacy" occurred at a higher rate than did asocial behavior problems, anxiety syndromes, and habit disorders. In Hsu's study no teacher complained of a single problem pertaining to the category of sexual problems, obsessive-compulsive symptoms, or toilet habits.

In the United States, however, it seems that the class teachers are as concerned with asocial types of behavior problems as they are with the acting out type of disciplinary problems (Bower, 1960). Basing his conclusions on the data gathered from 200 fourth, fifth, and sixth grade teachers on approximately 5,000 children, Bower found that "as perceived by teachers, 4.4 % of all the children in the classes were overly aggressive or defiant most of the time, while 6.1 % were overly withdrawn or timid most of the time." Analysis of the referral problems of children in clinic settings also indicates that asocial types of behavior problems are considered signs of maladjustment to much the same degree as are acting out disciplinary problems. In his analysis of the problems referred to the child guidance centers in four of the nation's five largest cities, Gilbert concluded that the most frequently cited reason for referral was "academic difficulties" (45 per cent) and that the relative frequency of the two types of problems differed little (30 per cent for aggressive and antisocial behavior and 22 per cent for asocial behavior problems).

The material from child guidance clinics in Thailand (Malakul, 1964) indicates that the referral problems most often cited are those in the category of academic difficulties. These difficulties comprised approximately one-third of all the problems presented by the 296 clinic patients. It also seems that aggressive and antisocial behavior problems were brought to the attention of the mental health profession more frequently than were passive, withdrawn, asocial behavior problems, with a ratio of approximately 2 to 1. The relative frequency of problems pertaining to the category of emotional instability and anxiety symptoms was almost the same as that reported by Gilbert in American clinic cases. Frequent somatized tension, headaches, sickness, vomiting, and the like were included in this group. The fact that the relative frequency of hyperactivity and motor symptoms was somewhat higher in the Thai clinic than in American clinics, together with the much higher frequency of aggressiveness in relation to asocial problems, may imply that the Thai culture is more sensitive to the acting out type of behavior problem and relatively less concerned with the asocial type.

The Taiwan data cited above suggests that also in Taiwan, where the child-rearing practices and the value system are considered much the same as in Thailand, society, as represented by middle-class schoolteachers, is more concerned with the aggressive type of behavior problems of the children than with the asocial problems. Worth mentioning in the Thai

clinic were the figures of 2.1 and 6.3 per cent for problems of sexual behavior and toilet training, respectively. These are similar to the figures given
by Gilbert, whereas in Taiwan the teachers reported no such problems. Perhaps in Thailand cases were investigated thoroughly in the clinic regardless
of the reports by teachers. Clarification of the implications of this finding
awaits further studies.

From these cross-cultural findings, it seems that American society
is equally sensitive to the aggressive and asocial types of children's problems, while Thai and Taiwanese cultures are more concerned with aggressive problems of children and less with asocial behavior. In the cultures
of both Taiwan and Thailand, quietness, politeness, and inhibition are both
expected and accepted.

Although no data have been obtained from the Philippine Islands,
whose people are predominantly Catholic, not Buddhist, Sechrest (personal communication) stated his impression that in referral problems the
ratio of the asocial type to the aggressive type is about the same as in Taiwan,
that is, 1 to 4. Terashima (personal communication) feels that in Japan
there are not nearly as many asocial problems as there are aggressive ones.

The mention of Catholicism is a reminder of certain religions other
than Buddhism which may influence child rearing in Thailand. The earliest
indigenous religion of Thailand, Animism, persists to the present in a large
section of the population, though its influence is weakening in educated
urban life. Five per cent of the Thai people are Christians, Hindus, and
followers of Islam. Although Thai people live according to Buddhist
ideology, in daily life Buddhist practices are mixed with traditions from
other ideologies, for example, the Hindu beliefs in Hindu gods, lustral water,
and so on; the Confucian extended family systems; and the superstitious
beliefs of Animism, the location of "spirit houses" within the compound,
and so forth. Thus Buddhism is not the only factor to have an effect on the
family and the emotional interaction of children.

No one yet has investigated the characteristics of Thai children
of different religions, but one has the impression that it would be hard to
differentiate between the Thai children of Buddhism and those of Christianity and Islam. They are alike in being polite, merry, obedient, and submissive. Sechrest has the same impression of Filipino children, who are
mostly Catholic. This similarity suggests that these characteristics may be
due to a basic similarity in family social structure throughout the Orient.

Apart from religion, certain other stabilizing influences may affect
the character of Thai children and adults, although research is needed to
verify these impressions and to demonstrate the mechanisms involved. For
instance, language also is a common factor. Dialects differ in different regions of the country, but each dialect is understood by all. The common
language may explain, to some extent, the unity of thought which is reflected
in the security of the family and of the children.

The institution of monarchy is also worth discussion, for in the society of Thailand it stands as a massive pillar. Monarchy has been for centuries identified with the country itself. During the time of absolute monarchy, the kings were "lords of life"; most of them ruled their people as a father rules his family, sternly perhaps, but with sympathy and understanding. There was a tradition of nearly selfless dedication to their people's good. Since 1932 the King has been relegated to the position of constitutional monarch. He is still beloved and still a guarantee of some sort of continuity with the past, and he helps to hold the nation together.

Political conditions also may be a factor to consider. Thailand is surrounded by Buddhist states, namely, Burma, Laos, and Cambodia. Only Malaysia, to the south, is a country of Islamic religion. Thailand differs from its neighbors in that it was never conquered or colonized during the period of imperialism but has remained independent since the birth of the nation 800 years ago, except for a very brief period of war with a neighbor which resulted in loss of sovereignty for a few years. Because of its long history of independence along with the institutions of monarchy and Buddhism, Thai culture and value systems are considered to have been well preserved and respected.

The economic condition of the country is considered more or less adequate. The country is agricultural, and the economic welfare of the country depends on rice, which is in surplus. Other products are rubber, tin, teakwood, and jute. Industry is developing steadily. The annual per capita income is $ 110 (U.S.). It is a country with potential resources still to be surveyed and exploited.

Any country with large areas not densely populated values highly the security of people and children. Thailand is facing a problem of rapid population growth at a fairly high rate of 3.2 per cent a year. Something must be done, for example, in terms of family health planning. For the time being, as in the past, people have enough space to live in with an adequate supply of food, and they therefore have a sense of security and stability. There has been no frustration to increase aggressiveness among the people.

In conclusion, I would like to make certain general remarks about religion before presenting my opinion concerning the effect of Buddhism on the rearing of the children of Thailand.

Religion, as a cultural factor, has distinct effects on society and child rearing in the family. Religion gives order to society. It brings man to terms with his environment. The status of interpersonal relations depends on the spiritual, psychological, and biological aspects of personality. The social effects arising from organized religious life tend to give social stability to the family. Religion transmits the best traditions, those moral and ethical principles which help keep families together. It also supports the individual as he grows up in his primary family group and, later, in the secondary family which is his own responsibility. The socially stabilizing influence of religion begins with the religious ceremony at birth and carries through various landmarks during a person's lifetime, so that he is aware of his place in the social order. Conformity to religious teachings reduces anxiety, and good mental health accordingly is to be expected. Throughout, man has to come to terms with problems of life and death. Religion, in this regard, too, brings comfort and security.

With regard to personality development, emphasis must be placed on the role of the family. The basic core of personality formation arises primarily from emotional interaction between a child and his parents and a child and his siblings. In this connection, religion is not likely to have as great an impact as is the family, but its importance resides in passing tradition through the family and creating a particular emotional climate. For example, religion reinforces the necessity of paying high respect to parents. In essence, then, one can say that, while the family is linked basically with emotional development, religion (while not denying its emotional impact) appeals at the intellectual level. In the relation between religion and the growing child, it also must be realized how negative attitudes may be produced, such as occurs, for instance, with the child who is in conflict with his parents and rejects religious teaching as an aspect of this personal relation. Extremely conservative and inflexible methods of religious instruction also may cause some antireligious attitudes among youngsters.

The influences on Thai personality are multifaceted, and Buddhism is one among others. Buddhism in Thailand, even though orthodox in its teaching, is not practiced by all the people in the conventional philosophical way; it is mixed with other faiths and traditions. The family structure and other socioeconomic factors involved in the production of Thai personality characteristics need to be further enumerated. My considered view, however, is that the Thai community, by and large, is in tune with the positive teachings of Buddhism; even in the present era when some young persons adopt negative attitudes the tendency is for them to come back to the teachings as they mature. The rituals have great significance for a majority of people, even those who intellectually are not able to understand the formal philosophical expressions.

Man is not meant to live up to only one specific, prescribed idea; just as man has to live, to eat, to possess, to love, and to be loved within his environment, he has to adjust himself to present-day life, especially in this time of rapid technical changes. The basic principles of his ideology, however, may temper to some degree his aggressiveness, jealousy, competition, and covetousness.

Thus the family value system in Thailand is marked by its persistent connection with the spirit of Buddhism. Buddhism, practiced by 95 per cent of the population, remains a very potent force among the common people. Their lives are still deeply touched by its compassion, even though one cannot tell whether it is deep enough to withstand the trials of a changing world. The Buddhistic influence still is pronounced in its effects on the mental health and emotional security of Thai children.

REFERENCES

Bower, E. M. 1960. Early identification of emotionally handicapped children in school. Springfield, Thomas.

Gilbert, G. M. 1957. A survey of referral problems in metropolitan child guidance centers. Journal of Clinical Psychology 13:37–42.

Hsu, C. 1966. A study on "problem children" reported by teachers. Japanese Journal of Child Psychiatry 7:91–108.

Malakul, S. 1964. Mental hygiene clinics' report. Bangkok, Thailand.

18. Westernization and the Split-level Personality
in the Filipino

JAIME BULATAO, S.J.
Ateneo de Manila University
Manila, Philippines

AT THE OUTSET let us assume the existence on this earth of an entity called the West, which has qualities of its own that set it off from the rest of the world, as Toynbee (1963) did in *The World and the West*. In general, it can be described today as Judeo-Christian in religion and ethics, industrial in economics, individualistic in sociology, democratic in political tendencies.

This was the West which in two main waves, Spanish and then American, joined in an encounter with a people now called Filipinos, but who at the beginning of the encounter were a set of scattered *barangays* (settlements of several families which served as units of government in ancient Philippines) speaking some 200 different tongues, fundamentally Malay in race, Animistic in religion, hunting and agricultural in economics, family centered in sociology, paternalistically despotic in political tendency.

When these two ways of life met in the Philippines, what was the result? Syncretism and Folk Catholicism (Lynch, 1956; Jocano, 1965) have been adduced as resulting from the encounter, but, within the individual himself, what happened? Was there a fusion like that of a new alloy, or was there merely a mixture of elements?

The hypothesis I propose is that within many, if not most, individual Filipinos, especially the urban and the more Westernized, two fairly distinct thought and behavior patterns exist, reflecting the two cultural patterns of their origin. The two have not fused organically into one but have created what may be called the split-level personality. The image is of two apartments at different levels, each of which contains a family, either of which communicates but rarely with the other. Some examples may serve to bring out this phenomenon:

1) Jocano (1965) described the simultaneous separate existence of two theologies in the town of Malitbog:

> [Roman Catholic saints] are conceived in Malitbog to have been so elevated to their present status because they possess power similar to those of the *enkantus* [environmental spirits] and that they could be manipulated for personal gains. . . . Many of the details of knowledge about their powers and how an individual can avail himself of their powers . . . are known to specialists . . . the priests. . . . On the other hand, knowledge concerning the *enkantus* and other environmental spirits are known to another group of specialists—the *baylans* or mediums.

> (The split: Two rival systems of "patron saints" as well as intermediaries are accepted simultaneously without feelings of inconsistency.)

2) A group of 36 workers on the lower managerial level were chosen from 30 companies for a training course in democratic management. Part of their training was a role-playing session demonstrating two leadership styles, the "coercive" and the "coactive." The word "democratic" was never mentioned. When asked which style they preferred, the vast majority chose the "coercive" because "the leader was strong." Later when asked in the abstract (independently of the role-playing) which they preferred, a democratic or a strong leader, they unanimously chose a democratic leader.

> (The split: On the level of words and abstract concepts, democracy is preferred, but, on the level of the concrete, the strong leader is preferred, and the inconsistency goes unnoticed.)

3) A group of teachers and guidance counselors (Bulatao, 1965), who insisted that they themselves always practiced democracy in their school system, attended a demonstration of group guidance techniques, where they sat in a half-circle behind a group of boys who were discussing the problem of barriers to parent-child communication. During the course of the discussion the teachers were angered by the lack of obedience of the young, by the fact that the young people thought they knew more than their elders, and so on.

(The split: Democracy is accepted as an abstract concept,
but, deep down, the teachers are as authoritarian as ever.)

4) A college student attending a leadership seminar addressed the guest speaker thus: "Sir, we now see that the main problem of youth is that the old people keep telling us what to do. They will not let us stand on our own feet. They will not let us think for ourselves. Sir, what can we do about this problem?"

(The split: On one level there is rebellion against dependency, on the other there is a deep dependency.)

5) In a prominent girls' school in Manila the girls in open discussion discovered that they cheated a great deal in school and that they cheated most in ethics class. They cheated to please their parents by bringing home good marks, and they helped each other during quizzes for fear of being labeled selfish or appearing not to join in *pakikisama* (a feeling of belongingness and ingroup loyalty).

(The split: The ethics they learn remains on the level of
concepts, while the ethics they follow is based on pleasing
the authority figure and meeting their own group norms.)

6) When Manila girls wearing short skirts sit down, they keep tugging at their skirts or else hide their knees with books or a handbag.

(The split: On one level the girls are modern and "liberated,"
but on the emotional level they are like their mothers.)

7) At a national student leaders' conference, whose theme was "The New Filipino," about 95 per cent of the delegates' time and energy was spent campaigning for a president.

(The split: On one level the young people look on themselves
as rebelling against the old Philippine ways, but on the other
level they conform completely to a value system which
emphasizes prestige rather than achievement.)

8) A civic organization was set up to protect civil liberties of Filipinos. When a bill came up in the legislature to make a certain book compulsory reading in all schools, the organization strongly supported the bill under the guise of nationalism, even though the reading of the book went against the conscience of a large segment of the general population.

(The split: Here there is sincere adherence to the idea of
democracy but a simultaneous adherence to old authoritarian
ways of imposing one's own values on others.)

9) A policeman in the downtown district in Manila goes fairly regularly to mass and considers himself a Catholic. Nevertheless, he col-

lects *tong* from the small stores in the district as protection money. He feels he has a right to it because he is their protector against gangsters.

> (The split: The modern Catholic principles of justice *vs.*
> a feudal attitude that the lord can tax those whom he protects.)

10) In an important research project upon whose outcome depended in great measure the revision of the language-teaching policy in the public schools, a group of teachers doing the research were trained in the latest refinements of the accurate handling of statistics. When pressed for time, however, they did not bother gathering any further data, but made up their own numbers and fed the manufactured data into the statistical mill together with the good data.

> (The split: The possession of the West's latest tools for accuracy alongside a value system where scientific accuracy has a low place.)

These illustrations indicate the existence of two systems at two different levels. The top level is made up of words and concepts borrowed from the West, appearing to have the same dictionary definitions (again verbal and conceptual) as in the West, though perhaps endowed with different meanings and apperceptions. The lower level is that of the native culture apparently unaffected by the veneer of Westernization. Furthermore, the two have not met each other in a real encounter, and it is only now and then that there is a weak attempt to try to reconcile the two by simple rationalization.

Characteristics

There is a real opposition or inconsistency between the two levels of the split-level phenomenon. The underlying gestalt or pattern of attitudes and behavior tendencies on one level differs from that on the other level as would harmonics from different musical pieces played simultaneously, one by the left hand and one by the right. Thus from the examples given above, one can draw up dichotomies such as freedom *vs.* dependence; need for scientific accuracy *vs.* need to get along without blame; need for honesty *vs.* need for loyalty to one's primary group.

The top level has a modern Western quality. Its elements are the norms and rites of Christianity, the teachings of democracy, and the techniques of science. Furthermore those seemingly affected by the split-level phenomenon are the segments of society which have been most exposed to Western influence—teachers, students, managers of businesses.

The two levels are different in the degree to which they are subjectively real. To use a college boy's phrase, one is "true" but the other is "really true." Thus, for instance, it is "true" that one should not cheat in class, but it is "really true" that out of a sense of *pakikisama* one must help a companion who asks for the correct answers to an exam. The "real truth" is the unverbalized reality of group belonging and group pressure, with all the "real" censures of ostracism which threaten one who is disloyal to the group. In the face of these "realities," the principle asserting the ethics of the other level fades into pallid hypothesis.

The incompatibility of both levels is in most instances either totally unconscious or taken as a normal phenomenon, *talagang ganyan* ("it's really like that"), and therefore accepted without too much awareness. Thus the young man in the example who asked "What can we do about this problem?" ordinarily never would notice his own dependent behavior. The members of the Civil Liberties Union are quite pleased with their own patriotic efforts to have the national hero's books read.

Although both levels contain norms for behavior differing in degree of explication, the lower level norm wins out more often than not. When such behavior occurs and is detected by a representative of the upper level, such as a Westernized teacher, priest, or foreign boss, the response is often an allegation of human weakness, *"Sapagkat ako'y tao lamang"* ("I am but human"). There is little, if any, real feeling of guilt, only a feeling of having failed an authority figure, a feeling which is in itself characteristic of the lower level norms. It is the absence of guilt which distinguishes the split-level phenomenon from that other phenomenon, seen all over the world, in which one goes against the dictates of conscience and suffers guilt as a consequence. Guilt is an inability to live with one's self. The split level is the ability to live on two different levels of the self, one part of the self overlooking what the other part is thinking or doing.

Historical Origins

It may be of interest at this point to speculate on the origin and dynamics of the split level in the Filipino. Historically, mention is made of a similar phenomenon by Phelan (1959), who showed how, in the process of Hispanicization of the Philippines, the Filipinos defended the integrity of their ancient culture by taking on the religious rites and external trappings of their conquerors while maintaining their old beliefs underground. In the course of time what may have originally been a political necessity evolved into a way of life.

The dynamism involved was that of defense, conscious or unconscious, against the felt encroachments of the authority figure. What Joseph and Murray (1951) said of the Chamorros of Saipan (who are of the same racial stock as most lowland Filipinos and have a similar religious history) is applicable to Filipinos, also:

> The attitude adopted by the individual Saipanese
> as a defense against fear is compliance. He conforms as
> nearly as he can to what he thinks is expected of him. On

the other hand, his underlying hostility and his need for the preservation of his psychological integrity confine this compliance to surface behavior. He does not allow the external pressures to penetrate his inner life, and in small ways which are not likely to lead to punitive consequences—delay, forgetting, misunderstanding, indifferent performances of tasks, and so forth—he indicates his largely unconscious repudiation of the superimposed authority.

The Filipino thus tends to create distance between himself and the authority figures—a distance serving as insulation from criticism. While this distance is mainly a psychological one, it can sometimes become geographic, too, as in the interview by Jocano (1965) with a man who had returned from Protestantism to Roman Catholicism, the reason being that:

> the priest does not have as many restrictions. He lets you alone, that is, to do what you like. He does not come here often and tell you "Don't do that," "Don't do this," and so on. He doesn't live here you know. But the pastor? He keeps coming to your house calling attention to whatever you do. Sometimes it is embarrassing because the neighbors talk. They know what you have done because the pastor preaches about them during Sundays.

The representative of the West is welcome provided he keeps his distance and does not criticize the other level, with which he has no business.

Social Dynamics

One way of conceiving the split-level personality is in terms of group membership theory. According to Freudian theory, a human being matures socially through a process of identification with the authority figures of his environment. Modern group theory has modified this view to extend it to group identity: one identifies with the group "spirit." The idea is that an individual "belongs" to a primary group and with lesser intensity to other groups. In each of these groups there are reference individuals who in great part wield the power to lay down norms of thought and behavior. The individual, under group pressure, patterns himself after these models and thus, as it were, takes them into himself.

In accordance with this view, one can explain the split-level phenomenon as the simultaneous allegiance to two groups or, more accurately, as the taking into oneself of surrogates of two groups which one can, in general, call the West and the traditional *barangay*. In other words, there are present in Philippine society reference models embodying the one or the other or, already in split-level form, even both simultaneously. It is these models which pass on their surrogates into the child and build up within him the split-level personality. The double membership then allows the child, like a man with double citizenship, to mix freely with two groups, at least as long as relations do not become too close and intimate. Perhaps it is for this reason that the Filipino can appear to get along so well with Westerners, even when in a Western country, until such time as he comes to realize that the other half of his split self longs for fulfillment and is not being fulfilled.

An interesting social manifestation of this "double citizenship" is the factionalization which occurs at the rare social gatherings in which representatives of the various social classes meet together, as on the occasion of a town fiesta or a big wedding in the provinces. Typically, the host places the Western foreigners, the mestizos, and the Westernized Filipinos in the parlor where they sip Western drinks and speak a Western language. He allows the others to locate themselves in another room or about the grounds, where they feel much more comfortable speaking the local vernacular. The Westernized Filipino, especially when politics demands it, can and does mix with the group about the grounds, and, while doing so, shows an amazing personality change. There comes an expansiveness of gestures, a flow of words, a surge of self-confidence. One is reminded of a truck which, after laboring up a hill in first gear, reaches the top and shifts into high.

Learning Theory

It is important to realize that the two levels are not of equal depth within the individual, or, as already stated, do not have for him the same sense of reality. Of course, one can, in broad sociological terms, explain this difference as one of intensity of group belongingness to the West and to the *barangay*. It is possible, however, even from learning theory, to account in great part for the difference by the quality of the things learned.

The contents of the level I call the *barangay* level generally are learned from early childhood experiences. It is at a very early age in Philippine society that one learns that only family members are to be trusted and no one else; that reasoning does not work while emotional ties do; that friendly relations to those in power are most important; that one is bound absolutely by such ties as *utang na loob* ("debt of gratitude") and *pakikisama* (a feeling of ingroup loyalty). A taxi driver from the provinces once told me: "I always tell my children that even though we are very poor I have passed on to them an inheritance of which they can be proud. My wife and I have taught them to be obedient and to kiss the hand of their elders. These are our riches." These are indeed some of the *barangay* values that are absorbed at an early age. This level is realistic ("really true"), learned from direct experience.

On the other hand, the contents of the second level, which can very roughly be called the Western level, are learned verbally or conceptually and do not have the same force as things learned from direct personal experience. Western words are just words, as is evident in the behavior of Filipino girls who have no difficulty singing "I wanna be kissed" but in reality will not let a boy hold hands with them. The words have no counterparts in the emotional reality of actual experience. Incidentally, up to very recent times the censors' norms for foreign films were quite different from their norms for local films, mainly because, despite technical crudities of Tagalog films, their words and situations projected a sense of reality, while those of foreign films remained harmlessly on the level of fantasy and did not involve the watching ego.

Accordingly, institutions, such as the school, which represent the West find that the material they teach remains on a verbal or conceptual level. Thus a school can teach Thomistic ethics and then discover that the students cheat most during ethics class, a victory of the *barangay* value of *pakikisama* and of the need to make a good appearance before the authority figure. A Lions' Club (another Western institution) may hold a Voice of Democracy contest where the young orators exhort their fellow youth ("the hope of the fatherland") to love democracy, freedom, and responsibility, but find that the young orators themselves had to have their speeches written by solicitous parents. There is here no hypocrisy in the Western sense. It is just that the ethics, the ideals, the platforms, the philosophies, the theologies of the West have been learned on a verbal level and have not been experienced in their existential reality.

Furthermore, there is a special difficulty with Filipinos coming from the remote *barrios* ("villages"). Their narrowness of experience very often prevents their grasping the precise meaning of representatives of the West. Take, for instance, the Western concept of respect for the individual, a concept which is the basis for the Western form of democracy. The Western speaker using the word "respect" may not even be aware that the image evoked by such a term is that of taking off one's hat to a superior or kissing his hand. Hence, to a Filipino villager the advice to "respect your children" makes no sense at all. So, too, when a Western speaker tells a parent-teacher association, "You must love your children," the message that is received very often is: "You must give your children what they ask for. You must be *mapagbigay* ['generous']."

The result is that verbal instructions are distorted to fit experienced actuality. To understand what the Westerner means by respect for the individual, one must have experienced such respect in all its qualitative nuances. To understand what the Westerner means by mother love, one must have experienced, in oneself or in another, the type of love the Western mother tends to give to her child with its goals of breaking dependency ties, which is quite different from the Filipino mother's type of love. In the absence of experience, there must have been a great deal of two-way communication between the Westerner and the Filipino.

One-way communication, especially when conducted in a foreign language, such as English, cannot help but lead to semantic distortion. The student will give back the correct words from the top of his mind while deep down he remains untouched by the foreign ideas behind the words.

Why Unconscious?

Why does the incompatibility of the two levels remain on the level of the unconscious? Why does the Filipino ego not integrate these two levels within itself? To answer these questions, I am reduced to further hypotheses.

The Filipino has not been brought up to do thinking of the problem-solving variety. His educational system is based mainly on rote learning. For instance, on such tests as the differential aptitude tests, the Filipino high school student may do better than the American in spelling but much more poorly in reasoning. The Filipino tends to give back by rote, without analysis, what he has been taught by rote and ignores problems of inconsistency.

The Filipino has been called a "hysterical personality" (Lapus and Reyes, 1963). Such a personality is extroverted and does very little reflexive thinking. Results on the Edwards Personal Preference Scale (Bulatao, 1964) show both the rural and the urban Filipino to be low on the "Intraception" scale, showing a low need to analyze feelings and reduce inner reality to conceptual terms.

The authoritarian set-up of most Filipino families and the *hiya* (a painful emotion arising from an experience with an authority figure or with society which inhibits self-assertion in a situation perceived as dangerous to one's ego) system make the individual very eager to please all authority figures. Hence, there is little motive for the ego to assert its own individual values or to try to reconcile conflicting claims of authority figures according to its own scale of values.

The colonial background of the Philippines has been such that the foreigner in power has imposed his own values and conceptual system in a somewhat one-way communication upon the Filipinos. The foreigner's authoritarian or semi-authoritarian ways have left little room for the Filipino to ask himself whether the new values and concepts apply meaningfully to him, or how they fit into traditional value systems. As long as the strong voice of authority was there, the pressure of authority prevented thought and self-awareness.

Process and Growth

From the above discussion and examples, the split-level phenomenon seems to be quite marked in urban areas and among fairly well-educated segments of the population, such as teachers, factory supervisors, and students. The rural inhabitants seem to be less affected and remain integrated within the pre-Western framework. They absorb the few, weak dribblings of Western culture in traditional syncretistic fashion.

Where the influx of the West has been not in driblets but in massive waves, the pre-existing system seems incapable of organically absorbing it. The culture cannot evolve fast enough to absorb the new influx in an organic, integrative way. Instead, the external structure of democracy and industry—*Robert's Rules of Order,* Civil Service procedures, mass elections, labor unions, and so on—are seized upon and allowed a place on the culture's surface, while deep down the personality retains an integrated system whose elements are predemocratic, preindustrial, and even pre-Christian.

The split-level personality can be seen as a stage in a process: the meeting of two cultures, but the absence of real encounter, at least up to now. In the meeting neither culture has been totally victorious or totally vanquished. Neither has a third something arisen to organize all elements into a relatively integral system (I say "relatively" because no culture is completely integrated). Such integrity comes only after much questioning and self-questioning, after much reflection on the Filipino personality. The past four or five years have produced a great deal of discussion on such matters, on values and culture change. All these discussions seem to be a part of a process leading toward the creation of a Filipino identity, a personality which is neither old Filipino nor foreign West but a new, creative fusion of the two.

REFERENCES

Bulatao, J. 1964. Personal preference of Filipino students. *In* Symposium on the Filipino personality. Manila, Psychological Association of the Philippines.
————. 1965. Conflict of values in home and school. Guidance and Personnel Journal 1:50–53.
Jocano, F. L. 1965. Conversion and the patterning of Christian experience in Malitbog, Central Panay, Philippines. Philippine Sociological Review 13:96–113.
Joseph, A., and J. Murray. 1951. Chamorros and Carolinians of Saipan. Cambridge, Harvard University Press.
Lapus, L., and B. Reyes. 1963. The practice of psychiatry in the Philippines. Journal of the Philippine College of Physicians. 1:161–65.
Lynch, F. 1956. Catholicism. *In* Area handbook on the Philippines. Chicago, University of Chicago Press for the Human Relation Area Files.
Phelan, J. 1959. The Hispanization of the Philippines: Spanish aims and Filipino responses. Madison, University of Wisconsin Press.
Toynbee, A. J. 1963. The world and the West. London, Oxford University Press.

19.   Philippine Culture, Stress, and Psychopathology

LEE SECHREST, Ph.D.
Department of Psychology
Northwestern University
Evanston, Illinois

FOR MANY YEARS there has been surprising controversy concerning the relation between culture and psychopathology. Although willing to grant enormous importance to culture in almost every other sphere of life, many writers—often quite sophisticated ones—have been singularly reluctant to suppose that culture might in some fundamental way alter psychopathology. Many other writers have been vociferous on the opposite side of the issue. The evidence for cultural influences on psychopathology has been reviewed elsewhere from various perspectives and very well (e.g., Lin, 1955, 1963; Opler, 1956a, 1956b, 1959, 1964; Parker, 1962; Wittkower, Chapter 27; Wittkower and Fried, 1959). Suffice it to say that if one takes the position that culture does not influence psychopathology a great deal of research must be explained away, and the explanations often are less plausible than the hypothesis they are attempting to impugn. Cross-cultural research often is rejected for methodological deficiencies (e.g., Berne, 1959), but one then must ask that equally rigorous standards be applied to research using other approaches. For example, careful reviews of genetic and biochemical research on schizophrenia (Jackson, 1960; Kety, 1959) justify little more confidence in these approaches than in cross-cultural studies.

Of even greater importance is the fact that the cultural hypothesis is not actually competitive with any other hypothesis. The cultural hypothesis and the genetic or biochemical hypotheses are not incompatible; rather they are complementary. Only the supporters of the most extreme genetic or bio-chemical position would suppose that environmental factors are of no consequence in determining either the probability of mental disorder or the form it is likely to take. The hypothesis I use in this chapter is that culture *influences* psychopathology, not that it determines it nor that it is the only influence which must be taken into account. As Opler (1964) noted, the paramount task is to discover how culture and psychopathology are related.

Culture can affect the phenomenon of mental disorder in a variety of ways, and also several aspects of psychopathology. Cultures can differ with respect to overall frequency of mental disorder, the range of psycho-pathological manifestations, the frequency of various psychiatric syndromes, the type of symptoms, and the content of symptoms. The present investigation focuses upon differences in symptoms between samples of Filipino and American hospitalized psychiatric patients and upon the relation of these differences to Philippine culture.

Most cross-cultural and intracultural studies of psychopathology have been at the level of syndromes or presumed "diseases" such as schizophrenia, obsessive-compulsive neurosis, and the like. In accounting for data presented or in suggesting the possibility of different forms of the same disorder, many writers have had to pay considerable attention to specific symptoms. Most investigators who have not emphasized traditional diagnostic categories (e.g., Leighton *et al.*, 1963) have studied *patterns* of symptoms. A few studies, however, have made specific symptoms the focus of the study. Zigler and Phillips (1961a) have studied symptoms of American psychiatric patients and have reported data on frequencies of specific symptoms. Schooler and Caudill (1964) have reported on symptoms of Japanese patients; Enright and Jaeckle (1963) have reported on symptoms of Japanese and Filipino schizophrenics in Hawaii (*see also* Katz, Gudeman, and Sanborn, Chapter 9); and Meadow and Stoker (1965) have compared symptoms of Mexican-American and Anglo-American hospitalized patients. I reported in an earlier paper (Sechrest, 1963) preliminary data on symptom frequency among Filipino psychiatric patients.

Although the study of broad categories of mental disorder certainly is justified and should be continued, there are also good reasons to wish for the simultaneous and complementary study of specific symptoms, both within a culture and cross-culturally. First, numerous studies have shown the un-reliability of psychiatric diagnoses (e.g., Ash, 1949; Mehlman, 1952; Zigler and Phillips, 1961b), and if low reliability is a problem within the psychiatric profession in the United States, it is likely to be even more of a problem in a cross-cultural comparison based not only on patients in different cultures but upon diagnoses by psychiatrists with perhaps very different orientations. Since symptoms are closer than diagnoses to behavior and to observations which are actually made, they should be more objectively ascertainable than are diagnoses. Leighton and his associates (Leighton *et al.*, 1963) have shown that it is possible to get good agreement between the ratings of symptom patterns by psychiatrists. At the very least, the study of symptoms extends and complements the study of diagnostic categories. If the specific symptoms found are consistent with expectations based on diagnoses, so much the better; if not, the finding is a useful guide for future research.

Second, many writers have complained about and demonstrated the heterogeneity within diagnostic groups (e.g., Zigler and Phillips, 1961b), the differences very often seeming to be about as great within as between groups. Thus, even if one finds the same proportion of schizophrenics in two cultures, there is no assurance that the schizophrenics are equivalent, and some investigators even have denied that the same phenomenon is being studied in two cultures in spite of the use of the same diagnostic label (e.g., Carothers, 1953). Again, the study of symptoms is quite likely to complement the study of diagnoses by revealing more clearly the exact nature of similarities and differences in psychopathological manifestations.

Finally, since symptoms are closer than diagnoses to behavior, because they are either observed behaviors, e.g., destructive, or first-order inferences from behavior, e.g., delusional, symptoms are closer to the cultural forms which underlie a society's behaviors. It is far easier to trace the cultural factors which produce an excess of delusional fears of being poisoned than it is to trace the factors which result in an excess of manic-depressive reactions. Understanding of the almost certainly intricate relation between culture and psychology will be furthered by the tracing of distinct lines of cultural influence. At the present level of technical and methodological development, greater tasks than this may be too ambitious. Thus the cross-cultural study of symptoms is amply justified. If granted that indubitably they do not give the whole picture (cf. Yap, 1952), they give at least part of it, perhaps with more clarity than is otherwise likely.

There are many cultural variations which may have some effect on the occurrence of psychopathology. Leighton and Hughes (1959) have suggested several very likely possibilities, among which are four to be considered here in special relation to Philippine culture. These are cultural stress, protection from stress, sanction, and facilitation, all of which are either explicit or implicit in the discussion of Leighton and Hughes.

Arsenian and Arsenian (1948) have suggested that cultures can be arranged along a continuum of "easy-tough" according to the demands made on individuals and the provision of reasonable ways to meet the demands. Though tough cultures are stressful to live in, the relation between stress of any kind, whether societal or individual, and psychopathology, is as yet far from understood. Evidence supporting a strong relation between stress and mental disorder is not common, and there is a good bit of negative evidence. Nonetheless, the hypothesis relating stress to mental disorder is difficult to relinquish on theoretical grounds and remains one of the most commonly invoked explanations for the occurrence of mental disorder.

Just as some cultures may tend to expose their members to stress, so may some protect their members from stress in some manner (Caudill,

1958). Such protection could take numerous forms; probably one of the most likely is support and help offered the stressed individual by friends, family, or cultural institutions, such as shamans, medical personnel, and legal authorities. Cultures also may protect their members from stress by benign attitudes and practices with respect to areas of behavior which are often fraught with difficulty, e.g., sex, dependency.

Cultures also may tend to foster various kinds of psychopathology by either sanctioning or facilitating attitudes and behaviors in critical areas, one notable example being suicide. Probably some societies permit if not encourage many other kinds of problem solving attempts which would be considered reprehensible and in need of suppression in others, e.g., somatic complaints, hostile aggression, paranoid projection, withdrawal, and the like. Similarly, cultures may encourage beliefs, such as in witchcraft, around which delusions may be formed.

This analysis of Philippine culture stems from a variety of research and observations carried out over a considerable period of time by several investigators. The study of symptoms of mental disorder is my own and represents an extension of research previously reported (Sechrest, 1963). A description of the study and the data are given below. For comparative purposes, data also are given for a sample of American state hospital patients and reference is made to the work of other investigators.

Stress and Frequency of Mental Disorder in the Philippines

Before presenting the data on symptoms, it is relevant to note something about the overall frequency of mental disorder in the Philippines. As I have noted elsewhere (Sechrest, 1964), there are several preliminary investigations in which different approaches to the estimate of frequency of mental disorder converge on an estimate of about one case per 1,000 population, a figure well below those usually reported for other cultures (Lin, 1963; Primrose, 1962). The estimate given is probably lower than would be found by more intensive surveys, but for reasons detailed in the earlier report it seems unlikely that it is off by a factor of more than two.

Certainly there are a good many sources of physical stress in the Philippines for the great majority of people in the working and peasant classes. Unemployment and underemployment are chronic conditions of existence for a very high proportion of the population, and economic privation is virtually the rule. "Folk" theories of mental disorder put considerable emphasis on the importance of physical stresses; it is common to find psychopathology of very serious proportions explained in terms of such stresses as going hungry, working too hard, and being cold (Sechrest, MS). Nonetheless, such stresses do not seem to be associated with an especially high frequency of mental disorder elsewhere, and their importance in the Philippines can be questioned.

Aside from physical stresses, the culture of the Philippines probably falls on the "easy" side of the continuum proposed by Arsenian and Arsenian (1948). As others have suggested (Guthrie, 1961), the demands on the Filipino by his culture are not extensive, and most probably are met relatively easily by passive acceptance and do not require active coping responses. Honigmann (1954) listed six cultural factors related to level of stress, only two of which seem to be of special significance in the Philippines. Moreover, there are several important attitudinal and value characteristics of Philippine culture which make possible a rather optimistic and non-anxious outlook on life (Guthrie, 1966). The strong family system provides the distressed individual extensive and important sources of emotional support, thus ameliorating many unpleasant circumstances. The stresses which are to be found in Philippine culture are discussed later.

A Comparative Study of Symptoms
of Philippine and American Psychiatric Patients

The data reported here are an extension of a study published in 1963, the number of cases having been increased and data from an American sample added. All the data for this investigation are based on psychiatric patients from two large hospitals: the Philippine National Mental Hospital (NMH), Mandaluyong, Rizal, Philippines, and Chicago State Hospital (CSH). Both hospitals are located in urban areas; NMH draws perhaps 30 per cent of its cases from rural areas; all CSH patients resided in Chicago or suburban areas at the time of their admission, but some of the Chicago patients had rural backgrounds. Because of the uncertainties of psychiatric diagnosis, no effort was made to equate the two samples on the basis of diagnostic categories. In order to make the two samples approximately equivalent, however, the CSH sample was selected so as to exclude patients with psychoneurotic, senile, and organic diagnoses, all three of which appeared infrequently or not at all in the Philippine sample.

In neither hospital was it possible to sample cases randomly, but attempts were made to keep the sampling nonsystematic so that no obvious biases intruded. NMH cases were selected from both active and nonactive files, but all the inactive cases had been discharged within the preceding five years. Thus there was some assurance that the sample would not be heavily biased in the direction of chronic, residual cases. All CSH cases came from active files owing to the unavailability of inactive files. The NMH cases were obtained by pulling out case folders, with as little regard as possible to characteristics such as name of patient, location in the file, or thickness of the folder. In CSH an IBM list was obtained of all active cases except for those with an inappropriate diagnosis, and every fourteenth case was selected until records of 100 males and 100 females had been examined.

The symptoms of each patient were written on a data sheet along with various other information. All symptoms were recorded, including the complaints that led to hospitalization, the symptoms discerned upon admission, and any other symptoms noted during the patient's hospitalization. In cases of multiple admissions, symptoms were noted for each admission. In addition, an attempt was made to determine the time of onset of the disturbance and any precipitating factor associated with the onset.

Since the present investigation concentrated on symptoms recorded in hospital records of patients, those associated with long-term hospitalization and deterioration almost certainly are underrepresented, because little in the way of symptomatology is ever recorded about a patient once he has been admitted to either NMH or CSH. Nearly all the symptoms available for study were those recorded in the presenting complaint and in the interview upon admission. After that time either the interest of the staff in symptomatology or their time to make note of it declines rapidly.

All symptoms first were recorded exactly as they were described and later categorized as in Table 1. Because of the large number of categories, the categorizations appeared likely to be reliable, and a check on agreement between two judges in categorizing 200 symptoms indicated 98 per cent agreement.

It is necessary to define some of the symptom categories employed:

Delusions: All delusions were categorized in a straightforward way as involving probable pleasant, satisfying feelings (e.g., delusion of wealth) or unpleasant, upsetting feelings (e.g., delusion of persecution).

Violent, dangerous: A physical or serious verbal threat to the welfare of other persons, including the possession of potentially dangerous weapons. Verbal threats, usually to kill, were in most instances associated with other threatening behaviors, such as carrying weapons or physical attacks. Any degree of physical attack was counted as violent.

Harmful to self: Behavior which caused or could cause minor injuries to the self, e.g., burning one's skin with a cigarette.

Somatic delusion: A belief about the anatomy or physiological functioning which is clearly untenable or bizarre from the standpoint of common consensus about the body, e.g., a belief that one's blood is turning to water or that one's insides are rotting.

Silly, bizarre: Behavior that is suggestive of especially poor judgment about social acceptability or that is markedly deviant, e.g., self-decoration, odd costumes, unusual mannerisms.

Primitive: Behavior at a low level of organization or representing a threat to survival through inferior judgment, e.g., hoarding of useless objects, swallowing inedible objects, smearing feces.

Nuisance behavior: Behavior which interferes with the normal course of other people's lives, but which is not actually dangerous, e.g., blocking traffic, petty theft, giving away family food.

Religiosity: Indication of excessive religious activity (excessive in the judgment of the person describing it), e.g., "always praying," "goes around preaching to everybody."

Homosexuality: Includes only indications of overt homosexuality.

Criminal activity: Indications that the patient engaged in serious criminal activity during the period just preceding onset, during onset, or at some later time. Criminal activities counted include grand larceny, narcotics offenses, interstate transportation of stolen motor vehicles, and robbery.

In Table 1 is a percentage distribution of the symptoms of the patient samples displaying the various symptoms noted in the records. The findings for NMH patients generally are consistent with those reported by other investigators (Mariano, 1962; Varias, 1965) for Philippine psychiatric patients, and, where comparable, the findings for the CSH sample are similar to those for other American samples (Meadow and Stoker, 1965; Zigler and Phillips, 1961a).

Because of my special interest in the nature of delusions and hallucinations, the Philippine sample was augmented by the selection of additional patients whose records indicated either delusions or hallucinations or both. The number of cases presented in Tables 2 and 3, which show percentage distributions of the nature of hallucinations and delusions, respectively, is thus larger than the samples for all symptoms. It also should be noted that the percentages given for each delusion or hallucination are the percentages only of those patients who had delusions *or* those who had hallucinations, not the percentages of the total sample, as given in Table 1 for all symptoms.

Interpersonal Stress and Symptoms

Almost certainly, the important stresses in the Philippines arise out of interpersonal relations, and there is good reason to believe that some aspects of interpersonal relations are more stressful in the Philippines than elsewhere. Although many observers have commented on the "smoothness" of interpersonal relations in the Philippines (Guthrie, 1961; Hollnsteiner, 1963; Lynch, 1964), one is probably quite wrong if one gets a picture from such writings of easy, tension-free intercourse that runs along nicely with little attention. In fact, interpersonal relations in the Philippines are no smoother than they are elsewhere; they may even be much more difficult. Any achievement of surface smoothness is through careful, constant monitoring and nearly transparent deviousness to obscure difficulties. For example, Filipinos are masters of euphemism, but they are so aware of its use that it fools almost no one. All it does is to preclude the occurrence of an immediate quarrel. The very emphasis in the Philippines on smoothness and care in interpersonal relations shows how difficult they are.

Behind a good bit of interpersonal difficulty in the Philippines is a strong sense of *amor propio* (Guthrie, 1961). The Filipino's self-esteem is extremely important to him, and for him there is a constant risking of it in situations that would be regarded as impersonal or trivial in other societies. Filipinos are easily humiliated, and they regard humiliation as an especially unpleasant experience. In some unpublished data of mine a sentence completion test containing the stem "To be humiliated _____" produced typically from Filipinos such responses as "is the worst thing," "would be horrible," and "must be avenged." American responses of a kind not found at all in the Filipino sample were "is not important," "is only a temporary blow to one's ego," and "can be a learning experience." The Filipino constantly is exposed to the possibility of being "put down" in some manner, but perhaps even more of a strain is imposed by the necessity of avoiding the humiliation of someone else. Thus interpersonal relations are characterized by a superficial aura of good will and an underlying strain and lack of openness.

Firm evidence is not abundant for my thesis that interpersonal relations in the Philippines are especially difficult, and much of what has been said is admittedly conjectural, but there are some indications which point in this direction. First, the homicide rate in the Philippines is unquestionably high. Bulatao (1963) has said that the rate in Manila is 11 times the rate in New York (an overestimate in all probability, since data which I am currently processing [Sechrest, MS] would place the rate at about double the rate for Chicago). Even more important perhaps are the motives for homicide in the Philippines. It is clear from my data that homicides involving friends and acquaintances are more frequent in the Philippines than in the United States and that they develop more frequently out of momentarily difficult interpersonal situations. Filipinos less often kill family members than do Americans, but they more often kill strangers, again in situations in which momentary difficulties in interpersonal relations develop. A fairly typical Philippine example of a situation leading to homicide involving strangers or acquaintances is one in which a Filipino on a drinking spree invites another to have a drink with him and is grievously affronted when the other refuses.

A second line of evidence comes from the stated precipitating circumstances involved in the onset of serious psychiatric disturbance in the Philippines as compared to those in the United States. In those cases for which some factor is either stated to be associated with onset or in which the connection is otherwise obvious, a larger proportion of Philippine cases (42 per cent) fall into the interpersonal category than do American cases (26 per cent).

CONFLICT BETWEEN STATUS AND MODESTY

Nearly everyone would agree that the emphasis on personal status in the Philippines is very strong (e.g., Minturn and Lambert, 1964). Titles are employed with abandon; great emphasis is placed on rankings in examinations, which are published in all the papers; much attention is paid to society news, and so on. When strangers meet, there is a good bit of social sparring until their respective status is determined; but once that status is learned all else in the relation follows naturally. Brothers and sisters are quite aware of age status, which determines so many of their interactions. Many more examples could be given. At the same time, one of the para-

Table 1: Percentage Distribution of Symptoms of Patients in the Philippine National Mental Hospital and Chicago State Hospital*

Symptom	Philippine National Mental Hospital		Chicago State Hospital	
	Male (N=105)	Female (N=105)	Male (N=100)	Female (N=100)
Impairment of Normal Function				
Sleep	71	80	33	44
Appetite	19	32	33	22
Appearance	23	15	18	19
Work	04	05	28	11
Speech				
Excessive	09	21	01	07
Talk to self	36	36	09	19
Incoherent	15	10	22	11
Mute, uncommunicative	18	22	11	15
Hallucinations and Delusions				
Hallucinations				
Auditory	59	58	49	48
Visual	33	29	07	07
Delusions				
Unpleasant	52	37	58	59
Pleasant	10	14	02	12
Other	03	06	01	—
Ideas of reference	10	14	38	24
Somatization				
Somatic complaint	19	23	27	15
Somatic delusion	06	04	22	15
Hostility				
Irritable, quarrelsome	22	31	44	33
Violent, dangerous	57	50	18	26
Destructive	28	21	11	04
Activity Level				
Sing, dance, and shout in public	30	29	06	11
Laugh, cry inappropriately	35	46	09	30
Hyperactive	14	13	13	11
Wander aimlessly	30	23	07	—
Underactive	17	05	11	04
Immobility	08	05	04	07

(Continued)

Table 1: (Continued)

Symptom	Philippine National Mental Hospital		Chicago State Hospital	
	Male (N=105)	Female (N=105)	Male (N=100)	Female (N=100)
Withdrawal				
Blank stare	22	17	11	11
Unsociable, seclusive	12	10	13	04
Withdrawn	04	04	09	15
Inaccessible	10	16	07	02
Dull	14	01	06	01
Depression and Self-harm				
Sad, depressed	03	10	22	38
Ideas of guilt	02	02	06	07
Suicidal attempt, threat, gesture	07	09	27	26
Harmful to self	10	10	04	03
Fear				
Fearful	06	10	39	37
Suspicious	03	06	22	11
Phobic	08	02	14	09
Inferior Judgment and Manneristic				
Silly, bizarre	15	07	04	15
Grandiose	05	02	11	–
Primitive	06	07	01	04
Obscene, sexy	07	07	11	11
Nuisance behavior	10	08	09	04
Denuditive	08	03	06	–
Mannerisms	17	14	06	07
Conduct Disturbance				
Use of alcohol	07	02	43	15
Homosexuality	–	–	06	11
Criminal activity	–	–	25	04
Miscellaneous				
Religiosity	09	08	04	07
Obsessions	–	–	05	04
Compulsions	01	–	06	03
Disoriented	01	02	04	02

*   Figures do not add up to 100 per cent because symptoms are multiply categorized.

Table 2:   Percentage Distribution of Nature of Hallucinations of Patients
in the Philippine National Mental Hospital and Chicago State
Hospital*

Nature of Hallucinations	Philippine National Mental Hospital		Chicago State Hospital	
	Male (N=171)	Female (N=225)	Male (N=60)	Female (N=60)
Auditory				
Unspecified or innocuous	57	45	50	43
Knocking, buzzing, or ringing	08	01	05	07
Animals, birds	03	02	–	–
Threats	14	19	08	07
Uncomplimentary remarks	11	08	43	30
Complimentary or				
pleasant remarks	02	07	02	07
Indecencies	01	01	03	10
Commands	19	24	33	30
Religious	09	20	10	15
Other	–	02	–	07
Visual				
Unspecified persons or things	17	15	12	10
Spirits, ghosts	09	11	–	–
Dead people	07	12	10	07
Devils, demons	02	04	05	03
Threatening	02	06	05	13
Bizarre	05	04	08	08
Religious	09	18	08	15
Fire, insects, animals	04	05	–	03
Living family member	01	02	02	03
Other	–	01	–	–
Olfactory	01	04	08	07
Tactile	–	–	02	07

*   Figures do not add up to 100 per cent because hallucinations are multiply categorized.

Table 3: Percentage Distribution of Nature of Delusions of Patients in the Philippine National Mental Hospital and Chicago State Hospital*

Delusions	Philippine National Mental Hospital		Chicago State Hospital	
	Male (N=123)	Female (N=201)	Male (N=60)	Female (N=60)
Threatening				
Threat of being killed, fear of being killed	28	16	35	47
Other threats, enemies	46	52	40	47
Fear of poisoning	07	08	02	12
Punishment, guilt	03	04	13	10
Others "angry"	11	05	02	02
Witchcraft	02	07	–	–
Pleasurable				
Grandeur				
Wealth and fame	11	13	08	05
Power	11	10	07	03
Other	01	05	02	03
Control				
External control of behavior	03	–	15	07
External control of thought	01	01	10	12
Thought diffusion	03	01	07	07
Other				
Sexual	03	20	07	07
Jealousy, infidelity	09	19	08	05
Uncomplimentary belief about another person	01	04	03	03
Somatic	07	06	33	23
Religious	07	21	10	18
Bizarre	15	09	15	25
Accusatory, i.e., of others	03	05	08	–
Homosexual	01	–	12	–
Miscellaneous	10	19	15	12

* Figures do not add up to 100 per cent because many delusions are multiply categorized.

mount values in the Philippines is personal modesty and a proper sense of *hiya* (Bulatao, 1965), an untranslatable term which has to do with an individual's recognition of his proper position with respect to others and his capacity to experience "shame" when he disregards that position. One should not be boastful, and one should not attempt to rise above one's peers in any way. One of the most scornful comments that one Filipino can make about another is that "he thinks he is too good for the rest of us." An individual who rises discriminably above the rest will find himself the object of serious attempts to cut him back to his proper level (Lynch, 1965).

One is supposed to strive for and attain status and recognition, and yet one is supposed to remain humble, unassuming, and capable of shame at being singled out in any way—a dilemma for many Filipinos, for they sense that their accomplishments will expose them to the envy and hostility of their peers but that a mediocre performance will not bring recognition from their betters, their family, or their peers. That the conflict engendered is of no small importance is attested to by the fact that several cases of serious mental disorder in the present Philippine sample began immediately following a promotion in employment and that a smaller number began following the failure to gain a promotion. In only one American case could the precipitating event be traced to employment, and that involved failure to gain a promotion.

SUPPRESSION OF INDIVIDUALITY

From very early childhood, tendencies toward individuality are suppressed in the Philippines (Bulatao, 1963; Guthrie, 1966; Hollnsteiner, 1963). In child rearing much emphasis is placed upon the absolute authority of the parent and the right of the parent to know and control all aspects of a child's behavior (Guthrie and Jacobs, 1966; Macaranas, 1966). In peer relations the child is expected to blend in and be inconspicuous. The young person is expected by his family and by others to behave and to think as everyone else his age does. Deviations in thought or action are condemned, and the sanctions which can be brought to bear against the deviant are severe. Teasing, for example, can be light and gentle, but it can also be quite cruel when necessary—and sometimes even when it is not. Guthrie (1961) studied interpersonal attitudes of Filipino and American college women, and some of the items Filipino women agreed with relatively more frequently were: (1) I prefer to accept suggestion rather than insist on working things out in my own way; (2) I often seek the advice of older persons and follow it; (3) I am easily hurt by the snobbishness or exclusiveness of others; and (4) I feel lonely and homesick when I am in a strange place. Filipino women relatively less often endorsed such items as: (1) I argue with zest for my point of view against others; (2) When in a group, I like others to pay attention to me; (3) I boast a bit about my achievements from time to time; and (4) I like to have people watch me do the things which I do well.

It is not necessarily and inevitably stressful to have individuality suppressed, especially when the suppression is a culture pattern carried out from birth. There are many suggestions, however, that conflicts do arise for Filipinos out of their desires to express their individuality in some way or to be different. Guthrie found some indication that Filipino college women are in conflict between their desire for the "society girl" role and their feeling that such a role is probably immodest or otherwise wrong. This points to one of the sources of the individuality conflict among Filipinos, the fact that in their transitional society thay are constantly being exposed to models whose behavior is at odds with the cultural pattern, e.g., in movies, the lives of celebrities, society news, and the like. Hollnsteiner (1963) gave many examples of the problems which arise for Filipinos who need under various circumstances to exert or express themselves as individuals but who must either bow to the will of the group or suffer criticism, teasing, ostracism, or some other painful consequence. Bulatao (1963) found Filipino male college students lower than American college students on measures of need for autonomy and need for exhibitionistic expression and higher on need for abasement and need for deference, but the probability of conflict arises because Filipino students are relatively higher than American students on need for dominance and need for aggression.

The Filipino finds his identity in his family connections rather than as an individual in his own right. In this connection it is interesting to note that Carothers (1959) suggested that among nonliterate Africans the individual does not develop a conception of himself as an independent, self-reliant unit, but rather views himself as only one part of a larger organism such as family or clan. While the Philippine culture certainly cannot be described as nonliterate, a good part of it certainly can be described as traditional (Guthrie, 1966); later some similarities between Philippine psychopathology and that found in other traditional societies will be noted.

There are not many systems for which one could make very specific predictions from the nature of Philippine interpersonal conflicts, partly because the problems described above are by no means limited to the Philippines. Filipino patients are not more likely than Americans to be withdrawn or seclusive, nor are they more likely to have unpleasant delusions, mostly delusions of persecution. When they do have persecutory delusions, they are considerably less likely than Americans to express explicit fear of being killed, but they are somewhat more likely to talk in general terms about "people out to get" them or about having "enemies." Filipinos are somewhat more likely than Americans to have delusions of grandeur involving either power or wealth and fame. Meadow and Stoker (1965) found their Mexican-American population to be lower than the Anglo-Americans on persecutory delusions, delusions involving enemies, and also on delusions of grandeur. Thus the Filipinos may depart in some degree from the Anglo-Americans in the latter respect. A rather curious finding is that Filipinos report more auditory hallucinations involving threats of harm but far fewer hallucinations of simple uncomplimentary remarks, e.g., "My, you are ugly." No ready explanation of such a finding occurs to me.

Finally, while it was hypothesized that suppression of individuality may be a source of conflict in the Philippines, it must be admitted that such is likely to be the case only for persons experiencing the forces of change in the society and that the majority of the population still living in somewhat traditional ways are not so subject to conflict on that score. Delusions involving control of thoughts by external forces as well as delusions of thought diffusion are all less frequent in the Philippines than in the United States, and hallucinated commands are also less frequent, especially for males. As I have suggested elsewhere (Sechrest, 1963), Filipinos may have less conflict about independence and thus have reduced symptomatology related to that problem. Varias (1965) reported the exceptional case of a Filipino professional man, a college graduate, who believed that his behavior was being controlled by an electronic machine by which his thoughts also were being broadcast.

Hostility and Its Management

Very evidently, the problem of hostility and hostile expression is an interpersonal problem, and it is such a salient problem in the Philippines that it merits special and separate treatment. Nearly everyone would agree that Filipinos are not given to open displays of hostility, and various observers agree that child-rearing practices stress the suppression of hostile aggression in all its forms (Abasolo-Domingo, 1961; Guthrie, 1961, 1966; Minturn and Lambert, 1964; Varias, 1965). Fights are broken up when they begin, and children are shamed about their aggressive behaviors. My own observations indicate that mothers will themselves deny and relabel the hostility of their children. Thus when a mother hears one of her children say that he "hates" someone, she is quite likely to shush him and to tell him that he is "tired" or that he "doesn't feel well" and attempt to pacify or distract him in some way. Guthrie (1961) found that upper- and middle-class Filipino mothers were much like American mothers in their responses to two "aggression" items but that the attitudes of lower-class mothers, who constitute the majority and who reflect more traditional Philippine attitudes, differed widely. The two items were: (1) A child should be taught to avoid fighting no matter what happens; and (2) children should not be encouraged to box or wrestle because it often leads to trouble or injury. On both items lower-class mothers were far more in agreement than either middle- or upper-class mothers. Nor are verbal expressions of hostility much more tolerable than physical ones. The exceptional sensitivity of Filipinos, presumably even Filipino children, to criticism and to threats to *amor propio* make even verbal aggression repugnant and possibly dangerous.

Varias (1965) reported the results of an investigation into acceptable and unacceptable ways of expressing or getting rid of anger, his subjects being graduate students in public health (presumably relatively Westernized). Among the acceptable ways named were: work, crying, bathing, whistling, praying, and going to a movie. Questionable ways were: fighting, getting drunk, and gambling, but also slamming the door, and shouting. The totally unacceptable ways were running amuck and suicide.

Despite the existence of such strong pressures toward suppression and inhibition of hostility, even to the point of inhibiting use of appropriate verbal labels for the feelings involved, hostility, of course, is aroused. Guthrie's (1961) report on attitudes of Filipino and American female college students showed that on some items indicating irritability Filipino females were higher than Americans, and Bulatao (1963) found that both male and female Filipino students were higher than American students in a measure of need aggression.

Since the expression of hostility is suppresed in several ways, some difficulties are almost bound to occur. One very likely difficulty is that hostile feelings may be inadequately labeled and poorly understood or poorly responded to. In fact, some of the newspaper stories involving homicides in the Philippines indicate problems in labeling hostility. For example, a battle was reported in which two men slew each other with bolo knives, and the police reported that "It is believed that the two men had a misunderstanding."

A second problem is that the suppression, but perhaps not the complete repression, of hostile feelings may lead to a great deal of projection of such feelings. The cues for the detection of hostility in others may be as lacking as the cues in one's own behavior and therefore there may not be a sufficient basis for inferring the existence of friendly, nonhostile feelings. Thus, especially with people whom he does not know, e.g., those whose subtle vocal and gestural cues he has not learned, the Filipino may be uncomfortable or even afraid, searching for cues to hostility against which he must defend himself. Moreover, when questions of *amor propio* arise and the Filipino does detect hostility, it may become important that he not be "put down" in some manner. A not infrequent occurrence in the Philippines is a "staring" duel, which occurs when one individual senses or believes that he is being stared at by another (Varias, 1965). At that point, particularly if he detects contempt in the stare, the Filipino must either stare right back or studiously avoid the other's eyes in such a way that no one can detect that he is refusing to be engaged. Risk is incurred when the staring contest begins because the first to avert his eyes will be the loser, and in proportion to the number of persons watching, the loser may be grossly humiliated. In such situations fights often break out, and the results are serious and even fatal in many instances.

A third problem is that for want of appropriate labels and because of great sensitivity and lack of practice, it is probably difficult for Filipinos to maintain controlled levels of hostility.[1] Once they start, there is an almost inexorable escalation of hostile gestures. Looks become gestures,

gestures become verbal statements, verbal statements become blows, and blows lead to the introduction of the ultimate weapons of the individual, knives and guns. In order for hostility to be manageable in society, it must be possible for people to express hostility at levels which are appropriate to the degree of offense and to keep the expression at that level. Some persons (e.g., Varias, 1965) have felt that hostility may occur at weak and intermediate levels until an individual finally explodes, an interpretation supported by some findings in relation to highly assaultive adolescents in the United States (Megargee, 1964). Even when hostility begins at a relatively weak level of expression, it may escalate because of inadequate practice at mild and intermediate levels of expression. In fact, teasing is one of the rare intermediate forms of hostility widely accepted in the Philippines (Guthrie, n.d.; Varias, 1965) and even teasing must be carried out with caution. The teasing may be vicious only when it is clearly understood by everyone that it is teasing that is taking place.

It is my conviction that problems in the management of hostility manifest themselves in distinct ways in Philippine psychopathology. The problem of homicide in the Philippines already has been mentioned. The rate is high in comparison with that in the United States, and there is a different pattern in the relations between assailants and victims (Sechrest, MS). Moreover, the proportions of males among both assailants and victims are higher in the Philippines than in the United States. Children also are less likely to be victims in the Philippines than in the United States, and, when they are, they are usually only incidental victims in multiple slayings. Such findings are congruent with the hypothesis that homicide in the Philippines stems in large part from problems in management of hostility. Even casual perusal of Manila newspapers shows that a very large proportion of homicides in the Philippines occur when two or more persons become involved in rapidly escalating arguments or when an earlier argument becomes the reason for vengeance.

Enright and Jaeckle (1963) reported that male Filipino mental patients are more violent and threatening than Japanese patients, and data reported above show that violent and threatening behavior and destructive behavior are more frequent among Filipino than among American patients. Moreover, the findings hold for both male and female patients. Fifty-seven per cent of male and 50 per cent of female Filipino patients were reported to be violent or threatening, while the comparable figures for the American sample were only 18 per cent of males and 26 per cent of females. These findings are not restricted to the sample studied here, for Mariano (1962) found that even private, paying Philippine patients had a high rate (46 per cent) of aggressive behavior, including 11 per cent considered homicidal. Meadow and Stoker (1965) reported somewhat higher frequencies of violent behavior for their sample of Anglo-Americans, the figures being 40 per cent of males and 25 per cent of females, both of which are well under the Philippine estimates. Mexican-Americans showed violence in 47 per cent of males and 40 per cent of females. The results were much the same for destructive behavior, defined as destruction of property. Twenty-eight per cent of Filipino males and 21 per cent of females were reported destructive in comparison to only 11 and 4 per cent, respectively, of American patients. It is of interest that Filipino patients, especially males, were not more often described as irritable and quarrelsome than were American patients. Only 22 per cent of Filipino males in comparison with 44 per cent of American male patients were described as irritable and quarrelsome. The corresponding figures for female patients were 31 and 33 per cent, respectively. These findings are in line with my hypothesis that the problem is rather one of management of hostility than of the level of hostility. An additional finding is in line with the supposition that the Filipino is likely to infer hostility in others without sufficient justification; 11 per cent of males and 5 per cent of females among Filipinos expressed delusional concern and even fear that others were angry at them. Only 2 per cent of American patients of either sex expressed such concerns.

Another aspect of hostility which it might be well to consider is the possibility of cultural sanctioning of hostile aggression. It already has been indicated that expressions of hostile aggression are interdicted in the Philippines, but whether aggression is strongly punished once it occurs is another matter. No data are available, but it is the writer's belief that the Philippine culture is one that pleads for innocence but is warm and forgiving toward the sinner. By and large, punishments for serious aggressions, even homicide, do not appear severe, especially for crimes which involve sudden flare-ups of passion without premeditation. Moreover, the deterrent effects of any such punishments depend at least in part on public knowledge of the punishment, and a seven-month survey of newspaper stories (Sechrest, MS) showed very little space devoted to crime. It is quite rare to find a news story dealing with the sentencing of a prisoner. Only in a few sensational cases each year in which capital punishment is the outcome is much newspaper attention given to the consequences of crime.

Sex and Psychopathology

Filipino sexual attitudes and behavior have not been studied much and are certainly not well understood. Some implications for psychopathology, however, are interesting. First, overt sexual expression at least through the years of parenthood is as strongly and definitely interdicted in the Philippines as is aggression. Filipino mothers agree much more strongly than American mothers that sex is a difficult problem in child rearing; Guthrie (1961) found that this agreement held across all social classes; fathers concur in regarding sex as a drive much in need of control (Macaranas, 1966). Filipino male and female students are both well below American counterparts in need for heterosexual expression, and Bulatao (1963) noted that in a culture where even holding of hands is considered taboo it made no sense at all to ask about kissing. In spite of the extensive suppression of sexual activity, attitudes of guilt about sex, ideas that sex is dirty, and the like do not seem to be engendered in Filipinos. As Guthrie (1966) suggested, it is control that is the issue. Sex involves proprieties, not prohibitions. As a result of suppression, even of stated interests, a very strong curiosity about sex is produced, and there seem to be very strong romantic interests fostered, especially among girls (Guthrie, 1966). Philippine news stands are filled with romance stories which young girls certainly read avidly, and informants have told me that college girls are well acquainted with and fascinated by pornography which they pass around and read rather openly—despite the fact that even with a roommate they will not expose themselves nude or talk about sex.

For the most part the Philippines is in the Latin tradition with respect to sex. Controls are maintained by chaperones, and, when chaperones are absent, anything goes. Rapists have been known to excuse themselves with the assertion that their victim must have wanted what she got, otherwise she would not have been walking alone on the street, and this excuse has been used for attacks which occurred in broad daylight! Also in the Latin tradition the double standard prevails, men being accorded great freedom and females almost none at all. That many men have mistresses, "second wives," or *queridas* is not only well known but also is joked about and accepted with the comment that "That is just the Philippine custom." Knowledgeable guides around Manila can point out the houses of mistresses of well-known political figures, businessmen, and celebrities. Probably no young bride seriously considers the possibility that her husband will take a mistress, but before they have been married many years it must become a question of some seriousness for a large proportion of wives.

Homosexuality certainly occurs in the Philippines, but it does not represent a special problem of any magnitude. Transvestites are not uncommon and are quite easy to locate. Moreover, overt homosexuals may be well known in their neighborhoods or places of employment, and their "boyfriends" may be equally well known, but there is little evidence of any conflict about homosexuality (Sechrest and Flores, MS), and the typical attitude toward homosexuals is one of fairly good-natured amusement. They are teased and bantered with but not detested and beaten. Although forms of deviant sexual behavior other than homosexuality must exist in the Philippines, none has come to my attention. Rape, a deviation in circumstance, certainly occurs with some frequency but apparently with little of the underlying morbidity that is so often encountered in the United States. Rape-murder is very infrequent in the Philippines, and I discovered no cases of child-molesting-murder. When rape occurs, it seems to be a straight-forward manifestation of masculine sexuality.

It is the contention here that there is relatively little *conflict* about sex in the Philippines. Given the proper circumstances, sexual relations occur without guilt or anguish. All that is necessary is that sex be controlled until circumstances are proper. It need not be inhibited completely, and it need not be repressed as a factor in one's life.

Sexual symptomatology, with two exceptions among females, is not common in the Philippines compared to the United States. In none of the cases studied was homosexual behavior reported as a symptom, whereas the frequency in the American sample was 6 and 11 per cent for males and females, respectively. No other sexual deviations were reported for the Philippine sample, while 5 per cent of the American sample of males showed one or more additional deviations, mostly exhibitionism. The auditory hallucinations of Filipino patients were less likely to involve "indecencies" than those of Americans, and in only 1 per cent of Filipino male patients did delusions concern homosexuality, while the corresponding figure for the American sample was 9 per cent.

The exceptions with respect to sexual symptomatology were the high incidence of ideation centering around infidelity of their husbands for Filipino females (19 per cent for Filipinos; 5 per cent for Americans), and the high incidence of delusions of a sexual nature for Filipino females (20 per cent for Filipinos; 6 per cent for Americans). The finding concerning ideas about infidelity closely approximates the results of Meadow and Stoker for Mexican-American and Anglo-American females, the comparable figures being 15 and 8 per cent, respectively. One must be careful about inferring that complaints of Filipino female patients about the infidelity of their husbands are delusional. I have heard similar complaints from women who were not patients, nor was it supposed at the time that they should be. The nature of the culture frequently makes ideas about the infidelity of one's husband not unreasonable. In fact, the figure given above excludes cases in which the wife complained about infidelity in which the husband either admitted it or a close relative supported the wife's contention. Thus among female patients complaints about infidelity of the husband are somewhat more frequent than is indicated by the figure given.

The higher incidence of delusions involving sex among Filipino women is accounted for very largely by the rather sizable number of women who claimed to have famous or powerful men as lovers or husbands. In view of the inferior position of women in regard to sexual freedom, it is understandable that some delusional compensating would occur. A small percentage of American women had similar delusions, but not a single male, American or Filipino, made the delusional claim to be the lover of a famous woman.

It is interesting to compare the management of sex and hostile aggression in the Philippines and their significance for psychopathology, since both seem to involve strong pressures for suppression. As shown, hostile aggression is apparently very relevant to psychiatric symptomatology, whereas sex seems only weakly relevant, at most, perhaps because only control is at issue for sex. For hostility there are no really acceptable direct outlets (*see* Varias, 1965), but for sex it is only a matter of the right circumstances. It may be that where merely control, without conflict, is involved in sexuality, its involvement in symptomatology is not especially frequent (e.g., Leighton and Kluckhohn, 1947, on the Navaho).

The issue of maintaining controlled levels of response is relevant to sexual behavior in the Philippines, where very little in the way of lower or intermediate levels of expression of sexuality is permitted. As with aggression, there is some indication of rapid escalation of sexual behavior to ultimate forms of response. While evidence is lacking, impressions of many observers support the contention that sexual intercourse in the Philippines can occur with rapidity and freedom when the circumstances are at all permissive.

Anxiety and Psychopathology

The Philippine culture is apparently not one strongly conducive to the development of anxiety (Bulatao, 1963; Guthrie, 1961, 1966; Varias, 1965). First, several attitudes characteristic of Filipinos probably are incompatible with anxiety. One such attitude Guthrie (1961) described as "optimistic fatalism," expressed in the untranslatable *Bahala na*—what will be, will be, and things will probably turn out all right anyway, and if they don't not much can be done about it. Events are controlled by forces outside the individual; therefore he need not worry much about them.

A second attitude is one expressed in the Spanish term *manana*—if things do not get done now, they will get done later; one day is about like another, and, when the last moment finally arrives, everyone pitches in and things get done anyway, at least well enough. As Guthrie noted, another factor important in Filipino behavior is the lack of emphasis on excellence. In few activities are Filipinos exhorted to do their very best, at least not in a serious, effective way. Poor workmanship is often the rule, and poor work is rewarded in about the same way as good work. Poor scholarship is tolerated, perhaps actually encouraged by peers, and few students are failed in classes no matter how poorly they do. A lack of emphasis on excellence may not be the way to achieve technological advancement, but it does not produce achievement anxiety.

In addition to the attitudes described above, the Filipino is probably protected from many sources of anxiety by the support given him by his family. Within the Filipino family—an extended family with bilateral kinship—the individual is likely to receive almost complete support should he become involved in difficulties of any sort. Extrafamilial sources of support, on the other hand, are limited or absent (Bulatao, 1963; Guthrie, 1961). Support in a physical sense, of course, is limited by the resources of the particular family involved, but, within their resources, support is very nearly complete. Emotional support is very nearly unlimited. Since a Filipino in trouble can call on rather distant relatives for help with the expectation of receiving it if it is possible, he is not limited by the resources of the nuclear family. Filipino mothers place emphasis on authority and control over their children, but they emphasize that control in the context of parental protection of the child (Guthrie, 1961). In my opinion, one of the important research questions which should be asked in countries such as the Philippines is just how and in what degree the individual is protected from stresses by the support available in both a nuclear and extended family. One of the practical issues is how the advantages of "familism" (Banfield, 1958) can be retained in a developing nation without suffering the obvious disadvantages.

That a generally low level of anxiety is reflected in psychopathology is evident, and I already have suggested that the frequency of severe forms of mental disorder in the Philippines is low. Unfortunately, it is extremely difficult to get evidence relating to mild forms of disorder. In a study of mental disorder done in 1959 by surveying 300 municipal health officers, the Philippine Mental Health Association (reported in Varias, 1965) found 1,768 cases, of whom only 101 seemed to be neurotic, and Varias (1959) studied 129 cases known to 39 graduate students in public health, of whom 34 were physicians, and concluded that only 5 of the 129 fell into the neurotic category. Present data indicate that Filipino patients infrequently show typically neurotic symptoms, such as obsessions, compulsions, and phobias, and that American patients are higher in all three categories. Thus, to the extent that anxiety is a feature of neurotic forms of adjustment, Filipinos seem to be low.

Among Filipinos, alcoholism and narcotics addiction also are infrequent; both of these often are thought to stem from anxiety which can only be mastered by drugs of some kind. Zarco (1959) studied narcotics traffic in the Philippines and concluded that narcotics addiction is not much of a problem among Filipinos, nor, from all the evidence, is alcoholism. Varias (1965) found very few cases of alcoholism reported either by municipal health officers or by public health workers. In this investigation of psychiatric patients only 7 per cent of Filipino males and 2 per cent of females were reported to drink excessively, whereas 43 per cent of American male and 15 per cent of American female patients were reported to use alcohol to such an extent that it was a problem in their behavior. The low level of alcoholism among Filipinos apparently is not peculiar to their native land, for in Hawaii, where they constitute about 16 per cent of the adult male population, only 1.9 per cent of patients treated at clinics for alcoholics are Filipinos (Hawaii Department of Health, 1961). That is not to say that Filipinos do not drink, nor that they do not drink excessively at times. Drunkenness is a problem of considerable proportions in the Philippines, for instance, many crimes involve the use of alcohol (although homicide is even more likely to be associated with drinking in the United States [Sechrest, MS].) Drinkers, however, seem not likely to become addicted to the use of alcohol, so that they escape classification as alcoholics. Chafetz and Demone (1962) believed that anxiety is a necessary but not sufficient condition for alcoholism and observed that there are many societies, mostly primitive or traditional, in which drunkenness, without alcoholism, is common. Note also the low frequency of excessive use of alcohol by Filipino patients.

Manis and Manis (1961) found that Filipino students reported fewer psychophysiological symptoms than did American students, a finding which could be interpreted as indicative of a lower level of anxiety, especially in the light of the rationale for use of psychophysiologic indexes of neurotic and other mild personality disorders (Macmillan, 1957). The adult psychiatric patients on whom data are being reported here did not differ from the American sample in frequency of somatic complaints, but they were much less likely than Americans to be described as fearful or anxious (8 per cent for Filipinos *vs.* 38 per cent for Americans). Much more work obviously needs to be done, but thus far the weight of the evidence suggests that anxiety is lower in the Philippines than in the United States. Finney (1963) believed that the stereotype of the Filipino in Hawaii is as an "hysterical" personality, and he viewed the symptoms of Filipinos as consistent with that stereotype.

Guilt and Psychopathology

The distinction between "guilt" and "shame" cultures (Benedict, 1946) has been called into question and criticized; indeed, there is serious doubt whether it is a valid and useful distinction (Ausubel, 1955; Piers and Singer, 1953). If the distinction has any validity, the Filipino culture is distinctly not a "guilt" culture. Whether it falls enough in the other direction to be classed as a "shame" culture is uncertain. For nearly all behaviors, the preponderance of emphasis is placed on the importance of external and social controls, and Filipinos themselves commonly voice the opinion that Filipinos believe that whatever one can get away with is all right. On this issue it may be safer to reason from psychopathology to culture rather than the other way around.

In his study of 129 cases of mental disorder known to public health workers, Varias (1965) described only one case as displaying self-accusation as a symptom. In the present investigation only 2 per cent of Filipino patients had symptoms involving ideas of guilt compared with more than 6 per cent of the American sample. Among patients having delusions, only 3 per cent of males and 4 per cent of females had delusions of guilt or punishment for sins, the comparable figures for American patients being 13 and 10 per cent, respectively.

Few Filipinos were described as sad or depressed (3 per cent for males and 10 per cent for females) compared with American figures of 22 and 38 per cent, respectively, a finding of interest from the standpoint of the concept of guilt, often taken to be at the basis of the depressive reaction. This very low level of depression is to be contrasted with the high level found by Meadow and Stoker (1965) for Mexican-American patients (40 per cent for males and 50 per cent for females). Whether diagnostic bias is all that is involved is impossible to say. Varias (1960) found 4 cases diagnosed as "reactive depression" among 50 seen at a Philippine mental hygiene clinic. It should be pointed out that manic-depressive diagnoses are uncommon in the Philippines and, probably, as elsewhere, are becoming less common as time passes (e.g., in the United States, Malzberg, 1959). The 1959 Philippine Mental Health Association survey (Varias, 1965) found 99 cases of a total of 1,768, of whom 1,009 were diagnosed as schizophrenic. A ratio of approximately 10 schizophrenics to every manic-depressive was the converging estimate for several investigations (Sechrest, 1963). This figure is well below that typically reported among Asians (Lin, 1963).

In understanding both guilt and depression, it is important to know that the suicide rate in the Philippines is very low. The city of Manila with a population of between one and a half and two million averages about 25 suicides per year (Mercado, 1960), and an average of about 10 of those is contributed by the 10 per cent or so of the population that is Chinese. In the present investigation suicide threats, gestures, and attempts occurred in 7 per cent of the male and 9 per cent of the female cases, the comparable figures for Americans being 27 and 26 per cent, respectively. Suicide is just not in the Philippine pattern. Moreover, when it does occur, it seems to be for different reasons than among the Chinese (Catuncan, 1959). The ascribed motives for Chinese are most commonly either illness or economic setbacks, but the three most common motives for Filipinos are said to be family quarrels, disappointment in love, and jealousy. The low rate of suicide in the Philippines probably is consistent with Naroll's (1965) "thwarting disorientation" hypothesis.

The data reported appear to be consistent with the hypothesis that guilt is not a common Filipino reaction, but much more work, and work of a direct nature, is badly needed on the issue of shame and guilt in control of behavior in the Philippines.

The Philippines Compared with Other Traditional Societies

It may be instructive to compare the appearance of psychopathology in the Philippines with its appearance in other societies of the traditional or even primitive sort. Opler (1956b) and Carothers (1959) described the characteristic appearance of pyschopathology among nonliterate groups as more resembling a general confusional state than the typical Western form of schizophrenia or whatever, in which a pattern of general excitability is one of the outstanding features. In the present sample such symptoms as impaired sleep; excessive speech and talking to oneself; singing, dancing, and shouting in the street; and wandering aimlessly (all of which are more frequent among Filipinos than among Americans) seem to fit into just such a pattern of general excitability. Enright and Jaeckle (1963) found similar symptoms characteristic of Filipinos in a comparison with Japanese patients in Hawaii. Meadow and Stoker (1965) found that their Mexican-American patients showed much excitable behavior, and that description applies also to the Formosan aborigines studied by Rin and Lin (1962). Opler (1956b) also reported that the mentally disturbed among nonliterate groups are likely to be characterized by overt, outwardly directed hostility, a finding again consistent with the present one and with that of Enright and Jaeckle (1963).

Still another symptom reported to be more frequent among non-literate and poorly educated groups than others is visual hallucination, which was markedly more frequent in this study among Filipinos than among Americans (31 per cent of Filipinos *vs.* 7 per cent of Americans). Meadow and Stoker (1965) found a similar difference between Mexican and Anglo-Americans, as did Rin and Lin (1962) between Formosan aborigines and Chinese. It has been reported recently that the apparent frequency of visual hallucinations is declining in Japan (Sakurai *et al.*, 1965), perhaps as a function of urbanization. It will be quite interesting to see whether a similar decline takes place in other developing nations.

In general, symptoms among primitive and nonliterate groups have been found to be less florid and delusions less systematized than among other groups (e.g., Rin and Lin, 1962). Although I have no relevant statistical data, it is my distinct impression that Philippine symptomatology tends to be less florid than American and that delusions are much less systematized. For example, visual hallucinations reported by Filipinos were likely to be only things seen. Only infrequently was it suggested that the things seen were engaged in some activity, that the vision was complex and more than fleeting. Several American patients, however, reported visual hallucinations in which complicated acts extending over considerable time took place, e.g., one was the slaughter of several members of the patient's family by monstrous figures. Delusions of persecution among the Filipino patients usually were expressed only as that someone wished to do the patient harm. Only infrequently was a delusion elaborated as involving a plot with any rationale. Several American patients, on the other hand, reported elaborate plots. The persecutors in Filipino delusions were usually "they" or "people" or else family members and townmates. No instance was encountered of persecution by remote and impersonal agencies such as Communists, a gang, the Philippine Constabulary, or the Army. A number of the delusional American patients reported that their persecutors were the Communist Party, the FBI, the Treasury Department, the Veterans Administration, and the municipal police.

Finally, it should not be at all surprising that delusions involving witchcraft occasionally were reported in the Philippines and were missing completely in the American sample. The concept of bewitchment is common in many traditional societies, and there are still places in the Philippines where beliefs in witches and sorcerers are prevalent (Lieban, 1960). The same general culture also accounts for more frequent visual hallucinations of spirits and ghosts among Filipinos than among Americans. Almost certainly a study would show that delusions of bewitchment and hallucinations of possession by spirits have been decreasing over time (Asai, 1963; Hasuzawa, 1963), such delusions presumably being more likely in traditional, poorly educated groups than in others.

ACKNOWLEDGMENT

This research was supported in part by Grant MH-07906 from the National Institute of Mental Health. The writer is indebted to Luis Flores, his assistant, in the collection of data, and to Drs. Anthony Rodriguez and J. Herbert Maltz for their kind co-operation in making their records and facilities available.

NOTE

1. The writer is indebted to Dr. John Wallace for assistance in developing the notion of controlled levels of expression of an impulse.

REFERENCES

Abasolo-Domingo, M. Fe. 1961. Child-rearing practices in barrio Cruz Na Ligas. Unpublished M.A. thesis, University of the Philippines.

Arsenian, J., and J. M. Arsenian. 1948. Tough and easy cultures. Psychiatry 11: 377–85.

Asai, T. 1963. The contents of delusion of schizophrenic patients in Japan: comparison between periods from 1941 to 1961. *In* Proceedings of the Joint Meeting of the Japanese Society of Psychiatry and Neurology and the American Psychiatric Association, Tokyo. H. Akimoto, ed. Supplement No. 7 of Folia Psychiatria et Neurologia Japonica. Tokyo, Japanese Society of Psychiatry and Neurology.

Ash, P. 1949. The reliability of psychiatric diagnosis. Journal of Abnormal and Social Psychology 44:272–77.

Ausubel, D. P. 1955. Relationships between shame and guilt in the socializing process. Psychological Review 62:378–90.

Banfield, E. C. 1958. The moral basis of a backward society. Glencoe, Free Press.

Benedict, Ruth F. 1934. Patterns of culture. Boston, Houghton Mifflin.

————. 1946. The chrysanthemum and the sword. Boston, Houghton Mifflin.

Berne, E. 1959. Difficulties of comparative psychiatry: the Fiji Islands. American Journal of Psychiatry 116:104–109.

Bulatao, J. 1963. Personal preferences of Filipino students. Philippine Sociological Review 11:163–78.

————. 1965. Hiya. Marketing Horizons 3(1):18–28.

Carothers, J. C. 1953. The African mind in health and disease. Geneva, World Health Organization Monograph No. 17.

_____. 1959. Culture, psychiatry, and the written word. Psychiatry 22:307–20.

Catuncan, M. M. 1959. The etiology of suicide in Manila and suburbs. Philippine Sociological Review 7(4):26–33.

Caudill, W. A. 1958. Effects of social and cultural systems in reactions to stress. New York, Social Science Research Council Pamphlet 14.

Chafetz, M. E., and H. W. Demone, Jr. 1962. Alcoholism and society. New York, Oxford University Press.

Enright, J. B., and W. R. Jaeckle. 1963. Psychiatric symptoms and diagnosis in two subcultures. International Journal of Social Psychiatry 9:12–17.

Finney, J. C. 1963. Psychiatry and multiculturality in Hawaii. International Journal of Social Psychiatry 9:5–11.

Guthrie, G. M. 1961. The Filipino child and Philippine society. Manila, Philippine Normal College Press.

_____. 1966. Structure of maternal attitudes in two cultures. Journal of Psychology 62:155–65.

_____. n.d. Philippine national character. University Park, Pennsylvania State University. Mimeographed.

Guthrie, G. M., and P. J. Jacobs. 1966. Child rearing and personality development in the Philippines. University Park, The Pennsylvania State University Press.

Hasuzawa, T. 1963. Chronological observations of delusion in schizophrenics. *In* Proceedings of the Joint Meeting of the Japanese Society of Psychiatry and Neurology and the American Psychiatric Association, Tokyo. H. Akimoto, ed. Supplement No. 7 of Folia Psychiatria et Neurologia Japonica. Tokyo, Japanese Society of Psychiatry and Neurology.

Hawaii Department of Health. 1961. Annual Report.

Hollnsteiner, M. R. 1963. Social control and Filipino personality. Philippine Sociological Review Vol. 11.

Honigmann, J. J. 1954. Culture and personality. New York, Harper and Row.

Jackson, D. D. 1960. The etiology of schizophrenia. New York, Basic Books.

Kety, S. S. 1959. Biochemical theories of schizophrenia. Science 129:1528–32; 1590–96.

Leighton, A. H., and J. H. Hughes. 1959. Cultures as causative of mental disorder. *In* Causes of mental disorders: a review of epidemiological knowledge. New York, Milbank Memorial Fund.

Leighton, A. H., T. A. Lambo, C. C. Hughes, D. C. Leighton, J. M. Murphy, and D. B. Macklin. 1963. Psychiatric disorder among the Yoruba. Ithaca, Cornell University Press.

Leighton, D., and C. Kluckhohn. 1947. Children of the people. Cambridge, Harvard University Press.

Lieban, R. W. 1960. Sorcery, illness, and social control in a Philippine municipality. Southwestern Journal of Anthropology 16:127–43.

Lin, T. 1955. A study of the incidence of mental disorder in Chinese and other cultures. Bulletin of the World Federation of Mental Health 7:55–58.

_____. 1963. Historical survey of psychiatric epidemiology in Asia. Mental Hygiene 47:351–59.

Lynch, F. 1964. Social acceptance. *In* Four readings on Philippine values. F. Lynch, ed. Quezon City, Ateneo de Manila University Press.

_____. 1965. Understanding the Philippines and America. Quezon City, Ateneo de Manila University Press.

Macaranas, E. A. 1966. Attitudes of fathers from two socio-economic levels. Paper presented at the Annual Convention of the Psychological Association of the Philippines.

Macmillan, A. M. 1957. The health opinion survey. Monograph Supplement No. 7 of Psychological Reports 3:325–29.

Malzberg, B. 1959. Important statistical data about mental illness. *In* American handbook of psychiatry. Vol. 1. S. Arieti, ed. New York, Basic Books.

Manis, J. G., and L. G. Manis. 1961. An exploratory study of culture change and mental health among certain Filipino college students. Mental Hygiene 45:389–93.

Mariano, L. D. 1962. Studies on needs for hospitalization: a statistical report. Philippine Journal of Psychiatry and Neurology 3:47–52.

Meadow, A., and D. Stoker. 1965. Symptomatic behavior of hospitalized patients. Archives of General Psychiatry 12:267–77.

Megargee, E. I. 1964. Undercontrol and overcontrol in assaultive and homicidal adolescents. Unpublished Ph.D. thesis, University of California, Berkeley.

Mehlman, B. 1952. The reliability of psychiatric diagnosis. Journal of Abnormal and Social Psychology 47:577–78.

Mercado, R. D. 1960. A review of suicides among Manila residents, 1954–1958. Philippine Journal of Public Health 5:135–51.

Minturn, L., and W. W. Lambert. 1964. Mothers of six cultures. New York, Wiley.

Naroll, R. 1965. Thwarting disorientation and suicide: a cross-cultural survey. Transcultural Psychiatric Research 2:89–22.

Opler, M. K. 1956a. Cultural anthropology and social psychiatry. American Journal of Psychiatry 113:302–11.

_____. 1956b. Culture, psychiatry, and human values. Springfield, Thomas.

_____. 1959. Culture and mental disorder. New York, Macmillan.

_____. 1964. Socio-cultural roots of emotional illness. Psychosomatics 5:55–58.

Parker, S. 1962. Eskimo psychopathology in the context of Eskimo personality and culture. American Anthropologist 64:76–96.

Piers, G., and M. B. Singer. 1953. Shame and guilt. Springfield, Thomas.

Primrose, E. J. R. 1962. Psychological illness: a community study. Springfield, Thomas.

Rin, H., and T. Lin. 1962. Mental illness among Formosan aborigines as compared with the Chinese on Taiwan. Journal of Mental Science 108:134–46.

Sakurai, T., Y. Shirafuji, M. Nishizono, T. Hasuzawa, T. Kusuhara, G. Yoshinaga, and S. Hirohashi. 1965. Changing clinical picture of schizophrenia. Transcultural Psychiatric Research 2:97–98.

Schooler, C., and W. Caudill. 1964. Symptomatology in Japanese and American schizophrenics. Ethnology 3:172–78.

Sechrest, L. 1963. Symptoms of mental disorder in the Philippines. Philippine Sociological Review 11:189–206.

_____. 1964. Mental disorder in the Philippines. The University of the Philippines Research Digest 3:5–9.

_____. MS. Patterns of homicide in the Philippines and the United States.

Sechrest, L., and L. Flores. MS. Handwriting on the wall.

Varias, R. 1959. Cases of mental illness known to a group of public health workers. Philippine Journal of Public Health 4:114–22.

_____. 1960. Cases seen at the Cubao Mental Hygiene Clinic. Philippine Journal of Public Health 5:130–34.

————. 1965. Introduction to mental hygiene. Quezon City, Phoenix Publishing House.

Wittkower, E. D., and J. Fried. 1959. A cross-cultural approach to mental health problems. American Journal of Psychiatry 116:423–28.

Yap, P. M. 1952. The latah reaction: its pathodynamics and nosological position. Journal of Mental Science 98:515–64.

Zarco, R. M. 1959. A sociological study of illegal narcotic activity in the Philippines. Unpublished M.S. thesis, University of the Philippines.

Zigler, E., and L. Phillips. 1961a. Psychiatric diagnosis and symptomatology. Journal of Abnormal and Social Psychology 63:69–75.

————. 1961b. Psychiatric diagnosis: a critique. Journal of Abnormal and Social Psychology 63:607–18.

20. Japanese Psychology, Dependency Need, and Mental Health

L. TAKEO DOI, M.D.

Department of Psychiatry
St. Luke's International Hospital
Tokyo, Japan

IN PREVIOUS PAPERS I have stressed dependency need as a keynote of the Japanese personality structure (Doi, 1962, 1963, 1964). I arrived at this conclusion from analysis of Japanese patients using the concept of *amaeru,* a common Japanese verb which usually describes what a small child feels toward his parents and also the similar feeling that may exist between two adults. The uniqueness of this concept and its usage seem to suggest that dependency need is quite accessible and acceptable to the consciousness of the average Japanese person. To put it the other way round, there sems to be a social sanction for dependency need in Japanese society. If this is the case for Japanese society, it clearly contrasts with the situation in Western societies where dependency need is looked upon as something that belongs to the child or the regressed patient and, hence, usually beneath the dignity of a grown-up person.

It is interesting that relatively few textbooks on child psychology written in Western countries refer to dependency need as such. They treat the emotional development of children at great length, but the dependency need which seems to the Japanese so elemental and basic for children is not given sufficient attention. In spite of a recent emphasis placed upon the mother-child relation and the importance of the child's emotional tie to the mother, the dependency need that should underlie such a bond is seldom mentioned. It may be true to the picture of such a cultural climate to state that it is as though a conspiracy eager to banish dependency need from the adult world had almost succeeded in eliminating it even from the child world.

Turning to psychoanalytic literature, however, it is apparent that in it the dependence of children upon their parents is duly recognized. Freud wrote in 1926: "The biological factor is the long period of time during which the young of the human species is in a condition of helplessness and dependency. . . . This biological factor, then, establishes the earliest situation of danger and creates the need to be loved which will accompany the child through the rest of its life." This need to be loved which Freud mentioned certainly seems to be the same as dependency need. It is interesting to recall, however, that dependence, as such, did not at first suggest the presence of a dependency need to Freud, for in 1915 he wrote that the primal narcissistic condition would not have come into being "were it not that every individual goes through a period of helplessness and dependence on fostering care, during which his urgent needs are satisfied by agencies outside himself and thereby withheld from developing along their own line." According to Freud, it is as though one could depend on fostering care without having a need on one's part for such a dependency; only secondarily would one develop the need to be loved because of the danger inherent in the state of dependency. Hence, in his thinking both loving and being loved came to be defined in terms of libidinal satisfaction (Freud, 1914, 1915).

Against this theory of Freud's, I propose that dependency need should be thought of as an independent drive, distinct from the sexual or aggressive drives, from which develops the need to be loved. In psychoanalytic terminology the sexual and aggressive drives usually are referred to as id impulses, whereas I believe that dependency need should be thought as deriving from ego; that is, it corresponds to the ego instincts in Freud's early formulation. I cannot help feeling that Freud discarded the concept of the ego instincts later, mainly because he could not appreciate the independent importance of dependency need. Now, though conceptually separated, sexual and aggressive drives, on the one hand, and dependency need, on the other, work together and are intertwined with each other in actuality. It can be presumed that object relations, which sexual and aggressive drives require for proper satisfaction, come into being by means of the operation of dependency need. It follows, then, that the pathology of dependency need comes first in individual psychopathology, and that either sex or aggression is secondary. This reasoning agrees with recent studies of animal behavior in which animals deprived of mothers from birth cannot develop proper sexual activities (Harlow and Harlow, 1962). Pathology must reside in ego first and foremost, whether in psychosis or neurosis, though id impulses greatly contribute to it. I feel also that such Freudian concepts as narcissism, homosexuality, masochism, unconscious guilt, and repetition compulsion, concepts which, though ill defined, are important for understanding the dynamics of psychopathology, need to be revised in terms of dependency need (Doi, 1965).

I have attempted to do with the concept of dependency need what Freud did with that of sexuality. He made it possible to conceive the whole development in continuum from infancy to adulthood in terms of sexuality, or more technically libido, by giving that concept adequate abstraction and generality. This procedure is what gives psychoanalysis the status of science, for, as Langer (1964) said, "The sciences are born under quite special conditions when their key concepts reach a degree of abstraction and precision which makes them adequate to the demands of exact, powerful, and microscopically analytic thinking." I think that this procedure can be applied to the concept of dependency need. I have no doubt been helped in so thinking by the fact that the Japanese language has many words like *amaeru* which express dependency need in its multifarious shades. Without such a cultural background perhaps even Freud, for all his genius, could not easily recognize the importance of dependency need. In his later years, however, he made the following statement (Freud, 1931) concerning his new insight into early mental development: "Everything connected with this first mother-attachment has in analysis seemed to me so elusive, lost in a past so dim and shadowy, so hard to resuscitate, that it seemed as if it had undergone some specially inexorable repression." This sentence is a good example of the great difficulty one would experience in identifying dependency need as such in Western societies, though it cannot be determined whether the repression of the dependency need is real or only apparent owing to the observer's lack of acumen, as Freud partially admits in the passage.

I have stated that dependency need should be thought of as an independent drive which makes object relations possible in the first years of life. It follows that the operation of dependency need initiates not only the process of personality formation but also the process of socialization. Heretofore, these two processes could not be integrated theoretically; hence, one was hard put to account for social and cultural factors in personality formation. For instance, Hartmann (1944) commented on this subject:

> Considering this complete dependence upon the care and protection of others, it is natural that man's need for love and his fear of losing the love of the object are especially strongly developed. It is evident that analytic findings of this kind are of great importance for sociology. At the same time when viewed from the angle of adaptation, maturation, and learning, they present an essential field in the biology of man. The relationship of the infant to his mother, the institution of the reality principle, the change in the types of instinctual

gratification, may all be described "biologically" as well as "sociologically."

Here, though Hartmann rightly has recognized the phenomena of dependence as a common area of study for sociology and biology, he has provided no working concept to mediate between the two disciplines. Faithfully following Freud, he has not regarded infantile dependency as involving a psychological need that through its own dynamism should promote the process of socialization. No wonder that he mentioned only sociology and biology, not psychology, an omission which probably betrays his hidden assumption that the phenomena of dependence cannot be studied psychologically. Thus in discusssing how man can be affected by cultural factors, he simply said: "They can, along with other influences, co-determine the central structure of the personality, by provoking, for example, the early establishment of specific reaction formations, or they can co-determine the degree of severity of the superego or the degree of mobility of the ego."

To be precise, one may argue, cultural factors cannot touch the central structure of the personality unless there is some need in the core of the personality which is responsive to and affected by cultural factors. This need is what I mean by dependency need, the need which first involves one's parents but through and beyond them extends to the wider world. I think Balint (1935), whose view is quite similar to mine, had the same thing in mind when he posited passive object love as a primary need and said: "Now I believe . . . that the different object relations do not succeed one another according to biological conditions, but are to be conceived as reactions to actual influence of the world of objects—above all, to methods of upbringing. Our therapy is the best proof of this." Thus, through the mediating concept of dependency need it becomes possible to relate social systems and personality systems, and I think this association will open a new vista for cultural anthropology and also for mental health.

In the light of the above hypothesis, let us consider some of the culturally conditioned personality types. I contrasted at the beginning of this chapter the attitudes of Japanese society and Western societies toward dependency need. I also suggested the possible existence of a certain bias against dependency need in Western societies—a bias which must be related to the Western ideal of personal independence. I cannot give here a detailed historical account of the reasons such an ideal came to exist in Western societies. Perhaps it has to do with the fact that the West has gone through more turbulent social and cultural changes throughout its history than has the East, thus creating a suitable climate for the spirit of personal independence. To state this spirit in dynamic terms, it means that one might just as well depend upon oneself or become independent, since there is nobody else to depend upon. In other words, personal independence is the dependency need turned upon oneself, and its viability as a defense presupposes the existence of a self worthy to be depended upon; this latter point is a crucial one for psychopathology. Furthermore, I think that the spirit of personal independence has been the driving force behind all the great cultural achievements of the West, rather than "the increase in autonomy of the ego" or freedom from instinctual conflicts which Hartmann, Kris, and Loewenstein (1951) have associated with the ability for higher mental functions. If anything, personal independence creates even more mental conflicts than does dependence, though it may subsequently check them successfully or unsuccessfully.

I now return to the discussion of the problem with which I started, that is, the ego-syntonic quality of dependency need in the Japanese personality structure, particularly with reference to remarks made by other Asiatics in this volume. For instance, Surya (Chapter 23) stresses the importance of dependent relations for Indians, but he cautions against the use of the word "dependency," because it has a bad connotation. According to him, the right words are bond, bondship, or kinship rather than dependency, and an Indian would not experience dependency but anticipation of closeness or bondship in the act of asking for a favor. This reasoning implies, it seems to me, that Indians share the same bias toward dependency need as do Westerners. Also, if Surya's interpretation is correct, what he describes as characteristic of Indians is intensive identification with one's group, and I am sure that the same group identification characterizes in good measure the Japanese as well. I feel, however, that, eager as the Japanese are to identify themselves with a group to which they belong, they also tend to think in terms of personal interests and often look upon allegiance to a particular group as a burden. They may even try to manipulate their group or others upon whom they depend, so as to turn their dependency into virtual control of others. In other words, the Japanese dependent relations are quite fluid, and the structure of these relations does not necessarily consist of the fixed social roles of a dependent and a superior. A person in a superior role may as easily experience dependency need as a person in a dependent role as part of the interaction. This structure is as it should be in terms of dependency need, for one establishes a close bond or a group identification more often than not at the expense of one's individual wishes, and I am inclined to believe that this structure is what distinguishes the Japanese pattern of dependency from those found in the rest of Asia.

The fact that the Japanese people have eagerly and readily welcomed Western civilization since the Meiji period is an indication of the value they place on the free play of initiative. I think it would be wrong, however, to infer that Japanese initiative is the same in nature as the Western idea of personal independence. Rather, I should say that their initiative has more to do with dependency than with the need to become independent, since it has been mainly motivated by the desire to appear acceptable and respectable in the eyes of others. In other words, the Japanese have accomplished the task of modernizing themselves by use of the surplus free energy of dependency need which is neither bound by any specific social relation nor turned upon oneself to make self-reliance workable. To prove this point, let us briefly examine the case of the recent war Japan waged against her neighbors. Without exhausting the list of the causes that entered into making this war, one could say that Japan wanted to be recognized as one of the world powers. Short of such recognition, she wanted to act as though she were a world power. In her eyes therefore the course of action she eventually took was an act of identification with the aggressor. Take also the case of the remarkable transformation which has come over the face of Tokyo during the past few years. It is no secret to the citizens of Tokyo that the change was made possible by the tremendous incentive that came from the honor of having the Olympic games there. Japan has always been like that. In fact, she made similar successful efforts in the past when she was confronted with a great civilization in China. From the Japanese example one may therefore hazard the thesis that a key to successful modernization of any country less developed than others lies in the inherent strength or relative health of dependency among its people.

At present the whole non-Western world is straining under the impact of Western civilization. While this social cataclysm goes on in the non-Western world, the West also is passing through a critical phase. For one thing, the West can no longer *depend* upon its cherished hegemony of the world. To maintain this hegemony, it preaches to or sells to or even forces upon the rest of the world the ideal of democracy, or whatever it may be, only to find more confusion created. It is little wonder, then, that at times the ideal sounds hollow even to the West itself. Thus the whole world rapidly is becoming one in political, social, and cultural confusion, for which the West has to take at least part of the blame. This situation also means, however, that conditions are hopefully again ripe for a rediscovery of the spirit of personal independence, the source of so much creativity in the West. I think that is why the people in Western societies are so eagerly seeking new meanings of emotional maturity and have to flock to psychoanalysts or to whatever promises them a complete self-realization.

As for the Japanese people, they also are not really content with their accomplishment of modernization. Since they have embraced Western civilization with all its dilemmas and conflicts, they are learning, almost despite themselves, the hard lessons that they cannot completely depend upon others whom they once looked upon as superior and that they have to acquire spiritual independence somewhere or somehow in order to cope with the cultural and social confusion. I think that the social instability now being experienced in Japan goes hand in hand with a recent increase in psychiatric casualties. What can be done to meet this emerging situation? Of course, all the facilities in the field of mental health will have to be mobilized and expanded, for it is the task of mental health workers to help those who stumble and fall by the wayside in this historical process of mankind. But how? With what philosophy? Or with what technique? Are we psychiatrists well equipped for the job? Does our work consist mainly in building more hospitals or producing an abundance of tranquilizers? I think the answer to this critical question which confronts us all today is obvious. It must be first and foremost to educate an increasing number of psychiatrists and other workers in the field of mental health toward a better understanding of the human mind, particularly to help them overcome their own sometimes unrecognized dependency need. Such education is essential because only those who are truly conflict-free in respect to dependency need, and therefore able to make use of it in creative ways, are able to understand and help others who suffer from the frustration of dependency need.

REFERENCES

Balint, M. 1935. Critical notes on the theory of the pregenital organizations of the libido. *Reprinted in* Primary love and psychoanalytic technique. M. Balint. New York, Liveright Publishing Company, 1965.

Doi, L. T. 1962. *Amae*—a key concept for understanding Japanese personality structure. *In* Japanese culture: its development and characteristics. R. J. Smith and R. K. Beardsley, eds. Chicago, Aldine Publishing Company.

————. 1963. Some thoughts on helplessness and the desire to be loved. Psychiatry 26:266–72.

————. 1964. Psychoanalytic therapy and "Western Man": a Japanese view. Special Edition No. 1 (Congress Issue) of the International Journal of Social Psychiatry. Pp. 13–18.

————. 1965 Seishin-bunseki to seishin-byōri. Tokyo, Igaku Shoin.

Freud, S. 1914. On narcissism: an introduction. *Reprinted in* Collected papers. Vol. 4. London, The Hogarth Press, 1950.

————. 1915. Instincts and their vicissitudes. *Reprinted in* Collected papers. Vol. 4. London, The Hogarth Press, 1950.

————. 1926. Inhibitions, symptoms and anxiety. London, the Hogarth Press.

————. 1931. Female sexuality. *Reprinted in* collected papers. Vol. 5. London, The Hogarth Press, 1950.

Harlow, H. F., and M. K. Harlow. 1962. The effect of rearing conditions on behavior. Bulletin of the Menninger Clinic 26:213–24.

Hartmann, H. 1944. Psychoanalysis and sociology. *Reprinted in* Essays on ego psychology. H. Hartmann. New York, International Universities Press, 1964.

Hartmann, H., E. Kris, and R. M. Loewenstein. 1951. Some psychoanalytic comments on culture and personality. *In* Psychoanalysis and culture. G. B. Wilbur and W. Muensterberger, eds. New York, International Universities Press.

Langer, S. K. 1964. Philosophical sketches. New York, Mentor Books.

21. Minority Status and Deviancy in Japan

GEORGE A. DeVOS, Ph.D.
Department of Anthropology
University of California
Berkeley, California

HIROSHI WAGATSUMA, Ph.D.
Department of Sociology
University of Pittsburgh
Pittsburgh, Pennsylvania

FROM THE STANDPOINT of socialization, it is pertinent to understand the effects of social discrimination as they tend to induce social deviancy and lack of respect for constituted authority. The following generalizations suggest themselves in examining conditions in American society. Minority group members often lack the incentive to internalize conformist attitudes toward the law, and there are also active personal and community inducements to flout in some form either symbolically or by actual behavior the rules of the majority society. Finding methods of trickery to outwit authorities is one of the basic defensive maneuvers of an individual in an exploited or discriminated role which excludes equal participation. By so doing, the minority group member salvages some aspects of self-esteem and "gets back" at an authority structure which is perceived as operating to maintain his degradation or to hinder his freedom rather than to benefit him in any way. What happens frequently in a minority role, therefore, is that the individual tends to become deviant in some way from the standards set by the dominant groups in the society. He may not identify strongly with formal authority, represented either by the school or the legal system. He may not subscribe readily to patterns of marriage stability set by the majority society. He may develop language patterns that distinguish him from the majority society. He may be less apt to exercise over either his aggressive feelings or his sexual urges standards of impulse control that are maintained by individuals more motivated than he by conformist needs, seeking to keep their social status in the majority society.

Generally, the majority society is less likely to exercise police powers over expression of impulses and sexual or aggressive activity among minority group members, since in its pejorative perception of a socially degraded group such behavior is expected and covertly condoned as long as the individuals injured are all within the group. There is sensitivity, however, to assaults on the persons or property of the majority group. In such situations legal sanctions are apt to be interpreted severely toward minority members, deepening the latter's sense of expected injustice.

In our cross-cultural research on delinquency and social deviancy in Japan, we were interested in determining whether a functional social parallel could be found to the high incidence of delinquency in certain minority groups in the United States. Four groups have minority status in Japan: the Ainu, Chinese, Koreans, and *burakumin*. The Ainu are a separate, aboriginal cultural group who have in many instances become assimilated with Japanese society. They are relatively insignificant in number and are only found in groups in Hokkaidō, the northern Japanese island. A second minority group, relatively small, consists of the Chinese (many from Taiwan)[1] living in Japan. This group is not easily studied, and very little research has been done regarding their adjustment. A third group, more socially viable than the first two, are the Koreans, some of whom are assimilating into Japanese culture to the extent of taking on Japanese names, but most of them are keeping their separate ethnic identity. They are recognized as constituting a social problem in Japan. So far, we have not had the opportunity to investigate this group to any degree. A fourth, and for us a more interesting, group is one which we were able to investigate using social anthropological methods. This group comprises the former outcastes, who were treated similarly to the pariah caste of India until 1871, when they were liberated, and as new citizens supposedly were accorded full citizenship. Through somewhat unusual circumstances, we were able to gain the trust and co-operation of some members of this group, a fact which permitted us to initiate our study.

The *Burakumin*

In present-day Japan, there are an estimated one to three million people residing in over six thousand communities, rural and urban, who are identified as *tokushu-burakumin* ("people of special communities"). In reference to these people one also finds the expressions, having a leftist connotation, *mikaihō-burakumin* ("people of unliberated communities") or, paradoxically, *dōwa-chiku-no-hito* ("people of integrated districts"). There are pejorative forms, seldom heard now, such as *eta* ("filled with dirt") or *yotsu* ("four-legged"). The neutral descriptive abbreviation, acceptable to all, is *burakumin*. The *burakumin* are the descendants of the outcastes or the untouchables, who are still socially and economically discriminated against as the result of prejudice by members of the majority society. The *burakumin* are not racially different from the majority Japanese; the only certain way that they can be identified is by the registry of place of birth and residence. Nevertheless, many Japanese believe that they are in some way or other visibly identifiable. The *burakumin* are considered mentally inferior, incapable of high moral behavior, aggressive, impulsive, and lacking any notion of sanitation or manners. Very often they are "the last hired and the first fired." Marriage between a *buraku* individual and a member of the majority society, while not impossible, is frequently the cause of tragedy and ostracism.

Historically, by the fifteenth century various groups of people appeared in Japan who were designated collectively as *senmin* ("lowly people"). Very roughly, they were classified into two large groups: (1) artisans, mainly engaged in working with leather or bamboo, dyeing, or serving as executioners, and (2) itinerant entertainers, prostitutes, and quasi-religious itinerants. The leather workers were engaged in the slaughtering and skinning of animals, the tanning of leather, and the making of leather goods, such as foot gear, saddles, and armor. Owing to the Shintō tradition of disdaining whatever was considered "polluting," such as the handling of carcasses, as well as to the proscription in Buddhism against killing animals, these leather workers were shunned by ordinary folk. The avoided (but certainly needed) artisans often lived in settlements on dry river beds (*kawara*) or on tax-free barren lands (*san-jo*), away from the communities of "decent" common people. The second group of *senmin*, the itinerant entertainers, were engaged in singing, dancing, acting, and puppet shows; or in fortune telling and other magico-religious practices; or in prostitution. Both groups of *senmin* were believed to have special magical power and to be "different"; they were objects of suspicion, fear, condemnation, and avoidance by the general public. The Japanese word, *iyashii* ("lowly") derives from *ayashii* ("mysterious and suspicious"). The *senmin* also included beggars, fleeing criminals, and the crippled. They also often engaged in cleaning roads and gardens, carrying baggage for travelers, and escorting and executing criminals and disposing of their corpses.

With the establishment of the Tokugawa government in the early seventeenth century, Japanese society was further organized into a rigidly hierarchical structure. At the top was a warrior-administrator-ruling class (*shi*), with numerous strata of subranks. The ruled consisted of peasants (*nō*), artisans (*kō*), and the merchant (*shō*) classes. Beneath this structure of accepted citizens were the outcaste or *senmin* class, into which all the lowly people of previous times were integrated. The two major outcaste groups were designated as *hinin* ("nonhuman") and *eta*. During the Tokugawa period, being an *eta* was inescapably hereditary; one was born, lived, and died as an *eta*, as was also the case, generally, with *hinin*. In principle, however, a *hinin* individual, by securing a respectable sponsor and paying a certain fee, finally could gain the status of a commoner. The practice was called *ashi arai* ("foot washing"). Commoners, in turn, were forced into *hinin* status as punishment for certain crimes, such as adultery, escaping the death penalty, and having attempted double suicide. In consequence of the slight mobility that was possible between "nonhuman" and "human" status, *hinin* was considered to be a higher status than *eta*. *Eta* and *hinin* maintained separate endogamous groups. They were made to live in particular parts of the cities and were forced to look different from ordinary citizens, by going barefoot, using straw to tie their hair, and, in many instances, wearing a patch of leather on their clothes.

Finally, in August 1871, a Meiji Government edict officially abolished the outcaste status and described the outcaste people as "new citizens" (*shin-heimin*). According to the governmental document, there were about 280,000 *eta*, 23,500 *hinin,* and 80,000 miscellaneous outcastes at the time of the emancipation. Their legal emancipation, however, had little effect upon continuing discrimination against the so-called *shin-heimin*. Around the turn of the century, a political movement against prejudice and injustice started the "integrationist movement" (*yūwa undō*), joined both by paternalistic *buraku* leaders of wealth and by the sympathetic elite of the majority society. The core of the integrationist movement was the Great Japan's Fellow Citizens Integration Society (*Dai Nippon Dōhō Yūwa Kai*), established in 1903. This group worked for "self-betterment" and "self-improvement" (*kaizen*) of *shin-heimin*, such as the improvement of their morals, customs, manners, sanitation. Discrimination, however, continued. For instance, when recruited into the Imperial Army, a new commoner (*shin-heimin*) usually was assigned to the transportation or maintenance corps, where he was responsible for making and repairing shoes and other leather goods. When assigned to the infantry, he had no hope of moving up, even to a rank of noncommissioned officer.

Following a series of "race riots" by impoverished peasants at the time of the inflation after World War I, a militant liberation movement was organized; in March, 1922, the National *Suiheisha* (Levellers' Association) was inaugurated, which adopted as its flag "a crown of thorns the color of blood against a black background of darkness." An early objective of the *Suiheisha* was "an eye for an eye" counterattack against discrimination, a cause of frequent bloodshed. From 1924 to 1930 the movement suffered from fraction and conflicts among anarchists, Communists, and nonrevolutionists. Then in 1930 it clearly took a leftist turn and established close ties with the union movement among laborers and farmers. Both in theory and strategy the fight against discrimination was incorporated into the broad context of class struggle and a proletarian revolution. For nearly ten years the Communist red flag and the flag of the crown of thorns flew side by side, but as the militarists took power and Japan moved into war, such movements, together with other leftist activities, were either rendered "harmless," forced underground, or broken by the action of special police.

At its last national meeting before final dissolution in August, 1940, the *Suiheisha* vowed loyalty to the Emperor.

After World War II, in February, 1946, the National Committee on *Buraku* Liberation was formed, which "inherited the revolutionary tradition of the *Suiheisha*." The Committee later changed its name to the *Buraku* Liberation League, known as the *Kaihō Dōmei*, and continues active in its attempts to end discrimination toward *buraku* people.

Burakumin Response to Discrimination

As discussed above, one basic means of expressing discontent with discrimination available to *buraku* individuals has been concerted political action. Many *burakumin* still find outlets for simmering discontent through leftist political organizations. Such political movements seek to change social attitudes by creating a different pattern of politico-legal sanctions within the society. Politically involved individuals may participate in politically deviant behavior rather than resorting to forms of individual extra-legal deviancy. Far-left political movements, while at times questionable from the standpoint of unrealistic assessment of possible influence and in some cases characterized by the overly emotional approaches taken by reformers, are socially integrative at least so far as they seek to find means of effecting change without denial of self-identity or resort to deviant mechanisms of expressing hostility toward authority through extralegal or unsanctioned behavior. The individual who takes political action is mobilizing his energy toward a cause rather than falling back from it in either resignation or apathy, as is the case with a great majority of the *burakumin*.

If we were to generalize about the forms of behavior likely among *burakumin* as a group subject to social discrimination on the basis of what we have observed in certain American minority groups with similar traditions, such as the Negro or the Mexican-American, we would anticipate that the *burakumin*, in addition to political activities, would show higher indexes of various forms of socially deviant behavior than the majority population (cf. Merton, 1959). First, we would anticipate a high incidence of apathy and aloofness in regard to education and public health and sanitary activities initiated by governmental authority. Second, we would anticipate some deviousness and dependent opportunism in respect to welfare programs initiated by the majority culture. Third, we would anticipate a higher incidence of antisocial attitudes expressed in behavior defined as delinquent or criminal in nature. The evidence from Japan supports these hypotheses.

BURAKUMIN ATTITUDES TOWARD EDUCATION

One striking parallel between the American minority group situation of the Negro and the Japanese situation of the *burakumin* arises from the fact that both American and Japanese cultures strongly induce and stimulate occupational and educational achievement in their value systems.

While a minority member is well aware of the fact that he "should" apply himself to his own training and education, he also knows he will be faced with a highly problematical situation when he applies for a job in a profession or skill for which he has trained himself. He has to be willing to face a number of self-deflations and rejections. Both American and Japanese cultures in this respect offer career blandishments, while at the same time offering a potential negative shock, should a goal actually be sought. For instance, Mahara (1960, 1961) reported that in March, 1959, 166 non-*buraku* children and 83 *buraku* children were graduated from a junior high school in Kyoto. Those who were employed by small-scale enterprises employing less than 10 workers numbered 29.8 per cent of the *buraku* and 13.1 per cent of non-*buraku* children. On the other hand, 15.1 per cent of non-*buraku* children could obtain employment in large-scale industries employing more than 1,000 workers, while only 1.5 per cent of *buraku* children could do so. Working conditions in large-scale industries generally are much better than those in small-scale enterprises. The average starting salary per month was 5,196 *yen* for non-*buraku* children, and 4,808 *yen* for *buraku* children. Ishida (1961) reported that at another junior high school near Kyoto almost all non-*buraku* graduates found jobs in April following their March graduation, or in May at the latest, while only 39 per cent of *buraku* graduates could find jobs by April and May. It is true that many *buraku* children are actually unqualified for jobs, but many employers are unwilling to hire *buraku* children even when they are well qualified.

The following story, told by a woman doctor (Kobayashi, 1962) who worked among *burakumin* for over ten years illustrates well the adverse effect of collective or family anticipations on the aspirations of individual youth. A *buraku* boy, who was a second son, completed a special high school for commercial and industrial training in Nara and found a job in a large company in Tokyo. This boy, the captain of a baseball team while in high school, was a promising, happy young man. Full of buoyant expectation, he left the community for a job in Tokyo. Everybody in his family and in the community was very enthusiastic about his prospects. During summer and New Year's vacations he returned from Tokyo and was his usual joyful self. About a year later, however, when the doctor dropped by the house of Mr. Y., the boy's father, she was surprised to find the young man present in a depressed state. The boy would indicate only that his health was not bad. Worried and curious, the doctor asked Mr. Y. what had happened. He told the doctor that he made his son quit his job in Tokyo and forced him to return home. The mother, who then joined them, said that when the boy had come home on his last vacation, both parents had told him not to go back to Tokyo, but he vacillated and finally went back. In the end he decided to quit and came back home; the mother said, "We feel relieved." The doctor asked Mr. Y. why the boy quit, since his job was a good one and he apparently had been happy in Tokyo. The father said, "It is better that a boy of the *buraku* comes back to his own community and learns how to make *zōri* ["straw sandals"]; that is a *buraku* industry." When the boy had told his employer that he wanted to quit, he was urged not to; also the employer kindly told the young man that, if he desired to leave in order to stay with his parents, he could be transferred to a branch office in Nara, to which he could commute from his own home. Nevertheless, the young man had quit. Mr. Y. then mentioned an individual, a brilliant graduate from the university who had earned a Ph.D. and become a professor. As a result no *buraku* girl was "good enough" to be able to marry this professor. Of course, he could not marry a woman from the majority society, and he therefore had to remain a bachelor. Mr. Y. remarked that the professor was a great man, but that he was very unhappy. Mr. Y. said that if his son became successful in his job in Tokyo and happened to fall in love with a girl from the majority society, it would result in serious unhappiness for his boy. The more successful the *buraku* individual becomes, the less happy he becomes. The father therefore wanted his son to quit his job and return to his family.

In the face of discrimination, the easiest solution is not to try, or to discredit the goal. A protective self-identity with a submerged group makes the necessity for trying unnecessary. Although numerous individuals from minority groups, nonetheless, have the strength of purpose and the ego capacities to survive in spite of discrimination, many react with general apathy and lack of involvement with the educational process.

We have an impression that the *buraku* children come out relatively poorly in school compared with majority group children. Their truancy rate is often high, paralleling the situation observed in California in respect to Negro and Mexican-American minority groups. The situation in Japan probably parallels that in America regarding response to education. The following paragraphs present some relevant evidence.

In Izumo (Shimane Prefecture) on the Japan Sea in Southwestern Japan, there is a long tradition of belief in fox possession. The potentiality of being possessed by a fox descends along the family line, and such families who are *kitsune-mochi* ("those who have a fox") are labeled as "black" in contrast with "white" families who do not have a fox. Marriage across the "black"-"white" line is tabooed because it is believed that if a member of a "white" family marries a member of a "black" family, all other members of the white family become "black." Needless to say, in this area, *burakumin* are treated even more stringently as outcastes, since they rank below the "black" families. Nomura (1956) compared the I.Q. of students in three junior high schools where members of all three groups matriculated: children of "white" families, of "black" families, and of *burakumin*. He used two different kinds of I.Q. tests, the nature of which unfortunately are not clear from his report. On both tests in all three schools, however, the results were uniform: "white" children averaged significantly higher than children from "black" families, and *buraku* children, while not markedly lower than the blacks, averaged lowest.

In the work by Mahara (1960, 1961) cited earlier, he compared a group of 247 subjects, 83 of whom were *buraku* children, at a junior high school in Kyoto on standard achievement tests devised by the Japanese Ministry of Education. The average in four subjects consistently showed higher functioning by the non-*buraku* youth than by *buraku* students. Numerous studies in the United States similarly have attested to the substandard functioning of minority group children from culturally underprivileged backgrounds. Racists would argue that this finding reflects innate differences in ability. We would argue that both in Japan and in the United States the results reflect early damage to social self-identity and self-respect vis-à-vis cultural expectations.

BURAKUMIN ATTITUDES TOWARD HEALTH AND WELFARE AUTHORITIES

Members of a minority group, having experienced a long tradition of discrimination, develop certain characteristic ways of handling their relations with dominant elements of the society. Not only do they develop defensive hostility in respect to the dominant groups, but they are also apt to develop ways of expressing ambivalent attitudes of dependency toward the economically dominant majority group members. Such dependent feelings are given an expediential tone by finding means of being devious in how one "takes." Deviousness is a balm to the ego and allows the individual to maintain his self-respect by not having his dependent needs make him feel completely helpless. Individuals from the majority groups sometimes are angered when they discover some form of cheating on welfare benefits. It confirms their prejudice concerning the worthless nature of the individuals who are being "helped" through the efforts of the more humane elements within their community. American society today expresses considerable division of opinion concerning the effects of its welfare policy in this regard, a subject too complex for this report. The Japanese evidence reveals analogously that the *burakumin* have developed certain expectations that they are "due" economic assistance from the majority society. They tend to see it as a right that goes with their minority status. The woman doctor mentioned before (Kobayashi, 1962) tells an incident which well illustrates the expediential-dependent attitudes of the *burakumin* toward welfare programs.

Mr. T., a very poor tailor living in the *buraku*, is not a *buraku* person, but his wife is from the community. She was working in a bar in a nearby city when Mr. T. met her. Mr. T. did not know that his wife was of *buraku* background, but he was not concerned when he learned about it. His wife, however, remained very much concerned, was always talking about it, and felt very inferior to other people. Mr. T. did not like his wife's attitude, so he went to the library of the town and started reading books on the history of the *burakumin*. With this knowledge he wanted to educate his wife, trying to free her from her prejudice, but he was not very successful, nor did he feel successful in getting her to believe that he was not prejudiced against the *burakumin*. As a last resort, he decided to move into his wife's community and now lives with her in the community where she was born. Once the doctor asked Mr. T. for his comments on life within the community. Mr. T. replied that he feels that the people of the community behave so as to cause social discrimination on the part of the general society. Within the community he, as an outsider, meets with discrimination. He is not accepted. About six months ago he wanted to take care of another man living in the next apartment who had wandered into the community from the outside. This man had no job and no money, so Mr. T. took him to a branch of the city employment security office. Mr. T. wanted them to register this man for relief; however, the public employees told Mr. T. that the number of people who could receive governmental unemployment relief money was limited and that they could not take Mr. T.'s friend at that time. He was told that they would have to wait for a while, so they waited, but nothing happened. Mr. T. then found that people of the *burakumin* community were being accepted and registered in the office. He found also that even people with considerable income were receiving relief money, some who even owned electric washing machines, telephones, and television sets. Mr. T. got very angry, went to the public employment security office, and criticized the employees severely. He was indignant that the man from the outside society could not receive relief, while people with *buraku* background could register and receive money even when they were well-to-do enough to own a television set or a telephone. Through Mr. T.'s efforts, his friend was accepted and registered for relief money, since minor officials at the office were forced to admit that they technically were wrong. They still did not reject the *buraku* people; they merely placed his friend on the rolls. According to Mr. T., in this community receiving unemployment relief is considered a kind of job, a job which people use all kinds of political pressure to obtain. If an individual has influential relatives, or simply many relatives, living in the community, he will have strong support and probably will succeed in getting relief funds. Mr. T. himself rejected strongly the clannishness of the *buraku* people and their exclusive attitude directed toward members of the majority society.

As another example of the expediential "take what you can get" attitude of the *buraku* toward the outside society, the same author writes that many families of her community, although relatively poor, use electricity liberally for cooking, warming up rooms, and so forth. They pay only the basic fee, however, having their own devices for using electricity without having its use register on the meter. Five years before the doctor wrote her book the Kansai Electric Company finally installed electric meters in each house, but the inhabitants found ways to reverse the meters, reducing the amount recorded. The people of almost every house do this, and they do not think they are doing anything wrong in cheating the company.

As the author was the only doctor living in this relatively poor community, she was accepted and well liked by the people. She had a hard time, however, making her patients pay her medical charges. The author herself was receiving a salary from the main hospital which owned the clinic she was operating. She was far from being exploitative; all she wanted was an amount of money sufficient to maintain the clinic and to pay for drugs and other supplies. The *buraku* people were very resistant and reluctant to pay even a little, although they had the money. The social apathy of the community was such that they could not "give" even to a cause of direct benefit to them.

Burakumin seem to be prone to more illness and endemic disease than are other groups. This situation does not seem to result from lack of efforts on the part of public health officials, but rather seems to stem from some resistance to governmental officials whatever their purpose. According to the same author, trachoma was common among the *burakumin*. In 1953 at the junior high school attended mostly by children from the *buraku*, 64 per cent of the 400 total students were suffering from trachoma. The district commission on education was alerted, and the next year the percentage dropped to 30 per cent. Nevertheless, the health programs initiated were met with a certain amount of apathy and resistance.

Inoue (1961), a well-known historian and active protagonist of *buraku* liberation movements, also has pointed out the frequency of "dependent-expediential" attitudes in older members concerning group efforts of the *buraku*. Inoue said:

> in their campaigns aimed at the prefectural or central
> governments demanding further administrative measures for
> *buraku* improvement, some of the older members of organized
> movements express the feeling that they have the "right" to
> demand things in compensation for a long period of
> discrimination, since they have not retaliated in any way
> against the majority society. People frequently fall into the
> mood that they have a special right to ask for governmental
> help for improvement because they are *burakumin* . . . but
> this is wrong. . . .

It is interesting to note that in leveling this charge against the *burakumin*, Inoue paid little attention to the fact that this demanding attitude is a consequence of social discrimination through a number of generations. Such underlying antagonism to legitimate authority is particularly disturbing to majority Japanese, since within the culture there is little tradition other than that of conformity to authority.

BURAKUMIN DELINQUENCY AND CRIME

The American evidence strongly associates delinquency problems with the social dislocations of mobility, migration, and ethnic minority status. In the state of California, for example, the Mexican-American youth are committed to correctional institutions approximately five times more often and the Negro youth approximately four and a half times more often than are whites of European background in proportion to the respective populations of these groups.[2]

To learn the delinquency rate among *buraku* children, we went through case files of a family court situated in one of the major cities in Japan with a population of over one million. When the case of a delinquent boy is first brought to the family court, his permanent address, home address, date of birth, nature of his delinquent behavior, and the kind of treatment received are all recorded on a card. The card is permanent, and if the same boy is brought back to the court for further acts of delinquency, these incidents are added to his records. These cards give a general impression of the distribution of delinquency in different residential sections.

From the records of all cases brought to the family court between August, 1957, and August, 1963, we obtained over 13,000 cards. We excluded cases of traffic violations, and then examined every tenth card. The resulting 1,044 cards included records of boys whose residences were unknown or outside the jurisdiction of the court from which we derived our sample. These cases were in turn excluded. We finally obtained a sample of 633 boys aged 14 to 19. Those who resided in districts known as "special" *buraku* areas were identified as "*buraku*" boys. Those living outside known *buraku* districts whether "passing" or not were *not* identified as *buraku* boys. This classification by residence in known *buraku* probably resulted in the inclusion of a relatively small number of non-outcaste children. Conversely, probably a larger number of children of outcaste families who were attempting to "pass" were misclassified in the "non-*buraku*" sample. Such probable misclassifications were unavoidable, since outcaste identity cannot legally be investigated or documented in official records. The 663 boys also included some Chinese, Koreans, and a small number of other foreigners. We obtained estimates of the total population of *burakumin* from the city's welfare department. The population of Koreans and other foreigners was obtained from the June, 1963, statistics of foreigners' registration. The total general population in June, 1963, was estimated from the census of October, 1960. The number of boys in each category was divided by the total estimated population for each group, thus producing a rough rate of delinquents per 10,000 individuals.

As shown in Table 1, youths of Korean background showed the highest delinquency rate—over six times that of Japanese youths living in majority areas. Japanese boys living in *buraku* areas showed a rate of over three times that of those in non-*buraku* areas.

In Table 2 a breakdown into first offenders and recidivists reveals that recidivism was significantly higher among Japanese living in *buraku* areas than among others. There was a somewhat higher proportion of recidivists among the Koreans than among Japanese living in majority areas, but within the numbers tested the difference was not significant.

The delinquent acts of the boys also were classified by offense.

Table 1: Delinquency Rate

Classification	Number of Cases	Total Population	Rate (per 10,000 population)
Japanese majority area residents	493	1,098,546	4.49
Japanese residing in ghettoed *buraku* areas	71	47,023	15.10
Koreans	63	22,365	28.17
Other non-Japanese	6	10,468	5.73

Table 2: First Offenders and Recidivists

Classification	First Offenders		Recidivists		Total	
	No.	Per Cent	No.	Per Cent	No.	Per Cent
Japanese majority area residents*	350	71.0	143	29.0	493	100
Japanese residing in ghettoed *buraku* areas	42	59.1	29	40.9	71	100
Koreans	42	66.6	21	33.4	63	100
Other non-Japanese	4		2		6	

* Majority areas versus *buraku* areas: $x^2=4.0$, df=1, p<.05
Majority areas versus Korean registrants: n.s.
Majority areas versus total minority categories: $x^2=3.4$, df=1, p<.10

Table 3: Percentage Distribution of Delinquency by Type of Offense

Type of Offense	Japanese Buraku Residents	Japanese Majority Area Residents	Koreans	Other Non-Japanese	Total City
Theft	41.4	55.5	44.8	41.7	52.6
Intimidation, extortion	42.9	22.8	26.1	16.7	25.3
Gambling, narcotics, prostitution, obscenity	0.7	2.2	1.9	16.7	2.2
Incendiarism, rape, robbery, murder	3.6	2.8	3.9	—	3.0
Fraud	0.7	1.4	1.3	8.2	1.4
Criminally inclined	9.3	8.8	8.4	—	8.7
Other*	1.4	6.5	13.6	16.7	6.8
Total	100.0	100.0	100.0	100.0	100.0

* Carrying guns and swords, petty crime, breaking the Alien Registration Law.

As shown in Table 3, those residing in *buraku* areas showed a very high rate of intimidation and extortion. In a number of these cases of threat and extortion, however, the delinquent boy involved, surprisingly, is much younger than the individual threatened. It is not unusual to find a boy 15 years old threatening a group of two or three older boys without the use of any weapon. In some cases by simply stating that he is from a feared *buraku* community, a boy can evoke fear in the minds of children outside the *buraku* and can obtain from them either money or goods.

Community control seems to operate to deflect delinquent activities outside the *buraku* community itself. Our informants generally agreed that violence, acts of stealing, or other forms of antisocial behavior rarely take place within the outcaste community itself, although the children are verbally aggressive toward one another, speaking in tough language. If some physical aggression seems to be in the offing, an adult quickly steps in and attempts to reconcile the quarreling pair. When a child is accused of delinquent behavior, the *buraku* people support the child rather than the outside authority. What is important, seemingly, is that the children obey their parents rather than that they show any allegiance to the outside. In court, the fact that children are obedient to their parents is cited as a mitigating factor by the parents.

Children placed on probation in Japan are supervised by a so-called *hogo-shi* ("supervisor") within their own community.[3] The delinquent children who are put under the supervision of the *hogo-shi* within the *buraku* community do not indulge in any delinquent activities as long as they stay within their own community. The *hogo-shi* therefore actually does very little in the way of supervision. He does not seem to be active in preventing the individual adolescent from leaving the community and committing delinquent acts elsewhere. The recidivism rate is disproportionately high for *buraku* children on probation.

The *buraku* community is not at all supportive of court decisions to place a child in a correctional institution. Sometimes when such action is taken, a large number of adults gather at the court building in an organized hostile protest. They may appeal to the court to cancel the judgment and instead place the child on probation so that he does not have to leave the community.

A general attitude of hostility is directed toward the buildings that house the prefectural offices, police, and court. These institutions represent for the *buraku* people the legal authority of the majority society, and the prefectural office represents also the place where birth records or registry of Japanese families and individuals are kept. For the *burakumin*, these offices symbolize the official records which are kept of their identity and background. Among the *burakumin* the police station and police system come in for considerable criticism. There is an implicitly understood regulation among policemen that, when a policeman wants to get married, the social and family background of the young woman is scrutinized carefully and reported to a supervisor whose permission is required for the marriage. One informant cited a story that he claimed was not unusual of a young policeman falling in love with a girl of *buraku* background, but his application for permission to marry was turned down by his supervisor with the reason stated that the girl had an unfavorable background and therefore could not become the wife of a policeman. When the police are brought up in conversation, such incidents readily come to the mind of informants, suggesting their readiness to feel hostility toward police authority.

For members of the *buraku* community a criminal career may be one method of "passing." If a *buraku* youth is successful in becoming a member of a criminal gang or *yakuza* group, his outcaste background discreetly is forgotten. It is a practice among professional criminals not to scrutinize an individual's past too closely. The *buraku* youth therefore may feel more readily accepted in this career than he would in attempting to face the overt discrimination that occurs in other occupational pursuits. In the same manner *buraku* women who become prostitutes find it an easy way to "pass" and to remove themselves from the *buraku* community.

Conclusions

Evidence from Japan suggests direct functional parallels between deviant trends in traditionally disparaged minority groups in the United States and Japan. An aggravated delinquency rate is but one symptom of a total situation influencing the internalization of social values. One must note, however, that the internalization pattern in minority groups is influenced not only by the external pressures of discrimination but also by the nature of the response to minority status in terms of the sanctioning methods available to families and the minority community generally.

Not all minority communities react to discrimination by producing socially deviant members or individuals who flout socially expected behavior. The tradition of discrimination has to exist for sufficient time to affect the socialization process of the young. Some minority groups acculturating to a new society undergo disruptive changes. The Puerto Rican immigrants to New York, for example, cannot sustain their previous community or family relations in their new setting. The Chinese in the United States, on the other hand, formed communities with strong sanctions that prevented any visible individual deviancy from the accepted standards of the majority that would bring them into conflict with the police. Some minority groups meeting a new situation of social discrimination maintain active defenses against legal authority based on previous traditions. The Mexican-American community as well as family groups, in socializing the young, develop attitudes of resistance to legal authority, which is perceived traditionally as an outside pressure boding no good to the individual. The Japanese, in contrast, meeting discriminatory attitudes in immigrating to the United States, socialize their young toward conformity to legal authority. Through a pursuit of strong Japanese values of education and achievement, the Japanese community, in contrast to other racially discriminated communities, has been able to maintain a significantly low delinquency rate.

Some minority groups are based directly on a disparaged caste position in the society to which the individuals must respond by some form of self-evaluation which in itself tends to incapacitate the individual from the ready assumption of social expectations. The parallel situation which we have documented in this paper attests to how a tradition of such social disparagement continues even after some alleviation of the discriminatory attitudes and practices themselves—another example of what might be termed a psychological lag found in a changing society, namely, that the effects of a particular social condition continue after the structural elements producing the condition have changed. This continuance occurs because an internalization pattern has been induced in individuals that cannot be changed readily, since internalized psychological mechanisms are involved. This internalization pattern occurs very often within the sanctioning practices of the primary family. In fact, the primary family itself may have been influenced seriously by certain types of minority status, as in the case of the American Negro, so that a serious disruption from the usual culturally prevalent family pattern has occurred. Although we have not discussed fully the evidence we have gathered concerning the freer sexual practices and more fragile family relations among *burakumin* than among the majority Japanese, we can cite a direct parallel on the basis of the impressions of some of our informants.

Individuals seeking to define social problems within a sociological framework sometimes tend to slight the psychological processes involved in socialization experiences within minority family groups. One cannot operate solely in terms of a theory based on social mechanisms to understand such complex problems as delinquency in society. The primary family and its functions in socialization are a meeting ground for psychological and social theory.

ACKNOWLEDGMENT

The substance of this paper also appears in modified form as Chapter 13 of a general volume on the Japanese former pariah or outcaste group by G. DeVos and H. Wagatsuma, *Japan's invisible race: caste in culture and personality*, Berkeley, University of California Press, 1966. The reader is referred to this volume for a full bibliography and review of previous works on the subject written in both English and Japanese. Our comparative research in delinquency and social deviancy has been sponsored by a grant from the National Institute of Mental Health, Bethesda, Maryland (MH-04087). We should like to acknowledge our deep appreciation for the able assistance of Mr. Yuzuru Sasaki, probation officer of the Kobe Family Court.

NOTES

1. Both the Taiwan-Chinese and Koreans in Japan legally were citizens from the time of the Japanese annexation of Formosa and Korea. They could keep their citizenship after World War II if they had resided in Japan for some time in a permanent capacity.

2. It must be noted that other minority groups have escaped a negative self-identity through the effects of strong, cohesive, well-integrated communities that do not bring them into conflict with the majority society. In California the Japanese-American and the Chinese-American minority groups have the lowest delinquency rates of any distinguishable groups.

3. In the Japanese court system under Japanese juvenile law, there are two different forms of probation. One is probation in the custody of Family Court probation officers. The second is probation under the custody of probation officers belonging to the probation bureau of the Ministry of Justice. Probation by the Family Court probation officers is called *shiken-kansatsu.* The second type of probation is called *hogo-kansatsu.* Usually when the prognosis of the delinquent case seems favorable, it is put under the probation of the Family Court. When the children involved are put under probation to the Ministry of Justice, they are at the same time put under the supervision and guidance of some person in the community who works on a voluntary basis. The qualifications of these volunteers are carefully examined by the probation bureau, and those who pass scrutiny are appointed to work in the capacity of supervisor of children. These are the so-called *hogo-shi.* Many *hogo-shi* are school-teachers; others are owners of small or middle-sized enterprises—small entrepreneurs. Usually the number of delinquent cases per probation officer is too large for him to handle personally. He therefore heavily depends on the lay volunteers for supervision. Very often the motivation for having a boy under supervision is that he will work at the factory or store of his supervisor.

REFERENCES

Inoue, K. 1961. Kaihō undō no rekishi ni manabu. Buraku No. 9:4–17.
Ishida, S. 1961. Shinro shidō to kōkō zennyūgaku mondai. Buraku No. 9:51–55.
Kobayashi, A. 1962. Buraku no joi. Tokyo, Iwanami.
Mahara, T. 1960. Buraku no shakai. *In* Buraku no genjō. Buraku Mondai Kenkyūjo, ed. Tokyo, San-itsu Shobō.
———. 1961. Buraku no kodomo to shinro shidō. Buraku No. 9:55–59.
Merton, R. 1959. Social theory and social structure. Glencoe, Free Press.
Nomura, N. 1956. Tsukimono no shinri. *In* Shūkyō to shinkō no shinrigaku. I. Oguchi, ed. Tokyo, Kawade.

22. On Getting Angry in the Society Islands

ROBERT I. LEVY, M.D.

Department of Anthropology
University of California, San Diego
La Jolla, California

The fateful question for the human species seems to me to be whether and to what extent their cultural development will succeed in mastering the disturbance of their communal life by the human instinct of aggression and self-destruction.

—Sigmund Freud, *Civilization and its Discontents*

THIS CHAPTER CONSIDERS the ways in which a group of people, the Polynesians of the Society Islands, deal with problems of aggression and self-destruction. Contemporary behavioral forms related to aggression seem to have deep historical roots for the Society Islanders, as evidenced in reports of the earliest Western visitors to the islands and in the similarities in behavior among closely related people, such as the Hawaiians. These behavioral forms are cultural forms, developed in the past, perhaps the ancient past, and transmitted and shared by successive generations. In the Society Islands, as seemingly in all changing cultural groups, many psychological traits have long survived such other aspects of the old culture as the religious and political systems to which they were adapted. Until very recently most Society Islanders, particularly those living in isolated rural communities, had been able, unlike other less fortunate acculturating people, to create a new culture out of the wreckage of the old under Western religious, commercial, and political pressures, a culture consonant with most of the persisting values, needs, and ways of thinking of the people. Since 1962, however, there has been a sudden, major acceleration in the rate of change of the conditions of life in the Society Islands, as a result of the opening of an international airport, the rapid development of tourism, and the development of a French nuclear weapons testing site in the nearby Tuamoto Archipelago, with major logistic, housing, and shipping facilities having to be developed on Tahiti.

The observations which are presented here are based on field studies which I made in June and July, 1961, and from July, 1962, to June, 1964, in two communities in the Society Islands. The studies (part of a larger project under the general direction of Douglas Oliver) consisted of household and community observations and psychological interviewing towards a general psychological description. Detailed discussion of methodology and of other findings will be presented elsewhere.

Historical Perspective

French Polynesia is a French Overseas Territory consisting of more than 100 islands scattered over a large area of the South Pacific from 7 ° to 29 ° south latitude and from 131 ° to 156 ° west longitude. The Society Islands are a subgroup within the territory, consisting of 7 large, high volcanic islands, 2 small volcanic islands, and a number of coral atolls. Tahiti is the administrative and commercial center, with most activities centered in the major town of Papeete. According to the 1962 census,[1] the population of French Polynesia was 84,550, of whom 68,245 lived in the Society Islands group. Of these Society Islanders, 19,903 lived in Papeete and 26,527 in other districts of the island of Tahiti. The Society Islanders all speak the Tahitian language and historically were members of a unified culture. In general "Tahitian" as an adjective is used to refer to the whole Society Island group, but it is sometimes used to distinguish the island of Tahiti from the other islands in the group.

I worked in two communities. One was a rural village, which I shall call "Piri" (population 284 in 1962) on the island of Huahine (population 3,214), about 100 miles northwest of Tahiti. The other was an urban enclave I shall call "Roto" in the town of Papeete. It had about 300 inhabitants in 1962. Most of the generalizations I present seem true of both communities, although they were gathered more systematically in Piri and often confirmed in Roto.

My main interest was in typical and shared traits, and their systematic relations. Thus I am interested here in aspects of anger which are in some sense Tahitian. I believe that the forms which I shall sketch are widely shared in the area, and one of my reasons for including historical notes and contemporary impressionistic reports is to suggest this. Further studies, of course, will be necessary to confirm or disprove, generalize or limit, these observational convictions.

The description which follows is arranged in a series of increasing magnifications: First, historical material; then general and official impressions of violence in the area; next, a description of styles of aggressive behavior observed in the two communities; and, finally, a consideration of cognitive forms, residues of childhood experience, and stimulus patterns which are associated with aggressive behavior and which are considered partial explanations for the forms of that behavior.

There is a relatively large amount of material descriptive of Tahiti and the Society Islands in the days and years following discovery by Samuel Wallis in 1767. Explorers, naturalists, sailors and mutineers, missionaries and commercial men described the attractive natives. A tough myth formed rapidly, or rather myths, for the romantic and missionary myths flourished in peculiar interaction. Both myths were woven around impressions of ethnic character. Fortunately, a large number of day-by-day interactions were described and embedded in the generalizations, and many glimpses of the behavior behind the generalities were preserved.

One of the most useful sources for information about Tahiti in the years subsequent to its discovery is the journal of James Morrison, a mutineer from H.M.S. "Bounty," who spent most of the time between October, 1788, and May, 1791, at Tahiti. He was neither a romantic nor a missionary but a sympathetic observer of considerable common sense. In his summary account (Rutter, 1935) of the Island of Tahiti he wrote:

> The people in general are of the common size of Europeans, the men are strong, well limbed and finely shaped, their gait easy and genteel and their countenance free, open and lively, never sullied by a sullen or suspicious look. Their motions are vigorous, active and graceful, and their behavior to strangers is such as declare at first sight their humane disposition, which is as candid as their countenances seem to indicate, and their courteous, affable and friendly behavior to each other shows that they have no tincture of barbarity, cruelty, suspicion or revenge. They are ever of an even unruffled temper, slow to anger and soon appeased and as they have no suspicion so they ought not to be suspected, and an hour's acquaintance is sufficient to repose an entire confidence in them.[2]

Other observers were in virtual agreement with this picture of the personal style of the Tahitians. As early as 1778 John Forster, who was with Cook on his second voyage, that of 1773–1774, wrote:

> In short, their character is as amiable as that of any nation that ever came unimproved out of the hands of nature. ... The natives of these isles are generally of a lively, brisk

temper, great lovers of mirth and laughter, and of an open, easy, benevolent character.

George Forster (1777), his son, also on the voyage, found the Tahitian's practice of infanticide puzzling: "When we consider the whole character of the Tahitians, when we recollect their gentleness, their generosity, their affectionate friendship, their tenderness, their pity. . . ."

The Reverend William Ellis (1829) wrote about the Tahitians of 1817 to 1824:

> Generally speaking, careful not to give offense to each other. . . . There are . . . few domestic broils; and were fifty natives taken promiscuously from any town or village, to be placed in a neighborhood or house—where they would disagree once, fifty Englishmen, selected in the same way, and placed under similar circumstances, would quarrel perhaps twenty times. They do not appear to delight in provoking one another, but are far more accustomed to jesting, mirth, and humour, than irritating or reproachful language.

Though fights and fracases were reported, it seems that it was often with some indication of their seeming rarity. Thus John Forster (1778) noted:

> Nor are the inhabitants of the islands in the South Seas [i.e., Tahiti and the Society Islands] quite free from a coarseness of manners, even to indelicacy in many respects, especially among the lower class of people; which appears from the disputes of many of them, wherein they fall to beat ing one another with the fist, and pulling one another's hair.

Morrison (Rutter, 1935) noted that "Private disputes between men relative to themselves only seldom produce a blow."

By 1784 the ship's doctor (Cook, 1784) on Cook's third voyage, during which four months were spent in the Society Islands, perhaps in reaction to French tales of Tahiti as the isle of love, inhabited by noble savages, noted:

> As the women, in such a life, must contribute greatly to its happiness, it is surprising that they should not only suffer the most humiliating restraints with regard to food, but should be often treated with a degree of brutality, which one would suppose a man must be incapable of towards an object for whom he had the least affection or esteem. It is, however, extremely common to see the men beat them most unmercifully. . . .

If this treatment were "extremely common," it was not so reported by other observers, although they noted occasional wife beating (and even husband beating by wives).

There was community sanctioned violence such as in human sacrifice and war, but the details of these institutions do not make them appear unnecessarily brutal. John Turnbull (1805), who had visited Tahiti in the first years of the nineteenth century, wrote:

> They certainly live amongst each other in more harmony than is usual amongst Europeans. During the whole time I was amongst them, I never saw such a thing as a battle; and though they are excellent wrestlers, and in their contests give each other many a hard fall, the contest is no sooner concluded, than they are as good friends as ever. Their frequent wars must be imputed to the ambition of their chiefs; and were it not for the restless disposition of these men, I am persuaded that war would be almost unknown amongst them.

Turnbull also generalized: "Their dispositions are gentle to an extreme. I never saw an Otaheitan out of temper the whole time I was in Otaheite." Morrison (Rutter, 1935) whom I quoted earlier as finding the Tahitians "slow to anger and soon appeased," recorded in his journal for March, 1790, the murder of one of the mutineers, Thompson, in revenge for Thompson's murder of another mutineer, Churchill. Churchill had been made the "blood brother" of a chief of a small district, thus gaining some chiefly status, and some of the natives of the district felt they had to revenge his death:

> The manner was this, Patire . . . being sorry for his friend's death, was determined to be revenged on Thompson, and having got five or six more, who when they knew the cause were equally enraged, they went to Thompson's house and saluted him . . . and told him that he was now Chief, and such like flattering stories till Patire got between him and his arms, and being a stout man, knocked him down. The others whipped a short plank, which happened to be at hand, across his breast, and placed one on each end, while Patire ran for a large stone, with which he dashed his skull to pieces. They then cut off his head, and buried the body . . . [cutting off the head was for ritual purposes]. I asked him why they had not brought him to us at Matavai, when he replied, "the distance is too great, and our anger would be gone before we could get there; and we should have let him escape when we were cooled and our anger gone so that he would not have been punished at all and the blood of the Chief would have been on our heads.

From the copious reports of early visitors to Tahiti, one gets the impression that in relation to European expectations acute, explosive, hostile behavior was rare and that prolonged, intense, sustained bad temper, grudge-holding, and revengefulness were even more rare. There are many anecdotes of individuals avoiding giving or taking provocation to anger and promptly seeking ways to make peace with each other as well as with the powerful Europeans.

The Reverend Mr. Ellis reported that, according to hearsay, there was some violent drunkenness in the early years of the attempts to convert the people to Christianity, a time of political instability prior to the establishment of hegemony by a missionary-supported chief. Ellis (1829) wrote that in 1814 some years before his arrival:

> Under the unrestrained influence of their intoxicating draught, in their appearance and actions they resembled demons more than human beings. Sometimes in a deserted still-house might be seen the fragments of the rude boiler and the other appendages of the still, scattered in confusion on the ground; and among them the dead and mangled bodies of those who had been murdered with axes or billets of wood in the quarrels that had terminated their dissipation. . . . It was not only among themselves that their unbridled passions led to such enormities. One or two European vessels were seized and the crews inhumanly murdered.

Whatever the objectivity of Ellis' report, though drinking continued, later reports presented it as nonviolent. For example, Jacques Moerenhout, a Belgian who lived in Tahiti between 1828 and 1845, noted in 1837 that there had been no case of murder in the islands since 1814.

The Tahitians were adjusting to their new situation, which was soon to be fully colonial.

Crime

The island of Huahine has only one French official, the *chef de poste* or *gendarme,* responsible for law and order, liaison between the island and various territorial administrative centers, and a limited variety of local judicial and administrative functions. Most of the people live in seven villages, and almost all the decision making and social control is at the village level. Serious crimes are reported to the *gendarme.* Disturbances which cannot be resolved in the village are supposed to be reported also but in practice seldom are. Violent behavior—murder, suicide, violent rape, maiming—is virtually always reported both in Huahine and throughout the territory. The *gendarme's* seat is in the port town of Fare, with a population in 1962 of 447, continually augmented by village people shipping and picking up goods, marketing at the Chinese stores, and drinking beer or wine at the town drinking places.

The *gendarme* who administered Huahine in the early 1960's had worked in Indochina, French Guiana, Algiers, and Morocco. For him the people of Huahine were "lambs" in contrast with the people of Morocco who were "hot tempered, easily angered, thieves, murderers, and rapists." Huahine, he said, is "the other end of the world." What surprised him, he said, echoing the early reports, was the lack of a revengeful spirit. Even though people occasionally were cheated or insulted by a visitor or a merchant, they did not seem to show any anger, any need to get even. There was, he said, no serious crime in Huahine, no violence, no forced theft. There were only very occasional and minor disturbances connected with drinking, and a few stern words usually easily controlled them.

The records for Huahine between 1940 and 1962 showed only one serious crime, a murder in 1953. (I use "serious crime" for the French legal designation "crime." These are serious offenses generally equivalent to felonies, requiring adjudication at a special criminal court, the *assise,* and entailing at least five years imprisonment.) The crime on record was a very violent, probably impulsive murder, although there was some question about the amount of premeditation involved. It concerned an 18-year-old man, a native of Huahine, who after an argument with a Chinese farmer killed him by stabbing him and hacking at his body with a bush knife. There had been previous arguments and exchanged insults and threats; apparently the assault grew out of the Tahitian's acute anger. For the period prior to 1940, only one other serious crime was known to the older people in Huahine. This had taken place in 1928, when a man, angered by his wife, had beaten and then drowned her.

The *Gendarmerie Nationale* at Papeete has published statistics for the territory for selected sample years (Bouvet and Iorsch, 1960). Table 1 shows the number of murders and total crimes (serious) committed in sample years between 1900 and 1959, not the number of criminals involved. Crimes recorded are artifically somewhat low, because for various reasons some offenses which would be handled as crimes in metropolitan France are handled as *delits* (misdemeanors) in the territory. Whether crimes were committed by Tahitians, Chinese, or Europeans is not indicated. Nevertheless, the figures suggest quite low rates. A supplementary report (Bouvet, 1962) gives total crimes (serious) for 1960 and 1961 as only 2 and 1, respectively.

In the years between 1900 and 1956 the population of the island of Tahiti increased from about 42 per cent of the population of the territory to about 50 per cent. For the sample years Tahiti was the location of 53.6 per cent of the serious crimes and of 73.5 per cent of the misdemeanors noted.

Informants remembered three suicides in Huahine since 1945. Two were natives of the island and one was an official from Tahiti, a *demi* (a French-Tahitian cultural half breed), temporarily assigned to Huahine. Of the resident cases one was a man who had been having intercourse with his 15-year-old daughter and had hanged himself on the day that the village policeman found out about it and decided to tell the *gendarme* at the port town administrative center. The other resident case was a girl of 15. According to the tale, her adoptive father, a Chinese, had died, and the girl was unhappy when her adoptive mother, a Tahitian, took a new man, who was much younger than the mother. The mother one morning became angry with her over something or other, threatened her, and then hit her. As the mother was leaving the house, the girl said, "You will never see me again." Then she laid out her white clothes (garments worn to funerals or as burial clothes) and hanged herself.

Officials believe that suicide in the territory is relatively common among Chinese, rare among Tahitians. Between 1958 and 1962 figures for the territory,[3] exclusive of the Leeward Island group which kept separate records, showed nine suicides. Of these only two were Tahitians, four were Chinese, one Vietnamese, one French, and one a tourist of unspecified origin. (The relevant population base for the reporting area in 1962 was 68,373, of which approximately 7,800 were Chinese or part Chinese, 44,453 Tahitians, and 7,197 *demis* or part-Tahitian and part-European; the remainder were Europeans.) The two Tahitians were both men who lived on the island of Tahiti.

Violent and Aggressive Behavior

Even when one has adequate statistics on rates for some types of violent behavior the question remains whether the high or low frequencies of behavior making up the rates have anything to do with the ordinary

Table 1: Murders and Total Crimes (Serious) in Sample Years in French Polynesia

Year	Total Population	Murders	Total Crime (serious)
1900	28,960	0	0
1910	31,770	0	2
1920	34,910	0	2
1930	39,480	4	8
1940	49,770	0	0
1950	61,270	2	5
1953	67,280	0	3
1956	73,201	0	0
1959	80,000 approx.	5	8

behavior of others in the population. To what degree are official crime and suicide rates related to the actual amount of such violent behavior? Is such behavior related to other forms of angry, aggressive behavior? If so, is it an index of conditions prevalent among the population which are widely shared, thus making the rate a comment on the population in general; or do these cases represent some discontinuous, mosaic population, thus providing no information on the remainder of the population? These are empirical questions. Similarly, behavior which in some cultural comparative sense seems hostile or nonhostile may have different import in the local culture.

In moving from general impressions of officials and foreign observers to observations in the community and then to closer investigation of individuals, perhaps I can begin to give structure to various social impressions.

My first impression of life in Piri was one of interpersonal restraint, and lack of hostile aggressiveness. (One needs such implicit comparative judgments to describe first responses.) As I learned more about the community, it was clear to me that the effective hostility mediated in small acts, such as gossip, teasing, and coolness, was stronger and more important both in discharge and hurting effect than I had been able to judge at first. In many ways life in Piri is low key in emotional and interpersonal intensity. The effectiveness of small acts may be related to a Weber's Law for cultural cases: The lower the initial stimulus level, the less an increment has to be to be perceived as an increment.[4]

There were very few physical fights in Piri, nor were those that did occur particularly violent. I saw only one physical fight there and none at Fare, the port town in Huahine, even during the July festival, when villagers from all of Huahine went to Fare for several days of sports, dancing, and drinking. During the twelve months that I was there three other fights reportedly took place at Piri, all among the same group of drinking companions, and involved mostly quickly terminated pushing and shoving.

In Piri the absence of fighting was evident particularly among children in public settings. Groups of children usually were playing near the schoolhouse, or on the wharf, or in the fields near the village. Their play was highly energetic, involved a good deal of joking, and, in same-sex play, body contact and often mock aggression, such as pushing or a tug of a girl's pigtail. (Cross-sex play was more limited, and did not involve body contact, except among very young children.) The mock aggression did not turn serious. Occasionally in a game a critical or irritated remark would be made, but the recipient would simply ignore it or, rarely, withdraw crying. He would disengage. There seemed to be few provocations, and a disinclination to pick up the provocations which were given.

In the two serious children's conflicts which I saw, the fashion of expressing a threat was carefully ineffectual. An offended boy would chase his tormentor but never catch him, while other children looked on with serious expressions. Giving up, the boy would throw a small piece of dry coconut husk at his antagonist and miss. Children were excellent marksmen in other kinds of throwing.

The village school in Piri had 85 children in it in 1963. The head schoolteacher said that in his two years at Piri he had never seen a fight among the older school children (8 to 15) in the school yard, where the children played before and after school as well as during regular play periods. Younger children (6 to 8) on rare occasions cried angrily or threw pebbles at each other over some disagreement.

Another teacher who had worked in Piri and in other villages in Huahine for nine years, contrasted the behavior of children in Huahine with behavior in Anaa, in the Tuamotu Archipelago, a group in the territory with marked linguistic and cultural differences. At Huahine, she said:

> the children do not fight much, and it is rare to have a bad child in class. In the Tuamotus the children are wicked. They fight and throw stones at each other, and sometimes threaten the teacher. When they play, it is not to have fun but often to hurt each other. In their language, they are vulgar and dirty, as are their parents. In Huahine it is very rare to hear dirty language even among the adults, and very unusual among the children.

Public hostile aggression, both among children and adults, seemed to have other general features. By "public" I mean that which took place in out-of-the-house village areas or within a house when there were visitors. Private household hostile aggression had some special features. This private hostility could be made public with a complex shift in its structure, by shouting, so that neighboring households could hear the argument. The general features are the substitution for or the restraint of physically hurting action directed at another person, dramatic form, dependence on an audience, audience anxiety and passivity until a certain threshold is reached, and exaggeration in the later reporting of incidents.

The following episode is illustrative. In 1963, during the Piri New Year's festival lasting eight days and involving a considerable amount of drinking, only one episode might be described as violent. This involved a deviant man named Tore who lived by himself in a small house in the far inland part of the village and stayed out of most village activities. He was regarded sometimes as a clown and sometimes as mildly frightening, and he seemed to encourage and enjoy generating anxiety. He usually wore sunglasses and a unique knotted handkerchief cap and effected dramatic mannerisms. The New Year's festival had started with church services to be followed for most people by an all-night prayer and hymn singing session. Everyone was dressed in his best clothes, except Tore, who made a point of walking through the assemblages outside the various church meeting houses, wearing only shorts, an old shirt, the handkerchief cap, and sunglasses. On the second day of the festival Tore appeared at a temporary dance shed where food and jugs of wine were set out. Tore rapidly drank three or four tumblers of wine. Immediately after, he began to stagger around exaggeratedly. Onlookers looked mildly anxious (it was generally said that Tore was troublesome and bad when he drank). He began to try to pick arguments with people, who ignored him, and after an hour or so of such attempts, the village policeman, who was also somewhat drunk, took hold of Tore, who made little resistance, and tied him up to a tree. He was left thus for about two hours. Many people ignored him; others commented that it really had not been necessary to tie him up. When it began to rain, a neighbor of Tore untied him. Sometime later Tore again entered the dance shed. Tamu, one of Piri's heavy drinkers who was slightly drunk, accused Tore somewhat angrily of "frightening people." They began to hit each other lightly. Tamu finally pushed Tore, who fell down. Then Tamu picked up the chastened Tore and, aided by Tore's sister, walked Tore, his arms about their shoulders, off to his house inland, where he went to sleep. The next day Tore claimed that he did not remember anything of the previous afternoon after his first drinks. He said that he had been drunk, that he had done wrong, and that he was through drinking for the rest of the New Year's festival. This was an accurate prediction. During the rest of the festival he was seen occasionally sitting at the edge of the dance floor and quietly watching the dancing.

This was a typical blow-up in that it was quite dramatic and relatively harmless both physically and socially, since it had no long-term, unresolved consequences. Note that drinking seemed necessary for Tore's argument picking and its consequences, but that his drinking did not produce particularly destructive behavior.

There were two general types of hostile-appearing behavior which did not involve physical hurting. First were the usual, daily hostile activities such as gossip, withdrawal, and teasing. These activities were overtly understood to be types of, or substitutes for, direct angry expression. They were widely used in socialization and village social control. Second were episodes in which a dramatic expression of destructive action turned out to be carefully limited in its effectiveness. (In contrast, for example, to the *amok* of other cultures.) Thus a man furious at his *vahine* [5] set fire to some coconut thatching sections lying on the ground at a safe distance from his and other houses. A group of men driven to exasperation after months of administration by a crudely interfering and destructive *gendarme* gathered one night and threw very small stones at a safe distance from his feet; when the time came for him to leave the post, he was given an exaggeratedly elaborate farewell feast, combining regret for the action and further indirect hostility. In actual fighting men do not hit each other very hard, and it is easy for bystanders to hold them back.

The presence of bystanders, of audiences, is necessary for these expressions. A main object of the explosion is to bring some tension from the private into the public realm, to express a dissatisfaction or to shame an opponent. Even when the outburst is only simple discharge of tension, the presence of the audience gives safety to the actor or actors in that they feel that controls will be exercised if the situation begins to look serious.

The lack of serious physical destructiveness is impressive just because of the showy, dramatic quality of the behavior. The usual bland, quiet, easy going style of life gives noisy or mildly destructive episodes a particular shock value (*see* the comments above on Weber's Law). Episodes which looked relatively mild to people familiar with forms of destructiveness in other cultures often were reported later in terms which seemed exaggerated not only because of culturally different weightings of the seriousness of the episode but also because of the extent of the injury sustained. People also frequently reported fear of possible physical harm from other people in settings in which the fear did not seem to be objectively warranted. They would say of themselves: "Tahitians are terrible when they get into a fight." "Tahitians could never play American football [with tackling]; they would kill each other." Some of the women stayed away from the dancing and drinking sheds in Piri during the New Year's festival because they were afraid "someone would get killed." One young man who had said that he was afraid to walk on the dark streets in Papeete (which were obviously safe), said that the only reason he wasn't afraid to walk on the path in Piri after dark was that no one would try to hurt him, for everyone in the village would immediately know who had done it. The fear of the consequences of anger, of hostility, of violence—with little apparent experience of such consequences—was noteworthy.

There also seemed to be little violence under conditions of personal breakdown,[6] including drunkenness. Drinking was common, particularly during two yearly festivals. With the exception of a few incidents, such as the episode of Tore, the people were as unhostile drunk as sober. Nondrinkers would continue interacting with the drinkers normally, indicating no uneasiness. The situation was different in private in-the-house drinking or in drunken behavior at home following drinking in a public setting. Then drinking was sometimes associated with arguments and the occasional hitting of a spouse or children. As I have said, one of the major Tahitian tactics against becoming angry is not to become seriously engaged emotionally or to disengage—tactics which are difficult in spouse and parent-children relations (although there are some culturally approved methods). Most tension therefore is expressed in the household. There are also, of course, the special tensions of child socialization, the hostilities engendered in teaching the children not to be hostile.

Concepts of Anger

The ordinary word for anger in Piri (where a standard Tahitian with a few regional features is spoken) is *riri*.[7] *Riri* is one of a number of terms which can be put in the sentence, *Ua————vau*, "I have become ————." "Happy," "fed up," "tired," "frightened," and similar words also are appropriate, and one may gloss the series as feelings—states which happen to one, which arise. *Riri* is located in the abdomen (or more rarely, chest) as are a variety of other feelings and can arise spontaneously or be stirred up by a thought or by something seen or heard. The verbal sequence in the latter case often goes, "My eye saw the event, and the anger grew (*tupu*, as a plant grows) within me." According to the general doctrine the *riri* once generated is thought over (*feruri*) in the head; some localize this further in the brain, others in the forehead. Then action or restraint is decided on. Inadequate *feruri* may lead to impulsive action.

Extreme rage is *hae*, which one informant defined as "The person is so extremely angry, he wants to devour you." Another term, *'iriā* refers to a state of irritability, a proneness to become angry, and is often used to refer to a type of person.

In the early days of Western contact the missionaries compiled a dictionary of some 11,000 Tahitian terms (A Tahitian and English Dictionary, 1851). At least 1,500 of these terms (Levy, MS) describe feeling states, character types, thought processes, and nuances of interpersonal relations. The fact that most of these "psychological" terms are not known or used currently seems to indicate comparative blunting of the categories of psychological and interpersonal discrimination. Even after deleting many of the missionaries' words as dialectical variants, nonce words, and the like, there remains striking evidence of a contraction of Tahitian vocabulary since the early decades of the nineteenth century. Of a total list of 301 items which seem to describe various feeling states, 47 referred to angry feelings. It may be significant and is congruent with contemporary forms that terms for anger were the most common in comparison with the number of terms in such ordinary sense-sets as pleasure, fear, longing, "agitation of the mind," sadness, tenderness, and shame. Of these 47 items, at least 12 seem to represent trustworthy terms for anger, probably carrying different nuances of meaning. Of these 12 terms, only 3 are in use in contemporary Tahitian.

In spite of the limited number of terms, anger is "hypercognated" in Piri and Roto, that is, relative to some other feeling states (for example interpersonal longing and loneliness, which may be interpreted vaguely as being out of sorts), there is a developed and shared doctrine of the forms of anger, its effects, and what to do about it. Many statements about anger were so similar from all informants in Piri and Roto that they were either shared doctrine or generated from similar experience or a mixture of the two. Anger is always a bad thing. I heard repeatedly that it can lead to knife fights, to injuries, to killing. (It is interesting that the common word for "beat up," or "thrash," *taparahi*, also means "kill," and that the word for "unconscious," *pohe*, also means "dead." Thus ordinary statements about strong violence do not distinguish "He will get mad and beat up somebody" from "He will get mad and kill somebody." Are these particular semantic spans both indicative of anxiety about violence and to some degree productive of it? One can make distinctions, for example, by saying *pohe roa,* "very *pohe,*" for "dead," but in a large number of cases, such as statements about violence, they are not made.) Statements concerning the violent effects of anger are made, as I have said earlier, despite little experience of such violence.

Just as anger generally is stated to be dangerous, it is also stated that once angry the thing to do is express it, preferably by angry words, so that one's anger can calm down. One man said, "The Tahitian people say that an angry man is like a bottle. When he gets filled up he will begin to spill over." It is thought that unexpressed anger has bad effects on the body and may give trouble in the head or heart and that people have died from anger—a combination of toxic effects and the will to die because of pique. (People are said to die only when they wish to in the normal range of deaths.) One woman in Roto said that unexpressed anger would turn one's hair white. In addition to the physical effects of unexpressed anger are the social ones: "If somebody doesn't tell me when he is angry at me, he'll go and tell somebody else. He'll gossip about me, and exaggerate, and then trouble will start in the village." People who did not express their anger at the moment it was aroused because they were chronically timid, *mamahu,* often had special characteristics, according to informants. They could not look you in the eye. They did not seem to get mad usually, but when they finally got mad they were violent.

All this reasoning was part of a general doctrine that undischarged anger takes substitute forms, clearly labeled as expressions of anger. People sometimes attributed punishing their children to their anger at a spouse who couldn't be hit. The anger was said to carry over to someone else. Another clearly labeled substitute form of anger was suicide. The one informant who admitted any suicidal thoughts said they had been occasioned in his childhood by anger toward his grandfather following a beating. When the grandfather asked forgiveness, his suicidal plans disappeared. Suicides discussed in the village usually were explained as a result of anger, and death in general was sometimes explained as a result of the person's willing himself to death out of anger toward someone in his family. (This was especially true of some women who died in childbirth.)

In general not all affective sets had such detailed psychological doctrine as was related to *riri.* Some were highly discriminated—e.g., anger, shame, fear; others were very poorly discriminated—e.g., loneliness and depression. This high discrimination of angry behavior, combined with strong, shared evaluations, facilitates social and psychological control.

Certain aspects of magic belief were closely tied in with beliefs about anger. It often was felt that angry threats of the sort, "You'll see what is going to happen to you," or, "You'll get your reward for this," might be magically effective. When someone had a serious accident, people often discussed who had been angry with him, yelling at him recently. It was generally felt that to be effective such a threat had to be made in words, not just wished, because the punishment was carried out by some ancestral spirit of the threatener who heard the threat. In effect, however, this belief meant that a wished threat or fancied hostility could not hurt the object (although as noted it could hurt the wisher). A man would not go fishing after an argument with his wife for fear of some accident. A mother-in-law who disapproved of a daughter-in-law would try to calm down and not talk about it for fear that the daughter-in-law might have a miscarriage or die in childbirth. (Unless her hatred was so severe that she wanted this to happen. This wish would have been extremely deviant. The ascription, however, of actual miscarriages to disapproving mothers-in-law was not uncommon.)

Since all magic in Piri needs the co-operation of an independent spirit intermediary, if a family had some powerful spirits, and thus *mana* in the family line, either a man or woman theoretically could perform effective magic threatening. In actuality all reported cases involved women as threateners. When such women were frequently effective they were metaphorically sometimes said to have "poison tongues." It sometimes was explained that when a man got angry he could always hit a women but that a woman had no alternative to threats. In fact, however, in the village a man rarely "just hit" a woman; it was said that as the stronger a man should not hit a woman.

There are several aspects to this asymmetry in regard to magic threats. Because of his more active life, a man has more accidents and mishaps needing explanation. He also has other resources besides threatening, for he can more easily withdraw from the household for work or for an important discussion down the village path. Apparently, also there are in general more inhibitions on a man than on a woman in regard to hostile aggression. When a woman's threat produces a minor accident to her husband, both she and her husband may talk about it to others with pride. It is a sign of *mana* in her family. The husband is not angry with her, because it was the spirit ancestor who caused the accident. He must have deserved it since it was worth the ancestor's trouble. Not only that (and this is a pervasive theme in the vulnerability to magic and other hurts) it was partially his fault that the spirit could get to him; he must have been afraid of the spirit and concerned with it, for when one is calm, unconcerned, and emotionally unexcited, neither ordinary spirits nor people can hurt one. All this stops the *reverberation* of the angry interaction.

Although women make most ordinary magical threats in the village, there is a level at which men are also threateners—in tales or legends and in stories about wicked sorcerers, *tahu'a,* who may be men or women, but are said to be mostly men. The actual *tahu'a* in Huahine are magico-medical practitioners, who are admired, possibly uneasily, and are helpful in a variety of disorders. The hurting ones are usually fantasies. Wicked *tahu'a* are said to initiate curses out of personal anger. They run dangers that the threatening women do not run. Their curses may turn back on them. They are likely to be cursed by other *tahu'a*. They die terrible deaths (the death of bad *tahu'as* is a favorite subject of conversation), and they go to hell.

Although these threats and curses were talked about from time to time with great interest and pleasure, they were not used in explanation of the ordinary range of troubles in village life—small injuries, ordinary sicknesses, failures, and disappointments. They were used to explain serious and unusual injuries and illnesses. For example, it was only after the third miscarriage that people might begin to give magic explanations. (An exception was when a severe argument was followed immediately by an injury, or violent parental disapproval of a marriage by a miscarriage.) It is noteworthy that with a magic system so well constructed to project blame, there was so little blaming and "paranoid" behavior.

In both Piri and Roto the main effect of magic beliefs associated with the effectiveness of anger was to make people wary of angering others—to provide pressure for conciliation. To a lesser degree, the potential threatener might have been inhibited by fear of injuring a liked person or of the curse turning on the threatener.

Mechanisms for Coping with Anger

It is convenient to separate for discussion the dimensions of behavior which are associated primarily with verbal symbolic behavior, rules, doctrines, and namings—those aspects closest to the thinking, calculating, rationalizing aspects of behavior, the cognitive aspects—from a residual of other culturally shaped behaviors, e.g., a general disposition to be fearful. Judgments about the latter forms are usually based on different kinds of behavioral clues than are judgments about cognitive forms. It is possible to make a maximized cognitive model which handles most of the other forms but this does violence, I think, to some useful distinctions.

Certain pervasive forms related to anger can be inferred from a variety of behaviors. An adequate discussion of these forms would require an extended treatment of child-rearing sequences even though we were only interested in formed adult behavior, for the only language we have to describe them in some complexity must use as one of its dimensions a model of the child-in-the-man.[8] Within the bounds of this paper, however, I can only touch on them in a schematic manner.

In illustration of child-rearing sequences, I shall narrate two episodes involving Toni, a two-year-old boy, the only child of young parents. Toni's parents divided their time between his paternal grandfather's garden lands, where the boy and his parents made up the entire household, and the same grandfather's house in the village of Piri, where the child was part of a household of 11 and the center of attention in their leisure hours. Nothing delighted the family more than Toni's aggressiveness; he would hit at people, pull dogs' tails, swagger, shadow box at command, and so on. A quiet, somewhat constricted boy of five was the next in age to Toni in this household. A year and a half before, when I had first known him, this boy had been as cocky, comical, and aggressive as little Toni and similarly made much of. One evening when Toni was performing as usual, surrounded by all the household, amused and encouraging his aggressiveness, he suddenly stumbled and fell. Immediately his father, and the children in the household said *"Aitoa"* ("It serves you right"), and *Tera ta 'oe ma'a"* (literally "That's your food," meaning "You've gotten what you deserve"). Toni lay on the floor crying energetically. His father picked up a broom handle and stood over him angrily telling him to stop crying. Toni cried, his father threatened, the audience watched. After four very long minutes, his father finally picked him up and began to distract him. A week later little Toni was performing in his cocky way to the full household. A nine-year-old girl (his father's half sister) was lying on a mat, her head near the leg of a wooden bench. Little Toni gave her head a hard shove, and it banged into the bench leg. The little girl did nothing, but Toni's mother hit Tony on the leg. He started to cry and ran to his father. His father joked with him and calmed him, saying, "Your mother was bad to you." Five or six minutes afterwards Toni, again playing actively, made one of his usual, usually rewarded, fighting gestures toward one of the other children. Suddenly his father hit him hard on his rump. Little Toni lay down on the floor and began to scream. His father stood over him repeating angrily, "Stop crying, stop crying." He sent one of the children for the broom and brandished it over Toni. Within a few seconds Toni just ceased crying and stood up. His father with obvious pride and pleasure said, "He is afraid." Then Toni began to play again, very much as before.

These sequences represent experiences which are recurrent for children in Piri and Roto. One can generalize some of the child's experience as it relates to hostility and aggression as follows: (1) A period of relative security and gratification lasts at least one and a half years, sometimes longer. Various socialization techniques are prefigured, but in a discussion of aggression and hostility one can stress the child as the center of attention, highly stimulated and cherished. He is considered a separate individual and is in a busy interaction network within a few weeks after birth. (2) As his motility develops his energy, playfulness, cockiness, and mischievousness are much admired and rewarded. He may even be coached in fighting gestures. (3) Short, acute expressions of anger by young children toward someone who is disciplining him, an older sibling or a parent, are reacted to with amusement; in older children they are quietly tolerated. (4) Two kinds of behavior, however, are strongly discouraged—expressions of anger lasting more than a few moments and "reverberation-causing behavior," interpersonal behavior which will not let the difficulty die out after its first expression. Thus from the start angry crying is discriminated from other types of crying, which can be called "need for care" crying. The infant crying angrily is ignored, if possible, and an older child is first ignored and then threatened until he stops. (The fact that he will stop, as did little Toni, is curious to Westerners who feel that you cannot win this kind of battle.) The prolonged anger which is most vigorously attacked is that which results from an act of discipline. The parents' anger attached to the act of discipline is usually small, but the anger related to the child's responsive prolonged anger is very much greater, as are the threats and sanctions. Older children are discouraged from returning the blow of a younger child who has hit them, and in general sanctions are directed more against the continuation of a fight than toward preventing its initiation. (5) In general, the parent attempts to avoid making a child angry.[9] The child is thought to have a strong, stubborn will of its own and is allowed to set his own timings and activities to a large extent. (6) The child having a will of its own, the problem is how to get it to obey when necessary. Although adults often attribute their motives for resolving conflicting behavior in a socially approved direction to "shame," or "sympathy," the doctrine for the childrens' acceptance of an unpleasant social command usually is said to be "fearfulness." It is considered important to create fear in children so that they will obey. Fathers will say that it is good for boys to lose a fight, so that they will not fight again, and for them to fall out of trees, so that they will not take such risks again. Parents seem pleased by injuries to their children which will teach them such lessons. (7) There is an effort to shift the locus of the act of control from a specific parent-child act or battle to a generalized source of control. The parent acts as part of the unbeatable system, which has two aspects: First, the entire family, particularly those in the household (affinal relations are relatively excluded), have socialization rights and duties, which they carry out with only a limited supervision from the parents. For little Toni, ten people, starting with a boy only three years his senior, told him what to do and punished him (when he passed the wide limits of accepted behavior). Second, accident and the universe in general continually are called in as punishers. Most accidents are said to serve the child right and to have been caused by his general naughtiness and daringness (not by a specific act). Thus the whole system was against him, not merely an identifiable person, who might be coped with. (8) The major fear-provoking technique is threatening— "You are going to get beat up"; "You are going to be in trouble." This is a very frequent line of patter from mothers to their younger children, as any stroll up the village path attests. Beating, on the other hand, is rare. People who know Tahiti and related cultures, such as Samoa or the Tuamoto Islands, say that beating of children is much more common in the latter places. The adult Samoan and Tuamoto Islanders are reputed to be considerably more violent than the Tahitians. Perhaps threats produce more generalized, persistent fearfulness in relation to violence than does actual, experienced, violent punishment—which also, by the way, provides models for violent hostile acting which threats do not.[10] (9) Threats and beatings are often more a function of the parents' or siblings' mood than of a specific breach of any rule. What is learned is a generalized caution rather than a set of specific acts to be performed and avoided, as exemplified, perhaps, by little Toni's punishment for a minor act, rather than the preceding major one. (10) When a child is three or four his parents and siblings become much less amused by his showing off than they had been. There is a general emotional withdrawal from children who have reached this age.

I shall comment upon some general consequences of these socialization modes. A frequent theme in interviews is a sense of fear in relation to others' hurting potential. An aspect of this fear is that others are often seen as bigger and stronger than oneself, even though to an observer this seems not so. Fear of being hurt by the other is used as an explanation for inhibiting fighting. The effect of drinking is often explicitly stated as "overcoming fear," which may consciously lead to an otherwise inexpressible argument or fight. The fearfulness is not a generalized feeling of fright about most aspects of life. One can speculate about the encouragement of effective aggression in the young child before its discouragement in terms of the formation of an "aggression hostility dynamism," which is then discouraged. Were this aggression discouraged from the start, one might expect more pervasive, diffuse, and perhaps dysfunctional coping mechanisms in response to threats. It is of interest that in the socialization of a cluster of affectionate and dependent responses in the child, there is a period of gratification and encouragement, followed by a strong discouragement of these reactions.

Not only are others viewed as larger but also as more dangerous than oneself—"you never know what they might do"—in spite of a lack of supporting evidence. This feeling may be partly related to parental capriciousness in punishment as well as the fact that almost all children are socialized and attended to a large degree, usually with little or no supervision, by slightly older children who are often very capricious and hostile to the younger ones. Others also are viewed as relatively unimportant; they have little power to frustrate and are easily disengaged from.

There are indications that intense angry and emotional feelings in general are felt to be particularly disruptive because of some general qualities of personality organization which are threatened by strong feeling. Adult involvement in hostile, sexual, and tender feelings seems to be related to suppression of the intense, more primary feelings and their replacement by a carefully controlled, inhibited, somewhat stylized substitute. It is possible that this type of organization can be threatened by any surge of feeling, which threat may explain the observable discomfort in situations which tend to generate strong feelings and the reports of anger as being bad for the body or as interfering with sleep.

Given these considerations, the coping strategy may be stated thus: Try not to get into situations which will make you mad. Do not take things seriously or withdraw, if possible. If someone is mad at you, try not to let it build up. If you do get angry, however, express it by talking out acute anger so that things can be corrected and so that you will not be holding in your anger. Express your anger, if possible, by verbal rather than physical means. If physical, try to use a symbolic, harmless action, not touching your opponent. If you do touch him, be careful not to hurt him.

The system seems to work to prevent gross hostile action without causing strong repressed hostility, unlike the situation in other cultures where soft, gentle personality facades frequently are associated with much violent behavior. There is little apparent muscular tension, violence when drunk, violent crime, or violence in the behavior of institutionalized psychotics. There do not seem to be strong residual pressures for discharge.

An essential parameter in any consideration of hostile behavior is the nature and extent of the frustrations endured in the ordinary course of life. It may be useful to separate "primary frustrations" which are presumed to be universally frustrating (e.g., shortages of resources, conflicting provisions in rules for obtaining a goal) and "secondary frustrations" related to specific local definitions of situations. An analysis of frustration in detail would require a general discussion of the social, cultural, and ecological aspects of experience in Piri. Grossly, there are the usual tensions of life in a small isolated village, where people must spend their entire lives getting on with each other. A few people were glad to escape the village with its gossip and close mutual observation, but most were able to live peaceably and even happily there. There were certain themes which acted to reduce the "frustration meaning" of events. Much of the world view, of the dominant value orientations, served to reduce "secondary frustration." For example: (1) Much of Tahitian socialization is directed, through complex strategies, against striving. It is felt that too much striving is bad, unproductive, or may even bring punishment from nature. When one is not ambitious, he has, of course, less chance of being frustrated. (2) Emphasis is on the substitutability of goals, the objects of which are assumed to be in adequate supply. If you lose one woman, you will get another. If you do not get fish one day, you will on another. (Incidentally, there are no good luck magic and love charms. It is assumed that magic is not necessary for success and that manipulations will decrease your chances. The best way to get ahead is to take it easy.) (3) To Tahitians the actions of other people seem in some degree to represent the working out of general forces, part of the system. To the extent that actions are seen as inevitable, natural, and not arbitrary, willful, and unnecessary, they probably produce less sense of frustration and irritation.

Conclusions

So far, I have limited this discussion to certain general factors to the shaping of hostile feelings and action without mentioning differential and varying factors. All the aspects that I have mentioned apply to both men and women, but with varying emphasis. Boys are considered potentially more violent, and therefore harder to manage than girls. There seems to be more stress on encouraging the naughtiness of small boys as well as on controlling the anger of somewhat older ones than there is for girls. As might be expected in a culture which stresses the suppression of angry behavior, boys and men give the impression of being more generally inhibited and restrained than are girls and women.

The picture presented holds true for the *Ma'ohi* (Tahitian-oriented, as opposed to mixed French-Tahitian-oriented) people of the urban enclave of Roto and can be presumed for the Society Islands in general. In Papeete there is a drift toward a Tahitian version of modern culture; however, just as the modern Christian and peasant life in Piri preserves many of the psychological features indicated in early reports of the immediate post-contact life, so does modern town life. Even in the historically related, but much more highly acculturated Hawaiians, there are, I believe, many related personality features (forms, for example, related to aggression, sexuality and homosexuality, meaning of love objects, and structure of behavioral controls). One aspect of this persistence may be that certain psychological traits become relatively critical for a variety of other cultural and psychological institutions. These traits have a large variety of shaping forces associated with them and tend to persist through time and space. In a sense, the need for the shape, as determined by its relations with other forms, provides a "strategy suction," so that a variety of techniques can be used and innovated in changing situations to produce roughly similar, shared, persisting personality forms.

For those interested in returning to these old questions, the task is to identify traits of the proper level of complexity for comparison, to develop models of specific mechanisms involved, and to find more objective ways to validate clinical impressions.

ACKNOWLEDGMENT

Field work was supported by Research Grant M-5567-A from the National Institute of Mental Health and by Research Grant NSF-G 23476 from the National Science Foundation.

NOTES

1.   These figures are taken from preliminary reports on the 1962 census of French Polynesia.

2.   In this and the following quotations from late Eighteenth Century and early Nineteenth Century sources, spelling and punctuation are modernized.

3.   The material on suicide comes from the records of the Gendarmerie

Nationale and from the records of the Palais de Justice at Papeete, Tahiti. I am indebted to Capitain Bouvet, M. Charles Waddy, M. Georges Raid, and M. Rene Gauze in this, and many other matters.

4. For a discussion of Weber's Law in perception, *see* Berelson and Steiner (1964), pp. 95–97.

5. *Vahine* means "woman," "wife," or a man's "temporary mate."

6. There was one known case of functional psychosis in Huahine, a middle-aged woman. She was teased, and sometimes pitied, but not overtly feared. Her dress and actions were bizarre, but not threatening. Patients at the territory's mental asylum at Papeete were said by the chief nurse to be generally quiet and well behaved. Visits to the asylum confirmed this.

7. Tahitian can be rendered in conventional orthography with the addition of the macron (⁻) to indicate long vowels, and an apostrophe (') or similar sign to indicate the glottal stop.

8. "The complexity and subtlety of adult aggression is the end product of two or three decades of socialization by the individual's parents and peers . . . and bears little resemblance to the primitive quality of the infant's action patterns, from which it developed" (Sears, Maccoby, and Levin, 1957).

9. This is congruent with the socialization strategy which Sears, Maccoby, and Levin (1957) found to be associated with the least aggressive children in their American sample. "A child is more likely to be nonaggressive if his parents hold the value that aggression is undesirable and should not occur. He is more likely to be nonaggressive if his parents prevent or stop the occurrence of aggressive outbursts instead of passively letting them go on, but prevent them by other means than punishment or threats of retaliation." For some distinction between the effects of physical punishment *vs.* threats, *see below.*

10. There is convincing experimental work indicating that the observation of an aggressive model increases aggressive behavior. Sears, Maccoby, and Levin (1957) put it "when the parents punish—particularly when they employ physical punishment—they are providing a living example of the use of aggression at the very moment they are trying to teach the child not to be aggressive." Reviews of laboratory studies of aggressive behavior, particularly in relation to the effect of models, are Walters (1966) and Bandura (1965). Learning from models, or "vicarious learning," has central importance in such settings as a Society Islands village.

Apropos of threats versus physical punishment Bandura remarked on the Society Islands (personal communication): "Ordinarily the inhibiting effects of verbal threats rapidly extinguish through repeated disconfirmation, but the parents intermittently reinforce the threats by capitalizing on accidental contingencies. Impersonal agents rather than parents are the aggressors. Since they are omnipresent, fear of punishment by impersonal agents is likely to produce generalized inhibition, whereas punishment by socialization agents tends to establish specific inhibitory effects and often only in the presence of the punitive agent." As noted above, socialization agents act as equivalent agents in a fairly large network; this must also have a generalizing effect.

REFERENCES

Bandura, A. 1965. Vicarious processes: a case of no-trial learning. *In* Advances in experimental social psychology. Vol. 2. L. Berkowitz, ed. New York, Academic Press.

Berelson, B., and G. Steiner. 1964. Human behavior. New York, Harcourt, Brace and World.

Bouvet [no initial]. 1962. Rapport sur la criminalité en Polynesie Francaise. Papeete, Tahiti, Gendarmerie Nationale.

Bouvet and Iorsch [no initials]. 1960. Etude sommaire sur l'evolution de la criminalité à Tahiti et en Polynesie entre 1870 et 1959. Papeete, Tahiti, Gendarmerie Nationale.

Cook, J. 1784. A voyage to the Pacific Ocean for making discoveries in the Northern Hemisphere. 4 vols. London, Stockdale.

Ellis, W. 1829. Polynesian researches. 2 vols. London, Fisher, Son and Jackson.

Forster, G. 1777. A voyage round the world. 2 vols. London, White, Robson, Elmsly, and Robinson.

Forster, J. R. 1778. Observations made during a voyage round the world. London, Robinson.

Levy, R. I. MS. A psychological analysis of *A Tahitian and English dictionary* [1961].

Moerenhout, J. A. 1837. Voyages aux îles du Grand Ocean. 2 vols. Paris, Bertrand.

Rutter, O., ed. 1935. The journal of James Morrison, boatswain's mate of the Bounty. London, Golden Cockerel Press.

Sears, R., E. Maccoby, and H. Levin. 1957. Patterns of child rearing. Evanston, Row, Peterson.

Tahitian and English dictionary, A. 1851. Tahiti, London Missionary Society's Press.

Turnbull, J. 1805. A voyage round the world. 3 vols. London, Phillips.

Walters, R. H. 1966. Implications of laboratory studies of aggression for the control and regulation of violence. Annals of the American Academy of Political and Social Science. 364:60–72.

23.   Ego Structure in the Hindu Joint Family:
Some Considerations

N. C. SURYA, M.D.

All-India Institute of Mental Health
Bangalore, India

WHEN I RETURNED to India from my psychiatric training in the United Kingdom and began to practice psychiatry in my home country, I found that many of the terms and concepts in psychotherapy and interpersonal action that I had learned abroad made little impact. (My basic medical training was in British India in 1940; my initial medical practice was in the British Indian, later Indian, Army, 1942–52, my formal psychiatric training was in the United Kingdom, 1952–58.) At first I had a sense of failure and frustration, but after considerable internal struggle I located the difficulty. I was an Indian dealing with Indian patients and Indian situations, but to all of these realities I was completely out of tune for I was striving to apply totally different value systems, alien both to myself and my patient. All that follows in this chapter may have some claim to attention because it has arisen from practical experience and need. The views expressed here are entirely personal and do not in any way represent an official position of the psychiatric profession in India.

Transcultural psychiatry is a concept that should yield dividends to the extent that it implies a real two-way transaction, if not integration, but for a variety of historical reasons it is all too possible for this transaction to degenerate in practice into a one-way induction of conceptual frameworks, axioms, and implications that have acquired prestige in the economically well-developed countries. Danger from this pitfall is even greater when the professional personnel participating in the therapeutic transaction all have had their basic training in these countries and when their very fitness to practice and expound their profession had to be certified in terms of teachers, textbooks, and concepts of the alien culture.

I say these things with no intention to preach chauvinism, only in order to pinpoint a fact of essential importance to transcultural transactions in mental health. Unless a conscious, sincere effort is made to overcome this basic problem, mental health concepts about whole masses of people will be manufactured by distortion at more than one level, beginning with the level of language whereby all real transactions with these peoples first is translated into a different language and then by tortuously analyzing the resulting material by means of concepts and terms that are presently acceptable semantic currency in the West.

It is no wonder that in economically backward countries quite a few psychiatrists (and other technologists as well) have a sense of frustration when their jargon fails them in their day-to-day contacts and when their newly learned value systems, lightly worn as one wears a suit, rarely apply either to themselves or to the patients with whom they do their clinical work. Father Bulatao's concept (in Chapter 18) of the split-level personality in Filipinos is relevant to this situation.

It is believed in many quarters that the many ills of the economically backward countries are due to some sort of cultural deficit and that we have the authority or the power to change this. It is sometimes taken for granted that technological progress induces large-scale changes in cultural and personality characteristics. This is very doubtful. It is only necessary to visualize the large-scale technologic progress of the West in the last few decades and the almost uniform level of their technologic status, while noting the very material differences in basic culture and personality that have persisted. Culture subdues and masters technology: technology merely touches the superficial aspects of behavior. It is true that many Indians today sit at a table to eat their dinner, instead of squatting on the floor. It is also true that many of them ride in a car instead of in a bullock cart, but it does not automatically make them Germans or Americans eating at the table or riding in automobiles.

The rapidity with which technology spreads in a culture depends on leadership which can consciously utilize the available cultural cues for adequate motivation. One cannot import leadership as one can import radar equipment. Not only for the purposes of psychiatric practice but for the larger purposes of leadership training, cultural studies are imperative. They also are imperative for transcultural integration and the creative resolution of transcultural conflicts.

Apparently scientific and objective papers in transcultural matters by Western authors are full of value-laden words, terms, and implications. This circumstance may be unavoidable, but it is indefensible and calls for some conscious efforts at rectification in the interest both of science and of transcultural understanding. Some examples can be given. Literacy is permitted unconsciously to be an index of positive cultural maturity, but events of World War II—for instance the brutalities, the psychopathic murders in the concentration camps, and the emergence of dictatorships—go to show that, though desirable, literacy may have little relevance to positive cultural maturity or even to sound democracy. The label "superstition" is applied too readily to beliefs that are not current in one's own culture. The basic fact that all normal perception both omits and adds objectively nonexistent data is denied and pushed away. For this purpose we use the respectable words "selectivity of perception," "mental set," "situational set"—anything but "hallucination." Each culture chooses its own areas of selectivity of perception and experience and its own criteria of reality. Great care is needed in using such words as superstition or hallucination in reference to cultures and to whole peoples. The word "primitive" is another which requires some care when it is applied to a people or culture as a whole or even to generations of the past.

Let us turn now to the methodology of transcultural psychiatry. Does the average or a random sample represent a culture? Some transcultural studies seem to be concerned mainly with the study of behavioral abstractions derived from the study of so-called average representatives of a people, of clinical populations, or of paranormal phenomena in the culture. This type of study would be an excellent thing in itself were some kind of observation its sole aim. When the aim, however, is to create abstractions, to extract principles that should be of help in everyday clinical work with the patient, then one should ponder the adequacy of this approach.

Each culture provides positive and negative cues and modes of reaction leading to integrative and creative behavior in that culture. Each culture also provides positive and negative cues on how to meet threatening changes. In all cultures, however, a majority of the people can represent only the negative or lower levels of behavior: a vast majority can be termed reflex victims of their own culture. Only a minority are the thoughtful, conscious representatives of the best in their culture, the leadership, so to speak. The cues are provided by the religion and philosophy and by other such structures.

There has been a tendency to avoid the study of the successful leaders and representatives of a culture. To say that only the rock-bottom average sample of a culture should be studied is sound statistically, but it is like studying the average parts of an automobile and neglecting to study its engine. The successful leadership in a culture and the ideals that have grown in the culture and have advanced that culture are the motivating forces of a culture. I humbly suggest that a concentrated anthropological study of the elite of a culture is an urgent necessity.

Most transcultural studies involve the use of questionnaires, drawn up in a Western setting to sample areas of behavior meaningful there. Such questionnaires then are applied to a different culture. A concession to the other culture is made by conceding a translation, often laboriously arrived at. Mere translation, however, does not solve the problem. Take, for instance, questions on psychosexual maturity, management of hostility, and so on; it is quite conceivable that a particular culture does not give equal emphasis or significance to that zone of behavior, and any interpretation with regard to pathology or diagnosis placed upon such grafted questionnaires is damaging.

Equally unhelpful are the studies that laboriously demonstrate the similarity between all cultures. Such spurious similarity is reassuring about the possibilities for transcultural co-operation and harmony, but hardly convincing in the face of the hard realities of our world today and the abundant evidence of differences murderous in their implications.

Because it is of utmost importance to our existence that real differences be apprehended and understood, let us seriously ask whenever a transcultural study highlights similarity: Is it an artifact of the questionnaire? Have any areas significant to a particular culture been omitted? When conclusions are arrived at by use of one-way loaded questionnaires, the situation is made worse by implying remedial action based on experience of the dominant culture. Although I know advice is all too easy, I should like to offer the following suggestions to anyone using a questionnaire for a transcultural study. When, let us say, an American psychiatric or psychological study of Japanese character structure is planned, let the same combined teams which conduct the study in Japan, study a comparable group in America, preferably by employing questionnaires which the Japanese team has drawn up. Whenever situations permit, this method would be the ideal way of extracting meaningful variables and differences.

The true value of transcultural studies will evade us when such studies occupy themselves with attempts to reduce all phenomena encountered to already accepted, familiar words and terms. The qualitative richness of phenomena is lost if some energy is not expended in attempting to understand the differences in the phenomena encountered.

In constructing or employing personality theories, it is highly uneconomical and unproductive, even definitely disadvantageous, to start with well-developed concepts imported from outside and then to attempt laborious amendment and annotation. The tardiness with which Indian technological leadership moves is because of this perpetual activity of altering borrowed conceptual plumage. One cannot afford to neglect the broad high roads of thought and action, the theories of personality which one's own culture has accepted; one has to travel these roads and by intensive and extensive interaction with the people of one's own culture learn to make the necessary amendments and deviations. One must walk amongst one's people before pretending to lead them.

I cannot overemphasize this point. To take but one example: the term "ego" is too important in current respectable use for one to challenge it as a concept. One should not forget, however, that all the uses and associations which this word has acquired are rooted in a sociocultural historic setting and in philosophies and practices relevant to that setting. The Sanskrit word *aham* is a dessicated equivalent, but an Indian operates with this word, its implications and anticipations. The Indian psychiatrist who tries to interpret Indian personality based on the word "ego" can hardly expect to influence questions of the mental health of his people. This distinction is no mere verbal jugglery; it has interactional reality. Yet the Indian psychiatrist (with the split-level personality) finds it both natural and incumbent upon him to measure laboriously his whole people on the Procrustian bed of the concept of ego, rather than to take equal pains to get the word *aham* and its implications across.

In a universe of possible experience, each culture seems to be influenced by definite sets. Within each culture there may be subgroups which share ways of experiencing with another major culture. It is unfortunate, but true, that cultural practices and modes of experiencing that acquire dominance tend to suppress other practices and experiences. The Malleus Maleficarum for a long span of history successfully suppressed scientific thought in Europe. Subtly but equally successfully, present-day scientific fashion blocks all thinking that is outside its technologic and methodologic sovereignty.

Some cultures are deeply influenced by experience of and belief in forms of consciousness and powers that may be beyond our sense-limited universe of perception. Serious students of mental health cannot avoid discussion of this area. Most researchers in transcultural fields, however, take it too easily for granted that such experiences are merely psychological artifacts; they limit their attention to reducing accounts of such phenomena to accepted psychological terminology. Naive as it would be to decry the scientific method, it is equally naive to ignore the heavy cultural bias that certain lines of scientific inquiry acquire during the course of history. It would be very detrimental to the progress of the scientific understanding of human behavior to ignore these biases. In the study of transcultural mental health, it is premature to lay down binding dicta relating to the criteria for calling a work "scientific." It is all too easy to deceive oneself into thinking that one's preferred mode of perceptual organization is the only valid one, especially when international organizations and the sources of research grants generally have a heavy bias toward the dominant trend.

As a continuing student of psychiatry, presently involved in teaching, I may perhaps be permitted to make the following criticism of my own profession. We psychiatrists have often pointed to the dehumanizing, pseudoscientific influences to which the medical student is subjected during his medical college years, but somehow, noting the zeal with which psychiatric research uses the words "detached," "objective," "statistical rigor," and employs such terms as exclusive criteria of respectability in such research, one wonders whether we are not letting the very devil whom we exorcise in public enter through our own back door. The orthodoxy of the newly converted is well known. This worship of the "detached observer" is having a baneful effect upon the trainees from the developing countries. Their medical education already had dehumanized them—the farther from their people they are the better is "scientific detachment." Their psychiatric training should help to correct this attitude, but psychiatry's new-found enthusiasm for "detachment" produces further grotesque departures. Consequently, when the young psychiatrists return to their operational work in the field, their respect for statistical tables and dry-as-dust formularies regarding human behavior is truly amazing. Their zeal for "getting into print" or "doing research" is hardly matched by the patience and perseverance necessary to understand and help their patients.

I have great respect for the "scientific method," but I also plead against the subtle implication that any worker, or work, in mental health which fail to fit in with this concept is somehow automatically inferior. Senior teachers in psychiatry have a duty to ponder seriously the sociology of research respectability.

The Sociocultural Setting

The observations which I am about to present may have no more validity than some of the early psychoanalytic formulations. Planned, prolonged research to refute or substantiate such statements is essential. In the culture I belong to, however, it is not considered essential for any particular scientist to be at any particular post for any particular length of time in order to implement certain tasks, nor have indispensability and essentiality any value as applied to a person or a task. My work and nerves suffered before I made a conscious dissection of my experiences—my real and practical interaction with our people, not just in my inpatient psychiatric practice but also in social and administrative situations. After I came to understand certain elements of our personality structure I believe that there was an improvement both in my work and in my mental state.

First, let us consider the general background of our culture. A people evolve a philosophy, and a philosophy conditions the people. A child in the family is exposed inevitably, though perhaps never persistently or systematically, to certain concepts about life, existence, death, and so on. Very rarely is a child excluded from participation in the full social life of the family—discussions, quarrels, compromises. A very deceptive permissiveness in the manner and method of exposure covers up the tenacity with which these concepts influence from birth to death, especially in moments of crisis. The *Gītā* and *Rāmāyaṇa* display the ideal. Pseudosophisticated denials of allegiance to this ideal or to concepts illustrated in these works, especially on the part of certain intellectuals in their contact with Western colleagues, do not alter the importance of these points of reference alike for the lowest to the highest in the land. Concepts of *dharma, māyā, karma, ātman,* or soul, god, rebirth, and the great legends of *Rāmāyaṇa* and *Mahābhārata* have great relevance to understanding of the Hindu personality—much more so than do Greek mythology or the Bible to understanding the British patient.

Important facets of the life of the Hindu joint family are: (1) *Diffuse social and interpersonal relations.* Exposure to social relations is spread over a number of persons—grandparents, uncles, aunts, parents, sibs, and so on. The parents do not have the explicit or implicit privilege of being the sole agents for structuring social relations and regulations for the child. (2) *Dependency relations.* As the individual grows up, he or she progresses through an unending series of dependency relations within a large kinship circle, although with varying degrees of intensity and duration. There is no point in time at which he can look forward to a relatively free and full individual responsibility. Marriage does not connote a landmark for the development of a fully independent unit, but marks the beginning of a new set of relations—the recurring decimal of dependency relations. (3) *Schism of status and roles.* The everlasting and ever-recurring dependency relations are governed by concepts of inherent status. A relatively rigid status concept is divorced from the concept of role. This dissociation between status and role runs through the whole social fabric. Status is sought after because of its inherent advantages rather than because of the individual's fitness to play the corresponding role. A father might like to send his son to a medical college because of the status attached rather than because of the son's essential fitness for such study. An attendant refuses to sweep; a sweeper will not act as an attendant. Total energy output is considerably limited by there being little incentive to play more than one role.

The Ego Structure

Let us turn now to the ego structure. Earlier I pointed out the disadvantages in describing personality structure in terms such as "ego" developed in a different frame of reference. I shall here content myself, however, with proceeding on the existing pattern.

The concept of "mine-not mine" is poorly developed in the Hindu individual. In an average large joint family what rightly belongs to one and what does not are never clearly demarcated. Such insistence would be branded as selfishness. In group life outside the family, such as in a school dormitory or a worker's hostel, two opposite trends come to the fore: very defensive hanging onto one's own self and possessions or very liberal misuse of one's own and others' property. This question of the "mine-not mine" boundary applies not alone to material possessions but also to intangibles, such as time, thoughts, and emotions. In group existence where all have similar expectations, this attitude can be quite stressful.

A corollary is that for the Hindu one's efforts need not be commensurate with the rewards. He feels no relation exists. You may earn more, but you may eat less. Those who work less and eat more are naturally more numerous. If you so choose, you need not work at all. A detached efficient approach to work, ungeared to its benefits, becomes the ideal. The culture enforces it; the philosophy supports it. If you work ten times harder than the next, it is no special virtue.

In the joint family, first the child and then the adolescent is a uniquely valued member. A child rarely is exposed to the need to wait for anything or to stand any frustration for long. Any educative frustration of a child attempted by one member of the family is soon mollified by the over-protective attention of another. Moreover, someone or other always is assuring a child that he is the best, or, when that is patently false, at least that the neighbor's children are no better.

Such a childhood leads to an adult inability to wait for any length of time without becoming anxious and irritable. Personal time flies fast; social time is eternal. Then, too, the ego requires for its stability a constant external supply of esteem. If no one has the time or patience to say that he is a good lad, then he himself has to proclaim it. Friends, events, and the like exist and are valued only to the extent they supply these narcissistic needs. Deep, durable friendships become difficult and threatening especially outside the family ingroup. Measurement of others according to some criteria or other becomes a trait and finding a deficiency in the other becomes a satisfaction. When the individual is left for any length of time without external approval, some degree of anxiety is bound to develop.

Infinite patience and absolute indifference to praise or blame then becomes a remote ideal represented by only a few.

Dependency Relations

I have already referred to dependency anticipations. These have great relevance with regard to psychotherapy. In the West—at least in the United States and the United Kingdom—the goal of maturity is an inde-pendent existence. There, unacceptable and unrecognized dependency long-ings become the focus of psychopathology, and psychotherapy attempts to resolve these dependency needs in a manner satisfying the requirements of a culture that idealizes individual independence. In the Hindu (Indian) environment the ideal of maturity is satisfying and continuous dependency relations. Independency longings can cause neurotic anxiety. The goal of psychotherapy becomes the resolution of those independency strivings in a manner that satisfies the requirements of a culture that idealizes individual submergence in complex interdependence.

In the use of the word "dependency," one already can discern the distortion of language and of interpretation. A Western value judgment unwittingly is thrust on the people. There is no really equivalent word conveying the same value judgment. One speaks of *bandha, sambandha, bandhavya*—bond, bondship, kinship—not of dependency. It would be hazardous to import this word dependency into the Indian psychotherapeutic scene.

If an Indian asks you for a scholarship or a favor on short acquaintance, sometimes even with angry insistence, he does not recognize dependency. He is only expressing his anticipations of closeness, bondship. One can reject the claim, but one will be misreading the action if the word dependency is used. This is more than a mere nuance—it could make all the difference to psychotherapy or even social and administrative relations between Indians themselves.

The word dependency is not palatable; as Doi rightly points out in Chapter 20, the Indian, as opposed to the Japanese, does not respect and acknowledge dependency but, in fact, idolizes independence.

Other Cultural Characteristics

There are some further matters of psychotherapeutic significance which I wish to point out. The constant interdependency environment also produces a great need for company. To be left alone for any length of time becomes stressful. Neighbors are required even if only to argue with. The intense need for people is such that it constricts other perceptions. For instance, neither solitary immersion in the beauties of nature nor the study of local flora and fauna ("bird watching") is popular. In any group activity relations with persons become more important than the objective for which the whole group was formed. To a medical student it is important to observe a patient's color, pupils, and temperature, but relatively less important than the supposed attitudes of the professor to the student himself. This characteristic may explain the frequency with which unsupervised work gets neglected. There is little readiness to accept individual responsibility for anything at all.

This intense personal involvement is offset by a most exaggerated public denial of all personal involvement in any work. Thus selection even to the most important executive posts in the country is conducted by committees—one of the basic qualifications of the committee being that all its members must forswear all personal knowledge of the candidate they are selecting for a particular post. One would adopt a completely different approach if one were appointing one's own cook or mason. In psychotherapy the therapist must be constantly alive to this and bring to the fore the positive, constructive aspects of relations.

The role of culturally idealized concepts cannot be underestimated except at the peril of superficial generalizations regarding the Indian, or assertions that the Hindu no more follows the *Gītā* than the Englishman does the Bible. It is not a question of following the *Gītā* or the *Rāmāyana* but of the concepts they clarify and the ego-ideals and lapses they portray and the identifications they produce in the Hindu mind. The gentleman in the Savile Row suit, whose daughter does the twist and who proclaims his disbelief in stupid Hindu fatalism (we Hindus are superstitious) especially in a club frequented by foreigners, will be consulting the astrologers about his next promotion. In a crisis the very emancipated young woman runs back to her mother for protection against unwanted and unforeseen troubles. This conceptual framework and its identifying figures are constantly kept alive in the popular mind; the Indian psychiatrist who neglects this aspect can touch but a fraction of the problem that faces him.

Briefly, the concepts are: (1) *Dharma*: A man is said to be good and mature if he acts according to set, objective codes. Acting according to one's conscience is a Western notion. The word *ātman* has nothing much to do with conscience in the Western sense. "My whole conscience tells me this is wrong, but I must do it, for this is my *dharma*." *Dharma* also implies appropriateness of action according to *kāla* (time), *deśa* (place), and *pātra* (person and fitness). (2) *Karma*: This refers to propulsions derived from a previous birth, the effects of present deeds, and the attractions of the future. Fatalism is not equivalent to *karma*. (3) *Māyā*: This refers to the illusion of real knowledge of the universe and its causes, whereas humans are limited heavily by their sensory systems. The concept of reality so readily taken for granted by the Western psychiatrist and patient in the setting of their culture cannot be forced on the Hindu scene. (4) Relative independence of the various personality functions is assumed. The various sensory modalities—emotional, connotative, reflective—and additionally the spiritual dimension of personality are granted some independence. Integration of personality functions is the Western aim, but some degree of dissociation and ideally a detachment of the higher from the lower functions is the Indian ideal. An Indian can say, "My body is suffering, I can only watch," or "I do not mind," or "My eyes weep but I am helpless." The witness function of the ego emphasized by Hindu thought is an important step in psychotherapy. One is encouraged to be first a nonparticipant witness of one's own reactions before corrections can occur. (5) The explicit and implicit acceptance of higher consciousness, or powers other than the human and of their capacity to influence behavior, and equally the potential capacity of the individual to be in contact with and guided by these means is another important point. The all-embracing psychobiological and psychological explanations of the Western psychiatrist which have acquired authenticity and respectability in a certain historic setting are not taken as axiomatic by the Hindu except as a polite formality.

In this connection I would like to mention a patient of mine, a young engineering student (the son of a very able and modern surgeon) who developed very schizophreniform symptoms. He used to worship in the temple of a snake-god, who also represented the chieftain of divine armies. One of his symptoms was a hallucination of a snake rising out of a corner in the room. He was sure that it was a sign of the god's anger. I suggested that perhaps this god was there to protect him and show his favor and would go away when the need was over. I merely took the other aspect of his own statement. Anyway, this boy who had been ill for three to four years, has gone back to his studies and is doing well. When I once mentioned this case to a psychoanalytically trained Indian psychiatrist, he said that the thing was a hallucinatory projection of an undesired symbol arising out of an original anxiety and so on. This explanation he thought gave a scientific angle while my explanation supported superstition. I merely avoided replacing one so-called delusion by another so-called scientific explanation.

Needless to say, all these concepts operate at different levels for different people. In fact the *Gītā* lays heavy emphasis on constitutional differences. In the vast majority of the less mature people these concepts act as powerful cushions against anxiety in critical times; in the more mature they have led to amazingly successful contributions to the development of highly creative individuals.

Mr. Gandhi's example can be given. When our political scene was rich with brilliant economists, constitution makers, and the like groomed in the West the results were very sterile and arid. Gandhi with his instinctive, direct, sincere understanding and practice of the positive cues and codes of our own culture introduced a massive motivational dynamism unprecedented in our latter-day history. The qualities of the successful leader have derived from the cultural concepts and family constellations. Such a leader has to have the characteristics of the successful joint family elder. Since, in and out of the family, anticipations and habits formed in the joint family continue to operate at all levels of life in the country, the leadership qualities, too, have to be studied from this angle. I might say that Western experts and advisers get quite perplexed when monetary rewards do not seem always to produce a better result. Their anticipations and expectations are very different. The complaints, often justifiable, of some Indian scientists that they are not well paid do not always correspond to facts; good pay in India does not necessarily attract a good man or produce a better result. The joint family does not produce a work-reward correlation. The most efficient and respected leader with the most powerful influence in a group is the very detached person, immune to praise or blame; ready to forgive, to accept, and even to protect all default; one who can forge ahead with like-minded others. The hard worker who seeks proportionate reward faces frustration till he learns the lesson. The negligent one looks surprised when anyone suggests that he does not belong on the bandwagon. Whenever a venture is succeeding, one confidently can seek the source in the concepts mentioned and in the very necessary background of our people, their anticipations and thoughts.

Ours is a complex civilization. Mere cataloguing of the numerous characteristics of our people from trait-questionnaires drawn up in the West will give a very contradictory and distorted picture. The Kiplingesque importunate, docile, dependent, untrustworthy Indian and the firm, gentle, but stern and unflinching Gandhian Indian are two facets of the same coin. Very close studies are needed, however, for psychotherapeutic purposes, as well as for understanding group dynamics in India in the present era of technologic and other co-operative ventures between different cultures. Such work is being done; its systematization requires very close cross-cultural work.

Conclusion

Before closing this chapter I must clearly state that all this discussion has reference only to what can be considered cultural determinants of personality and illness. It does not deny, but merely complements, our understanding of other more universal determinants, such as physiological mechanisms of anxiety, response to tranquilizers, and so on. When one speaks of Western and Eastern, it would be ingenuous to ignore the common biological heritage of all humanity.

From the standpoint of statistically minded scientific discussions, mine is very unsatisfactory. Even as an impressionistic document, it does not convey as much coherent thought as could extended description of individual cases and concepts. I hope, however, that it may serve to impress, upon those who are interested, three points which seem to me most important for transcultural research in India. First, the growth of a good corps of Indian psychiatrists trained intensively in the local setting is necessary. Second, whenever possible both learning and teaching of psychiatric interactions should be conducted in the language of the people. I have one group of students who work entirely in Hindi and are not allowed to use any English words, especially technical terms. How tongue-tied they can become even with each other when bereft of their borrowed defenses has to be seen in order to be believed. How ineffectual they would be with the vast masses of patients who know no English easily can be imagined and how equally ineffectual even with the English-knowing but highly cultured Hindu patient. A third essential is the presence of interested, experienced, open-minded transcultural observers, also participating in actual teaching, clinical work, and research. When these three points are followed, research in the true sense will have commenced.

24.   A Preliminary View of Family and Mental Health in Urban Communist China

EZRA F. VOGEL, Ph.D.
East Asian Research Center
Harvard University
Cambridge, Massachusetts

EVEN had adequate research been conducted in Communist China since 1949, it would be extremely difficult to attempt to generalize for the entire nation. In some ways Communist China is more like a continent than a nation. It has approximately 700 million people, far more than either Europe or Africa, and perhaps as much variety. There are enormous cultural gaps between the cities and the rural areas, from the arid desert land to the snowy country in the north to the semitropical country in the south. There are approximately 40 million members of minority groups in various mountain areas in China with patterns of living far different from those of people of the major majority group, the Han group. Furthermore, there are enormous regional differences among the dominant Han group: between people from the Peking area, the Hunan area, the Szechuan area, the Canton area, and elsewhere.

It is true that the Communists have introduced more homogeneity than had ever before existed in China. Because they have developed a highly disciplined and uniform organization throughout the country, there would be considerable validity in generalizing about Chinese Communist organizations: party organization, governmental organization, and organization of economic institutions, schools, mines, and so forth. The same kind of uniformity found in these organizations, however, is not found in family life and family organization. Although the regime has had considerable impact on the family, family life is still subject to enormous variety.

The problem of generalizing about the family in Communist China is further complicated by the very limited nature of research by outsiders which has been possible. Communist literature in newspapers and magazines can be read (*see* Yang, 1954). Their women's magazines and short stories reflect family life. Other sources of information are foreign visitors who have been to Communist China and Chinese who, for one reason or another, have left Communist China. In my opinion these data are far more extensive than most foreigners realize, but, nevertheless, their quantity and objectivity, and above all, the opportunity for first-hand observation and research are limited seriously.

Despite these limitations, I think there is sufficient consistency in the information at hand to state in a preliminary way a pattern of life that is found in many families in China. On the basis of data from these various sources, I feel that there is much greater consistency in family life in the cities, particularly the east coast cities, than in the rural areas. Obviously, good survey data are not available on all the cities in Communist China, but the available information suggests that certain common family patterns are fairly widespread. What I shall attempt to describe, therefore, is merely a modal pattern; while I myself would guess it to be in many instances the dominant pattern, this conclusion cannot be adequately documented.

Ascetic Patterns

Western reports of the disappearance of the Chinese family have virtually no foundation. Even in the communes no serious attempt was made to house people in any other way than in their family units. Even if the regime had hoped to achieve a communal type of organization in a very brief time, it could not have had the capital to build the radically new kind of housing which would have made possible the breakdown of the family. Although the regime has been concerned about breaking down clan organizations that interfere with its political and economic organizations and policies, it has profited from the U.S.S.R. experience and never has attempted seriously to break down the nuclear family.

Yet, as Talmon-Garber (1965) has argued in the study of a different part of the world, revolutionary fervor is fundamentally antithetical to the expenditure of time, interest, and effort in family life. When pressures of revolutionary fervor are at their strongest, they demand a kind of commitment that does not permit or encourage thorough-going devotion to the family. Even in pre-Communist China, it was not uncommon for a father to be absent for a period of time, but such absences reached new heights in revolutionary China. During the whole revolutionary struggle in China, ordinary soldiers were not allowed to have wives and lived apart from their parental families. Large numbers of youths nowadays are sent away to the countryside or to border areas for development and mass labor projects, and those that are married may well be separated for a period of time from their spouses. This kind of commitment ordinarily is required in the West only in national emergencies, such as wartime. In periods of great excitement and revolutionary fervor, such as the early period of the Great Leap Forward, Chinese men and women were expected to devote themselves so much to their work that they had relatively little time for family life. During campaigns, for example, men in important governmental or party positions are expected to sleep overnight in governmental offices, rather than returning home to their families, and this arrangement may continue for several weeks or months. The family thus is relegated to a position of secondary importance, and during busy times family affairs are relatively neglected.

Even aside from such extreme occasions, people are expected to spend a large portion of their time in the public as opposed to the private sphere. In addition to the long hours at work, most people are expected to attend meetings, study sessions, extra voluntary work projects in the evening or after work—all of which reduces the amount of time available for family life. Men and women frequently are mobilized for special literacy training. Already literate adults have been mobilized for further study of current events and for political training. Those who are suspected of disagreement or disloyalty toward the government are mobilized for special discussions of their thoughts.

Apart from the relatively little time available for family activities, there is also an asceticism which plays down sentimental behavior and large expenditures for family affairs. In China displays of affection in public always have been rare, and these customary attitudes have now been canonized. Literature, art, and music are expected to reflect ascetic rather than sentimental or romantic standards. Any music or literature which is sentimental or romantic in tone is stigmatized as "yellow" (as in "yellow journalism") and forbidden. In music, for instance, love songs are virtually unheard of; to play even Western marches is preferable to playing Chinese love songs. The opportunities for prostitution have been virtually eliminated by the very tight controls which were established within two or three years after the Communists took over. While premarital and extramarital relations have been described by numbers of people, they play a relatively minor role and are conducted relatively quietly and discreetly so as not to interfere with the public obligations and demands placed on the people involved.

Family celebrations have been reduced to a bare minimum and involve virtually no expenses. Wedding ceremonies, which had previously been quite lavish in some circles, have been reduced to very brief ceremonies often conducted at a place of work where husband and wife simply take the vow in front of some of their closest associates in a program seldom lasting more than 15 or 20 minutes; brief statements are made by their friends and by some representative of the local party organization or work unit, and the couple involved proclaim their commitments to the regime.

Refreshments are hardly anything more than tea and peanuts. Similarly, funerals have been simplified greatly. As with weddings, the gatherings are not large nor are the expenses great in contrast to some of the pre-1949 patterns. Very little land is taken up with ancestral graveyards, and the new pattern is almost exclusively cremation. Some graveyards have been retained at the family's expense, but it is not uncommon for graveyards to be removed and for the family to take their ancestors' bones or plaques for keeping elsewhere.

Another encroachment upon family life in the last several years has been the encouragement of young people not to marry before they reach fairly advanced age. The common age now for the man is 30 and for the woman 28. This represents an attempt by the regime to deal with the problem of an overly high birth rate by preventing matches among young people during a considerable portion of their highly productive years. Among those of high school age, dating is virtually nonexistent, and even among young people later on the amount of time and energy that can be devoted to courtship is limited by the commitments that each of the partners has to his own social group and by the limitations on spending for leisure-time activities.

I think it important not to overstate the general point I have been trying to make. The regime has in many ways encroached upon family life and increased the demands of public participation as opposed to the time and energy for private and family life. Yet most people in their childhood and after marriage continue to live in the family, spend a portion of each day with other family members, and have considerable intimacy within the family. Expenditures for family celebrations or development of comfortable and attractive family possessions are highly limited; yet in many ways family life goes on as before.

Changes in the Economic Organization of the Family

Economic activities have been virtually removed from families, and hence the economic authority of certain family members over others has virtually disappeared. Shortly after the Communist takeover in 1949, the wealth of private individuals was absorbed largely through bond purchases, bank deposits, confiscation, control of foreign capital, and so forth. Anyone who wishes to withdraw sizeable amounts of money from the bank will have to convince a tough-minded official of the value and importance of the expense for which he plans to use the money. Houses have been taken over essentially by the government; although many families are allowed to live in houses which they previously owned, when houses are large the government usually has managed to limit the family to two or three rooms and to rent the rest of the space to lodgers who pay rent directly to the government.

Furthermore, virtually all private enterprises were taken over by the government in the period of 1955–56. Large enterprises were taken over in the form of joint public-private organizations, and, in a small minority of cases, people who had owned these large organizations still receive a certain amount of interest, although their interest is deposited automatically in a bank, and they are subject to the same controls as other people in justifying withdrawing money from the bank. Small enterprises have been taken over in the form of co-operatives, and the former owners have become employees of the state. Even when the former owner has become the manager, he typically finds it difficult to run the enterprise as a family organization, for he no longer has the freedom to employ and direct members of the family that he had before. Before 1949 in many of the poorer families to which production jobs such as sewing and other small handicrafts were "let out," handicraft production was a family-directed activity. Now these small family handicraft activities have been absorbed almost completely by neighborhood co-operatives. Sewing machines which were formerly used by a single family have been brought into small sewing shops run by the Neighborhood or Lane Committee organized in the form of a co-operative. Thus the machine and the productive activities are no longer organized and run by the household but by a committee of people on the street supervised by a governmental agency.

The fact that inheritance is typically of no importance (compared to holding a governmental or co-operative position) for gaining an economic livelihood means that economic livelihood is controlled by the state, not by the family. In this regard, socialism has brought about changes which also have been occurring in nonsocialist countries, but it has brought about these changes more rapidly and completely. The passing of enterprises from family control has weakened greatly the authority of the elders in the family who previously had control of family finances. As one common joke on the mainland puts it, the 24 stories of filial piety are now reversed; instead of having piety toward elders, one has piety toward youth.

Furthermore, young people are encouraged and given the economic opportunity to strike out on their own, regardless of the advice of their parents. With the rapid changes in society, parents are not often in a good position to give advice to children who have a much higher degree of education than they and who are being prepared for a far different society. In fact, most youths say that they do not turn to parents or elders for advice about questions of schooling and obtaining employment. Furthermore, all these matters are now discussed openly at the school or the place of work, and the state consciously has taken over an important role in socializing youth on matters formerly handled by the family.

There is also a tendency to split up households, for young married couples to live separately from their parents, partly because the regime has taken over the management of housing and gives strong incentives for people to live close to their place of work rather than to relatives. This arrangement obviously cuts down on transportation demands and permits tighter social integration of the work community. New housing is built surrounding a place of work. Since rent in these dormitories or small apartments is far below cost, it is profitable for people to live near the place of work, and generally people live in very small housing units with room only for the nuclear family, plus perhaps an aged parent or sick relative.

Considerable effort also has been made by the regime to get women out of the home and into productive labor. Women have been encouraged especially to work in small Neighborhood or Lane Committee enterprises, which are usually small handicraft industries. The common pattern is for a married couple to live near the husband's place of work and for the neighborhood to adapt the smaller-scale enterprises to the availability of women living in a given neighborhood. The proportion of women working has varied considerably from one time period to the next. During the period of 1955–56, and even more during the 1958–59 Great Leap Forward, considerable effort was exerted to find employment for women and to encourage women to work outside the home. Since 1959, however, with the economic retrenchment, fewer jobs have been available, and many working women have had to return to their homes. Since the economic retrenchment, campaigns have been mounted to show that working in the home should also be considered socialist labor and that women should not be disappointed if they cannot go out to work. In fact, the financial advantages of employment and the desire to get out of the home generally have made Chinese women very receptive to taking jobs outside of the home and greatly disappointed when such jobs have not been available.

For working women, one common pattern is to have grandparents or old ladies in the neighborhood look after their children, and, in the bigger and better factories and higher class neighborhoods, special nursery schools and crèches are so expensive as to be beyond the reach of the ordinary laboring housewife.

A high proportion of children of primary school age are now enrolled in school; they, too, are encouraged to participate in youth activities in the cultural centers and through youth organizations, so that they, too, spend less time within the family than in the pre-1949 period.

Working mothers, especially those who work near the husband's place of work and are housed in large dormitories, commonly eat lunch and sometimes even supper in community mess halls. Sometimes the family goes together to eat in these mess halls, and sometimes one family member goes down to the mess hall and brings food back to the family. Because of the limitations on coal balls (usually made from charcoal) for cooking and because of the difficulty, at least up until the last year or two, in finding the necessary food on the market, many women have been willing to eat in mess halls. Furthermore the standard of food in mess halls generally has been at least as good as food available on the market.

Because family relations generally involve no questions of economic power (for the family has virtually no economic power), since few instrumental tasks are performed in the house, and because the furniture and other facilities within the home are so limited, the household involves few authority relationships. Indeed, as in the kibbutz in Israel, it is common for life in the home to be relatively relaxed, because family relations involve almost no obligation or responsibility, and the time spent within the home is almost completely free and easy. Because family roles are stripped of power, family members have few obligations to each other, and the constraints of authority between family members are weak at best.

The breakdown of authority relations and of the power of men over women and parents over children is perhaps best expressed in the changed kinship terminology used within the family. The husband and wife do not refer to each other by title nor commonly by name. Rather they call each other *ai jen*. This term (which means simply "lover") commonly has been used by a couple before marriage, but the fact that these terms are not only encouraged by the regime but widely used suggests the lack of authority relations between husband and wife. Furthermore, the wife ordinarily keeps her maiden name after marriage, and the parents may pass on to the children either the mother's or the father's name. Although in many families, children, influenced by the traditional concepts of filial piety, continue to have respect for their parents and to obey them, they nevertheless have considerable freedom in departing from the arbitrary authority of their parents and may enlist the help of their friends and political activists in resisting their parents' arbitrary claims to authority. In brief, then, the area of family activity has been reduced greatly and involves very little obligation, a change which has reduced greatly the authority nature of relations within the family.

Community Involvement

In mainland China the individual typically is tightly integrated into a small nonkin group. Ordinarily he belongs to such a group at his place of work, but women or children who are neither employed nor in school are integrated through the neighborhood. These small groups, composed of about 8 to 15 people, typically meet about once a week to discuss everything from current events, governmental policy, and examinations of individual ideology to attitudes toward housekeeping matters. These small groups are under the direction of an activist who is in turn under the direction of the Communist party, and the leader aims to ensure that the group follows the party's policies. The group serves as the transmission belt for communicating ideas from the regime to the individual and for ensuring that individual thought and behavior are in accord with party policy.

This multifunctional group which absorbs an enormous amount of an individual's time and energy may well be the only group outside the family to which he belongs. Ordinarily, this small group is composed of individuals with whom a person interacts most, even apart from group meetings. In school, for example, the small group also serves as the residential unit in a dormitory, and members commonly attend classes together from admission to graduation. In the factory the small group is composed of workers who are in direct contact with each other while on duty. In the neighborhood the small group is composed of neighbors. Other voluntary groups—aside from party, Communist Youth League, and affiliated and sponsored mass organizations—generally are discouraged and virtually non-existent. Discouragement is effective because of the suspicion and questioning that would accompany contacts with other groups. To use the concepts of Bott (1957), each member of the family is integrated into a separate social network, and there is little or no overlap between the groups to which family members belong. Family members do not share participation in these other primary groups. In other words, there is very little opportunity for husband and wife or for mother and child to take part in group activities together. Furthermore, to avoid political problems, virtually no one visits a friend's home. Such private activities are suspect, and therefore most group activities take place in public facilities.

These small groups also intrude into individual family affairs. The wife must be prepared to discuss her family matters with other members of her group, just as the husband may be called upon for similar comments in his group. At times, these groups can be manipulated to correct family situations. When, for example, a wife feels that her husband is treating her unfairly, she may encourage others in her group to express their opinions on the rights of wives. It is not uncommon for a woman's small neighborhood group to make representations to her husband or even to call him before the women's group to denounce him for his misbehavior to his wife. If he is unco-operative, the local party officials may be mobilized to assist in getting his co-operation. The impact of these groups is to separate further the spheres of the respective family members and to minimize the extent of overlap in their social and community activities.

Politics

The regime has highlighted strongly the importance of political distinctions between those who are more progressive and those who are less progressive, between those who come from working and peasant family backgrounds and those who come from bourgeois or landlord family backgrounds. Indeed, political attitudes are so important that people commonly associate with others of essentially the same political backgrounds and persuasions. A woman who is a party member is likely to be married to a man who is also a party member, or at least a member of the Communist Youth League. Bourgeois and landlord children may have great difficulty in finding spouses because no one wants to be contaminated with the opprobrium of their social status. Furthermore, people who are not particularly active in politics usually are cautious and reserved around those who are for fear that they might give out information which will later cause difficulties in their own careers. Hence, there is considerable reserve in communicating feelings to those with or near political power, and people are likely to marry within the range of people of similar political and social background.

The close tab which the local police station keeps on political activities of the family makes family members cautious, in order to avoid involving their relatives in trouble. The political attitudes of the regime also are reflected in their treatment of such matters as divorce. If a person seeking a divorce can find political grounds, divorce is relatively easy. If, for example, the husband has been criticized in a political campaign, it is simple for the wife to obtain a divorce by saying that she finds it necessary to divorce him because of his poor political attitudes and behavior. Similarly, a divorce usually can be obtained with ease if it can be argued that a pre-1949 marriage was based on some form of exploitation. Hence, a wife can claim that she married because of family pressure, or a husband that he was coerced into marriage. If the wife had been a child bride or if her capitalist husband had abused her, she need anticipate no difficulty in securing a divorce. But a person wanting a divorce who cannot make such convincing political arguments may find divorce difficult, since considerable effort ordinarily is made by governmental or party representatives to keep a family together.

Furthermore, minor political differences between husband and wife can lead to serious problems. Questions such as how enthusiastically one should participate in a political campaign, how frequently one should volunteer to attend political meetings or to stay late at work, may be regarded differently by the more politically active spouse than by his partner. Of course, the person who is the greater political activist has the advantage that he or she will be on the side of the regime and can get outside support if the other person does not follow his wishes.

As to division of labor within the family, there is generally little work to do within the home, and, although it is more usual for the wife to take care of the children and do the cooking, it is very common for the husband to help out. There tends at present to be less sharp segregation of husband and wife roles in the household. Who does what is now more determined by convenience of working hours than upon any sharp patterning of expected roles of men and women.

Child Rearing

Again, while limited opportunity for first-hand observation prevents a careful scientific formulation, it is my impression, based on reports by respondents, that child rearing in Chinese urban families tends to be relatively matter of fact in comparison, for example, with that in similar Japanese families. Although Chinese mothers devote considerable time to the children, dependence is not encouraged or rewarded in the same way that it is in Japan. On the contrary, the child is encouraged to become relatively independent at a fairly early stage. The mother often criticizes him or indicates by what she does or says that she can be unpredictable. The child learns very quickly that for many things he must rely on himself and cannot expect a great amount of indulgence. The lack of indulgence is reinforced by the regime's manuals on child rearing and articles giving advice to parents. The regime is deeply concerned that children not come to expect a soft life. Literature advising parents on child rearing recommends withholding comforts and reducing aspirations to avoid spoiling children. Children are encouraged to learn how to work hard within the family, for example, to wash and sew their own clothes and clean their rooms, so they will not have to rely on others. Such advice is directed especially to mothers in the higher income brackets and from bourgeois backgrounds.

There is relatively little distinct "child culture" in China. Children may accompany parents to most places (including restaurants, amusement centers, theaters, and the like), but there are relatively few amusements or playthings which are exclusively for children. A child generally is told no bedtime stories, and there is commonly no physical contact with adults before retiring at night. A child who cries is as likely to be criticized and ridiculed as picked up and comforted, and he soon learns that there is generally no point to crying or making a fuss.

Although Chinese mothers, like mothers in other countries, are not eager to separate from their children, still as a whole they seem to have considerable capacity for being parted from them for long periods of time. Most mothers who leave their children in crèches or nursery schools do not seem terribly upset and are better able to tolerate separation than is, for example, the Japanese mother. The mother-child relation is much less symbiotic and more neutral than in Japan. To slightly overstate the case, the Chinese child is not babied and is expected to behave much like a small adult fairly early in life.

One of the main concerns of parents in mainland China is that the child stay out of political trouble and difficulty. Parents really cannot control the child's future by determining his schooling or his employment, for such matters are now decided by the regime. There is little they can do to secure his economic future, and the regime's decisions about such matters have not been easy to predict. Parents can urge a child to study and prepare for examinations and, perhaps even more important, to avoid criticizing the regime or making other errors which would only cause one difficulty. Since children commonly are placed in some form of baby-sitting pool, nursery school, or kindergarten before grade school, considerable peer group authority is generated. This peer group pressure is mobilized consciously by the teacher or the nursery schoolteacher, and the study of the manipulation of peer group pressures is very useful to the aspiring young official. The impact of the guided peer group, like that of parental behavior, is to encourage responsible semi-adult behavior rather than to encourage prolonged dependency.

The regime's handling of problem children reflects little psychological awareness. Children who have nightmares may be assigned a different kind of diet. Children who wet their beds are likely to be dealt with by criticizing them in front of a group of their peers; if the problem becomes more serious, the bed-wetters may be treated by acupuncture (a complicated treatment procedure involving the application of needles to certain parts of the body). Little emphasis is placed on getting to know the personality of a child and adjusting to his needs and desires; instead, the needs and desires of the child are likely to be treated in a fairly simple and direct manner but never indulged in any event. If the child needs something within reason, he is ordinarily given it, but, unless he is very young, he is expected to accept considerable responsibility for looking after himself and his own belongings and for behaving as a responsible member of the group. In a sense the period of prolonged irresponsibility connected with childhood is reduced to a bare minimum, and the carefree life of a child is replaced very quickly by work and group responsibility.

Problems

One of the most serious tensions within the mainland Chinese family is that associated with political campaigns. Political campaigns arouse considerable anxiety and fear of punishment. The rights of the individual and the types of punishment are not defined. A person may be punished for any "incorrect" act or "improper" thought. In cases of serious criticism at the time of a campaign, a person may be denounced by all his friends and acquaintances, and these denunciations may include the most personal of attacks, incorporating any information (and possibly even incorrect rumors) about one's past. A great deal of diffuse anxiety which can be terribly crippling, builds up as a result. In times of campaigns ulcers are common, and in serious campaigns suicides are not rare.

A person who is criticized in these campaigns is isolated from his friends and peers because they are afraid to communicate with him. Even a person in a small group who is in some ways less responsive to the regime than the other members of the group is likely to be made a scapegoat by the group and criticized strongly because of the importance of his involvement in the group and because of the demands and pressures from political higher-ups. Such criticism can be total and incapacitating.

Discussion is limited in the family as well as among friends. First of all, one must be particularly careful not to discuss any problems in front of children who might communicate these ideas to the outside. Children who intentionally report on their parents are extremely rare, but, in their group discussions or in their essays in school, children reveal things incidentally or without thinking which reflect badly upon the family and cast certain political doubts. Furthermore, most husbands and wives try to avoid saying anything critical of the regime to each other lest somebody overhear or their partner incidentally or in an angry mood purposefully reveal some of these confidences; a spouse at best would have the psychological burden of hiding something. As a result there is no relatively unconditional base of support to which an individual can turn when he is being criticized or made a scapegoat.

As all individuals are relatively carefully regimented, a person's problem is less likely to stem from *anomie* (a "sense of alienation") than from overly tight integration into a group. Intellectuals and government and party employees especially are subject to continuous surveillance through group meetings, and those who are especially vulnerable may suffer from chronic anxiety and depression.

Still, the typical Chinese person is a very distinct and very determined individual. Although stress may cause some to become bland and washed out, it does not appear to debilitate a very large proportion of the population. The average Chinese person still has considerable inner resources of his own which make it possible to withstand some criticism and to survive in changed and stressful environmental surroundings. There is a reservoir of individual pride and determination that makes it possible for many to withstand considerable pressure, although many sensitive people show the strains of tight political controls.

REFERENCES

Bott, E. 1957. Family and social network. London, Tavistock Publications.

Talmon-Garber, Y. 1965. The family in a revolutionary movement; the case of the kibbutz in Israel. *In* Comparative family systems. M. Nimkoff, ed. Boston, Houghton Mifflin.

Yang, C. K. 1954. The Chinese family in the Communist revolution. Cambridge, Massachusetts, Technology Press.

25.   Changing Perception of Neurotic Illness

G. MORRIS CARSTAIRS, M.D.

Department of Psychiatry
University of Edinburgh
Edinburgh, Scotland

IT HAS LONG BEEN believed that the populations of industrially un-developed communities have relatively low rates of neurosis. Until very recently no systematic observations could either support or controvert this belief. On the one hand, every human society has evolved codes of behavior which impose restraints upon the gratification of instinctual drives, and some of the most oppressive restraints are found in quite primitive com-munities; this would lead one to expect evidences of repressed conflicts in every society. On the other hand, we know from the reports of survivors of concentration camps and from military psychiatry that when men find themselves in situations of considerable physical hardship and mortal danger neurotic complaints show a tendency to be forgotten; based on this analogy, low rates for neurosis might be expected among the poorest sections of our populations—but this is decidedly not the case.

Leighton and his colleagues have shown in Nigeria, as have Lin and his colleagues in Taiwan, that neurotic and psychosomatic symptoms are far from rare among the relatively uneducated populations which they surveyed, and this, too, was my impression during my two years of field work in Indian villages (Carstairs, 1955).

I must admit, however, that several months elapsed before I began to recognize the true measure of the frequency of emotionally determined illness in the Rajasthani villagers I studied. The delay was due to the high prevalence of recognizable physical diseases, such as intestinal infections, chronic bronchitis, severe anemia, and, above all, tuberculosis. Having seen many such cases, I was not surprised when patients complained of a general malaise, of feeling run-down and weak: even if I could not identify the specific cause of their states, it usually seemed appropriate to prescribe a course of iron to counteract anemia. It was only when I was consulted by a strapping, obviously robust farmer who begged me to give him an injection to counteract his weakness that I realized that his symptom might have a psychological basis. Accordingly, instead of hurrying to comply with his request, I asked him to tell me more about his weakness and how it had come about. He did so, and I had my first introduction to a whole system of interrelated beliefs about health-giving and debilitating foods and about behaviors which would enhance or endanger a man's bodily strength, respectively. Good food and right action would, over a period of time, lead to the creation of pure semen, as rich as cream, which is stored in a reservoir at the vertex of the cranium; but eating foods which are ritually condemned or indulgence in sacrilegious behavior (which included the infringement of any of a multitude of social taboos, from eating in the company of lower-caste friends to indulging in frequent sexual intercourse) is believed to cause a man's precious store of semen to deteriorate and leak away, leaving him feeling weak and out of sorts. In the case of my farmer patient, the cause was soon apparent: he admitted to extramarital sexual activities which aroused considerable guilt and, in turn, brought with it a hypochondriacal belief that his strength was wasting away.

Once alerted by this case, I found that many others who complained of weakness were also indirectly expressing anxiety and guilt about their violations of the rules of right conduct. Concern over spoiled semen was, in fact, the commonest form of presentation of an anxiety state among my village clients (Carstairs, 1956).

Subsequent analysis of my daily records of medical consultations showed me that symptoms of anxiety, hysteria, and psychosomatic illness came second only to endemic infectious disease as a cause of ill-health in these village communities, but, of course, these complaints were rarely considered to be susceptible of medical treatment. The great majority of my village patients regarded their malaise as having a spiritual origin and consulted the priest of a healing shrine rather than a medical man in order to seek their remedy.

It is not only in village India, however, that emotionally determined disorders find diverse modes of expression. In my own hometown of Edinburgh, Scotland, a Medical Research Council unit has been studying the epidemiology of psychiatric illness, and one topic of research has been the incidence of attempted suicide in the city. The frequency with which patients are admitted to hospital after having swallowed a poisonous substance or a dangerous overdose of drugs has been increasing very rapidly since 1948, when the beneficent National Health Service made drugs available free, on a doctor's prescription, to everyone who was thought to need them (Fig. 1). Since 1948 barbiturates have far outstripped all other methods of self-poisoning, as shown in Fig. 1, although during the last few years the use of antidepressants and other psychotropic drugs also has been rising very steeply. My colleague Neil Kessel, in reporting these findings, drew attention to the disturbing fact that it was doctors who, through injudicious prescribing, had put dangerously large doses of drugs in the hands of the great majority of these patients.

Here then is one pattern of neurotic behavior which has shown a marked increase over a relatively short period. By calculating rates of occurrence of attempted suicide for each of the 23 electoral wards of the city, it was possible to demonstrate associations of particular social and demographic factors in high risk sections of the community. Clinical and social investigations of the patients threw additional light on the circumstances of the event (Kessel, 1965a, 1965b).

It is clear that among the relatively poor and ill-educated members of the city population—especially among those of this group whose lives are complicated by abnormal personalities, with frequent recourse to alcohol and its attendant social handicaps—the act of taking an overdose has become a familiar mode of publicly announcing that one's personal problems have become unmanageable.

No one would think of calling attempted suicide a disease; it is a pattern of self-endangering behavior which may be precipitated by a wide variety of factors, singly or in conjunction. Nevertheless, it has proved highly informative to identify and count its occurrence as well as that of other forms of behavior which readily can be counted. Several indexes of social disorganization have shown a distribution similar to the rates for attempted suicide, viz., arrests for drunkenness and petty crime, arrears in rent, instances of gross neglect of dependent children, and the like. Where attempted suicide rates are high for adults, they are high also for adolescents, and juvenile delinquency is also high; in marked contrast, however, it is in these same communities that the *fewest* adolescents are referred for psychiatric consultation.

Counting the occurrence of these various patterns of disturbed behavior has drawn attention to factors in the environment, which seem to be of etiological significance.

I suggest that precisely the same technique could be adopted profitably in the very different social setting of village or small-town life in a developing country. One can, for example, learn a great deal by systematically observing village shamans and their clients. Sasaki and Lebra, respectively, give in this volume analyses of the personalities of a number of shamans in Japanese and Okinawan communities. Although shamans had not been a focus of inquiries in my own field of work, their findings at once provoked the recognition that each of several Rajasthani shamans

Figure 1: Hospital Admissions for Self-poisoning from the City
of Edinburgh, 1928–1963, Showing Method Used*

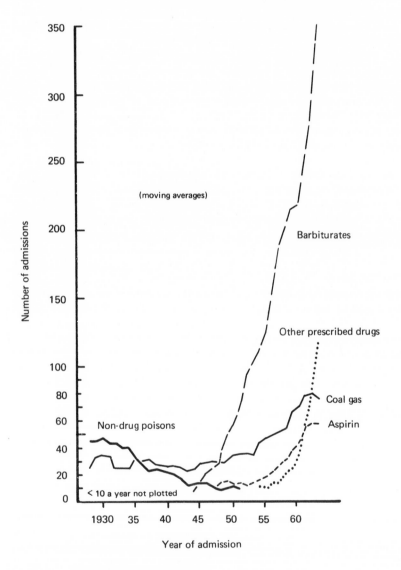

*Reproduced from Kessel, 1965.

whom I had come to know fairly well had been conspicuously unsuccessful in life until the assumption of his sacred role gave him new prestige. One, I recall, was an exceptionally impoverished member of a very low-ranking caste; another was a crippled orphan who had been robbed of his inheritance by unscrupulous relatives; and a third was a severe alcoholic until the "breath" of a local deity entered into him.

My own interest, however, lay in observing the type of complaints brought before the village shaman and the therapeutic procedures which he prescribed. There was a striking preponderance of young women and children among the clients of the Rajasthani shamans; the children, of course, were brought by their anxious parents, whereas the young wives came of their own accord. Their symptoms were diverse, often recognizable as gross conversion hysteria, and in the social context of their occurrence one could often detect echoes of sexual or interpersonal marital disharmony, just as in psychiatric outpatient clinics in the West; but there the situation was complicated by the stern authority of the mother-in-law, in whose extended household the young bride was compelled to live. It was noticeable that older married women, now the heads of their own households, seldom were seen consulting the shaman.

Scientific repudiation of superstitions should not be allowed to prevent recognition that shared beliefs, however erroneous, are social realities. In unsophisticated communities, for example, it may well prove rewarding to study the ecology of ghost-hauntings and accusations of witchcraft (cf. Spiro's chapter in this volume). At the earliest opportunity, I hope to see a team composed of Indian psychiatrists and social scientists carrying out a systematic analysis of the clientele of Indian village shamans and the social circumstances in which the clients' complaints occur to supersede my own crude observations and perhaps help to plan future mental health interventions which will be geared to the emotional realities of village life.

As is known, throughout the vast masses of humanity in Africa, Asia, and South America, insanity is still usually regarded as caused by the intervention of angry or evil spirits; taking the world as a whole, it is probably true to say that many more mental patients are treated by rites of exorcism than by electroshock or psychotropic drugs. Spiritual healing of this kind may be based upon quite ill-founded theories of the causation of disease, but it has two striking advantages over supposedly scientific reliance upon physical treatments: first, the patient is not exposed to the undesirable side effects of many of the newest psychotropic drugs; and second, spiritual healing requires the participation of other persons in addition to the patient and thus helps to reintegrate the mentally ill patient with the rest of his community from whom he has become estranged.

Even today, Western doctors differ very widely in their ability to recognize and in their willingness to treat emotional illness. Shortly before the British National Health Service came into being, Blacker (1946) tried systematically to assess the size of the need for specialist psychiatric clinics. An early finding was that some doctors were as much as ten times less likely than their average fellows to use these services. His finding since has been confirmed repeatedly, most recently in a large-scale survey of psychiatric morbidity in English general practices (Shepherd *et al.*, 1964), whose authors were obliged to attribute the very wide differences in the rates of recognition of minor psychiatric disorders to personality factors in the doctors themselves.

My colleague Henry Walton recently has been carrying out intensive studies of medical students and of doctors returning to the University for postgraduate courses in order to throw further light on this question. His research has confirmed an earlier finding by Knight Aldrich, of Chicago, that some medical students are temperamentally antipathetic to psychiatric illness and are uncomfortable in their relations with psychiatric patients. It generally is known that relatively few students graduate with the intention of specializing in this field (reported figures have varied from 1 per cent in one school to 25 per cent in another). In some countries, of course, psychiatry may not offer very tempting prospects in terms of career advancement or financial reward, but in others the reasons for low recruitment must be sought in students' attitudes toward the subject.

My colleagues and I examined this question by testing the opinions of a recent graduating class in Edinburgh (Walton, Drewery, and Carstairs, 1963). Just under half of the students (48 per cent) expressed a lively interest in psychological factors in illness, while the other half admitted to being more interested in organic factors. These two groups did not differ from each other in measures of factual information, whether of psychiatric matters or other areas of medicine; differences were apparent in their attitudes toward the psychiatry course, and, not surprisingly, in their readiness to contemplate a psychiatric career.

In a subsequent more detailed study of the same population, Walton, Drewery, and Philip (1964) employed the statistical technique of delegate analysis which singled out four different patterns, each typified by a group of students. Two of these groups were oriented organically, but whereas the larger of these was composed of doctors who had a positive or neutral relation with patients, the smaller group was frankly hostile toward all emotionally ill patients and far from relaxed in relating to patients in general. The remaining doctors all declared an interest in the social and emotional aspects of disease; in the third group this interest was associated with attitudes of scientific inquiry and a research orientation, whereas the last group were "patient-centered," predominantly interested in contact with patients and in therapy.

If this school is typical, it can be assumed that only half of the young doctors graduating in Britain today are actively interested in the psychological aspects of disease. The percentage was raised to nearly two-thirds by introducing a new curriculum giving students additional experience in interviewing patients and discussing their findings with tutors in small groups. This finding suggests that in medical schools where little emphasis is placed upon psychiatric teaching graduating doctors will have correspondingly little interest in psychiatric patients. Discussions with my colleagues from leading Indian medical schools have taught me that, with few exceptions, this pattern tends to be the rule in Indian medical education. In India, as in Britain, it is essential that psychiatric concepts be infiltrated into the thinking of every doctor if the neglected psychiatric needs of the ordinary patients are ever to be met.

There are thus three major obstacles to the recognition of neurotic behavior patterns. First, the existence in a society of long-established alternative ways of defining such behavior, in terms of supernatural intervention. Second, the Western-trained physician's bias toward seeing as illness only those disorders which have a physical basis, associated with demonstrable physiological or pathological changes. Third, the influence of changing fashions in sickness. This last factor deserves further elucidation.

Differences in the rates of presentation of particular neurotic syndromes in different communities may be due not only to the doctor's attitude and perceptions but also to those of the patient. It is known that there are fashions in illness, sometimes clearly associated with medical enthusiasm (as, for example, in the waves of appendectomies, tonsillectomies, and "lumbo-sacral discs" which have severally dominated British hospital practice). Other changes are not directly attributable to suggestion on the part of doctors; their origins are complex and must be sought in the improved educational level of the mass of the population, together with changes in their level of nutrition, their work habits, and their mode of life. It is in this realm of interacting personal and social factors that epidemiologists have sought the explanation of major changes in the incidence of psychosomatic diseases, such as gastric and duodenal ulcer, and of the rising incidence of lung cancer and coronary thrombosis in the last decades (Halliday, 1948; Morris, 1964).

Not surprisingly, neurotic illness also has shown itself susceptible to these socioenvironmental changes. It is common knowledge that conversion hysteria (euphemistically termed "shell shock") was the most usual form of psychiatric morbidity among ordinary soldiers on both sides during World War I, whereas the officers, who were highly educated, were more likely to suffer from anxiety states. In World War II, presumably because of the higher general standard of education, gross conversion symptoms were much less common in the European theaters of war, save one. The Partisans who fought with Tito in the mountains of Yugoslavia were tough but simple men, and they, when their capital of emotional reserve was exhausted, still tended to exhibit hysterical symptoms.

In recent years Indian and Pakistani military psychiatrists have made several contributions to the literature on army psychiatry, but an earlier monograph by Williams (1950) is of particular interest because it compares British and Indian casualties in the same campaign. From 1943 to 1945 Williams worked as a front-line psychiatrist during successive periods of very savage fighting in Burma. He became interested in studying the reactions to severe stress of British and Indian troops, exerting himself to study Urdu so that he could dispense with interpreters when he talked with his Indian patients. He found that psychiatric casualties occurred at roughly similar rates in the two armies, but that the character of the illnesses differed markedly. More than half of the British casualties presented symptoms of anxiety, whereas the Indians showed predominantly hysterical reactions, with no less than 15 per cent of acute psychotic states. Indian soldiers, particularly those drawn from communities with warlike traditions, excelled in hand-to-hand fighting, but they did not tolerate defensive warfare where the individual soldier was denied the relief of fighting back against an identifiable opponent. Williams noted that after the heat of battle British soldiers were able to express their fears quite openly but that Indians were prevented by traditional formulations of manly behavior from experiencing this emotional abreaction.

In a particularly interesting passage Williams discussed the factors which appeared to promote resistance to psychiatric breakdown in the Indian soldiers. He noted their proneness to homesickness and their tendency, when sick or wounded, to abandon themselves to despair at the thought of dying far from home and family. They revealed, in fact, the same strong element of familial dependency to which Surya draws attention in his contribution to this volume. It was noted that Indian soldiers displayed the best morale when they were led by officers whom they could regard as good parents. Such officers were expected to be disciplinarians, provided that their punishments were not such as to humiliate the offender personally and cause him to lose face; they were also expected to be responsible for the welfare, and to share the dangers, of the soldiers under their command. Wisely, the author concluded by pointing out that sound planning for the mental health of Indian troops must be based on full appreciation of the relevant medical, geographical, social, economic, and cultural factors in the different communities from which they come.

This study, in which the severe stresses of battle showed up strengths and weaknesses in the personalities of large numbers of ordinary British and Indian men, inevitably posed the wider question: In countries like India, where the benefits of curative and preventive medicine are changing the lives of millions, will there soon be dramatic changes in the presentation and recognition of neurotic illness in the population as a whole? There are some indications that this change already may be occurring. I personally have had occasion to witness the phenomenal growth of the demand for psychiatric treatment in one of India's leading medical schools, the King Edward Memorial Hospital in Bombay.

When I visited this hospital in 1949 it was still relatively new and had no inpatient facilities. During that year some 200 new cases were seen at the biweekly clinic sessions. When I visited the hospital again in 1964, the scene was transformed. Now, two large treatment teams, each headed by junior and senior consultants with supporting medical, nursing, and social work staff, daily man a teeming outpatient department whose orderly bustle resembles that of a railway terminus on a bank holiday. During 1964 over 5,000 new cases were treated as outpatients, while 200 or more were given short-term treatment in the psychiatric ward now provided in the hospital: similar numbers were reported from the rival medical school in Bombay.

During this relatively short period, the clientele has changed not only in numbers but also in diagnostic composition. Sixteen years ago many of the patients were suffering from severe brain damage or chronic schizophrenia; today, the majority are suffering from minor psychiatric disorders, including many cases of psychosomatic illness, anxiety states, and reactive depression.

From my detached position as an intermittent onlooker, I have been impressed particularly by the emergence of the awareness on the part of patients and their relatives that to suffer painful degrees of anxiety or depression is not simply an act of god, an affliction to be borne as best one may (unless the god can be appeased by an appropriate offering). These complaints are beginning to be perceived as illness, susceptible of medical treatment. My Indian colleagues tell me that this tendency is still more marked among their private patients, who tend to be more sophisticated than the clinic clients. It seems, therefore, that in India and perhaps in other developing countries the relatively new specialty of psychiatry very soon will be confronted by a mounting tide of demand for attention and help. At least for several decades, there will not be nearly enough psychiatrists to take over the role which has hitherto been filled by spiritual and magical healers. I suggest, however, that the new public awareness of emotional causes of disease be capitalized upon to place great emphasis on this aspect in teaching medical undergraduates to enable the general physician of the next generation to recognize the neurotic basis of emotionally determined illness in whatever guise it may present.

REFERENCES

Blacker, C. P. 1946. Neurosis and the mental health services. London: Oxford University Press.

Carstairs, G. M. 1955. Medicine and faith in rural Rajasthan. *In* Health, culture and community. B. D. Paul, ed. New York, Russell Sage Foundation.

————. 1956. Hinjra and Jiryan: two derivatives of Hindu attitudes to sexuality. British Journal of Medical Psychology 29:128–38.

Halliday, J. L. 1948. Psychosocial medicine: a study of the sick society. London: Heinemann.

Kessel, N. 1965a. Self-poisoning. I. British Medical Journal 2:1265–70.
————. 1965b. Self-poisoning. II. British Medical Journal 2:1336–40.
Morris, J. N. 1964. Uses of epidemiology. Second ed. Edinburgh, Livingstone.
Shepherd, M., B. Cooper, A. C. Brown, and G. W. Kalton. 1964. Minor mental illness in London: some aspects of a general practice survey. British Medical Journal 2:1359–63.
Walton, H. J., J. Drewery, and G. M. Carstairs. 1963. Interest of graduating medical students in social and emotional aspects of illness. British Medical Journal 2:588–92.
Walton, H. J., J. Drewery, and A. E. Philip. 1964. Typical medical students. British Medical Journal 2:744–48.
Williams, A. 1950. A psychiatric study of Indian soldiers in the Arakan. British Journal of Medical Psychology 23:130–81.

26. Sociocultural Change and Value Conflict in Developing Countries: A Case Study of Pakistan

S. M. HAFEEZ ZAIDI, Ph.D.
Department of Psychology
University of Karachi
Karachi, Pakistan

ONE of the features common to many developing countries is sociopolitical instability. Pakistan has had her share of this instability during the early years of her existence. My point of departure is a set of assumptions about the transitional state of Pakistan society. These assumptions were formulated in an earlier paper (Zaidi, 1964) and are recapitulated here briefly. It is assumed that: (1) Pakistan society is under stress, stress being defined as a condition of conflict or frustration leading to the disturbance of homeostasis in an individual or group. (2) Social mobility in Pakistan since independence in 1947 has been very much out of harmony with the temper of a traditional society. (3) Pakistan society is facing a conflict between its own culture and the culture imported from the West along with Western technical tools and skills.

The present social situation in Pakistan seems to support these assumptions. A society in transition can be characterized as one which is still in the process of determining national goals and objectives, where the value systems are not uniformly stabilized, where there are regional preferences and narrowly circumscribed loyalties, and where the ultimate national outlook and character are still to develop. In Pakistan almost all these characteristics of a still immature society are found. In addition, on the eve of its independence from colonial rule this society was jolted by the immigration of Muslims from India and has not yet recovered fully from its aftermath. Not all the subgroups that came to Pakistan have been settled properly. Furthermore, frustration has been created by economic insecurity and early political instability. Political parties lacking any definite program, leadership, or following have mushroomed. The fight for Islamic as opposed to Western democracy continues. Values and concepts of the East and the West also are in conflict. In brief, the sociopolitical fabric of the society is being transformed into something which is neither Pakistani nor truly Western. The leaders of thought have not succeeded so far in resolving any of these conflicts. These conditions are clearly indicative of a society in transition in search of ultimate goals. Given this situation of sociocultural conflict, many reasonably accurate predictions about the mental health problems of the society can be formulated.

This chapter is an attempt to substantiate assumptions by analyzing the effects of technological and social change on the value orientations of Pakistan society. Value orientations broadly can be conceptualized as generalizations through which different acts of the members of a group can be related and through which a particular activity can be seen as part of a larger setting. My analysis will be based on historical facts, government statistics, and empirical observations on Pakistan and other developing countries. Very little social research has been done yet on Pakistan society; what is said here therefore is both impressionistic and inferential. What follows is divided into four parts which present: (1) social change in Pakistan in historical perspective; (2) conclusions from social psychiatric studies conducted in developing countries other than Pakistan; (3) government statistics indicative of the nature of social change in Pakistan; and (4) discussion of areas of value conflict in Pakistan village society.

Historical Perspective

Pakistan as an Islamic state was carved out of former British India on August 14, 1947. The early years of the new state were so beset with economic and political difficulties that many doubted her survival. Pakistan has survived, however, and her present economic viability is nothing short of a miracle.

Immediately upon coming into existence Pakistan faced communal crisis and political destruction. In addition, millions of Muslims from the remotest parts of India began pouring into Pakistan and the government had a huge task of refugee rehabilitation on its hands. In one of the biggest population migrations in history, people with different habit patterns, stereotypes, linguistic variations, and local belief systems chose Pakistan for their future home. The host population welcomed the newcomers, but welcome wears down, and familiarity often breeds conflicts. Economic pressures and the increasing scarcity of opportunities created tensions and misunderstanding. Host and the immigrant groups soon were competing with each other for jobs and business opportunities. The result was a complicated psychological problem of accommodating a variety of subcultural groups into an integrated sociocultural system. The preindependence social structure was shaken seriously by the onrush of the refugees. These people brought with them their own notions of right and wrong behavior, their own social myths and legends. The social dislocation thus caused gave rise to clashes of regional traditions, social and individual maladjustments, and intergroup tension and disharmony. Other problems also beset the new nation. A wave of urbanization overtook Pakistan from her start. Most of the immigrants went to cities and swelled their populations manifold. Karachi, with a population of 300,000 in 1947, had a population of nearly two and a half million in 1965, and similar population increases occurred in Dacca, Lahore, and Hyderabad. Smaller district towns also were affected by this population pressure. Most of the immigrants came originally from villages and small suburban towns and found it difficult to adapt to urban life. The result was an ill-adjusted urban population with decades of rural background. Social psychiatric research dealing with their adjustment would have been valuable. There seem to be increases in juvenile delinquency, theft, larceny, and sex crimes.

No statistics exist on the incidence of mental diseases, although adults parading naked on the busy streets of big cities and causing commotion in traffic are a common sight. Almost every village has a number of hysterical women who are supposedly possessed by genii and witches. Such people should be institutionalized and looked after by state psychiatrists, but, unfortunately, only four very ill-equipped mental hospitals exist in the country, and they are no better than jails where patients are not treated but isolated. Psychosomatic diseases are quite common, although they are rarely diagnosed as such. In a report on human relations problems in an industrial center in East Pakistan, it was noted that for symptoms such as the recurrence of headaches, fever, restlessness, and lack of interest in work the medical officer's diagnosis was "diseases of the nerves" (Zaidi, 1959).

Another reason for assuming the presence of factors causing mental ill-health in Pakistan society is industrialization. At present Pakistan has a fairly large industrial complex, an attempt is being made to pattern the economic and social life after Western industrial society. The semiskilled labor force which has been created now draws improved wages with which to buy the amenities of modern life. The general atmosphere of modernization has kindled in these workers the desire for more material comforts. They question and disregard some of the basic values of the village society of their origin. This drift has not yet gone far, but the symptoms of conflict and dissatisfaction with the old order are clearly visible. The rural youth who comes as an industrial worker to a town or city goes back home, if he does return, with a dislike for his parents' way of life. He begins to question traditional morality, the joint family and its baneful effect upon his own happiness, the state of rural sanitation, and other aspects of village life. A recent survey of industrial workers' adjustment in Khulna (East Pakistan) indicated clearly the value conflicts and social maladjustments which workers from the villages have to face (Husain and Farouk, 1961).

In this context, another significant influence is the launching of the government's community development program for village agricultural industrial development. Pakistan has been an agricultural country for centuries, and the tools and techniques of agriculture also are centuries old. The villagers are used to a certain way of life. There is resistance therefore to any change in the traditional and indigenous local methods. The government, however, is determined to bring about socioeconomic change in the villages. Family planning, the use of power pumps, tractor cultivation, adult education, sanitation, and animal husbandry are some of diverse elements in schemes of change. A change, however, in any of these respects is a long leap forward, for which the villagers are neither prepared nor equipped. The result is their passive acquiescence, probably without real willingness to effect any change.

In order to add validity to the above observations, I randomly interviewed eight persons (one army officer, one college teacher, one religious leader, one housewife, two civil servants, and two small businessmen) about their awareness of, and reactions to, the changes taking place in society. Their views, though not representative of the entire population, indicate the general atmosphere of disillusionment and frustration inevitable in a society which has had to face serious economic, political, and psychological difficulties during the short period of its existence. A summary of their views follows:

> Society is undergoing change at a great speed. Some changes are for the better, while others are for the worse. They do not feel happy about the way religious obligations are being overlooked. In education there is only a craving for a degree; in social life, indulgence in extravagance, physical pleasures, and display of riches and status are the virtues. Simple and happy households have become mad for status symbols, resulting in unnecessary stresses and strains in the family life and an unhealthy trend in society. To meet the demand for physical comforts and social status, people try to gain more and more wealth by fair or foul means. Politics is no longer clean. Cheating and flattery are the keys to success. The girls no longer are interested in rearing and looking after children. They are more given to social life outside the home. Ostentation and hypocrisy in interpersonal behavior has spoilt the basis of social life.

These causal factors are presented here with a view to setting the proper historical perspective for the observations that follow. Psychologists in general have made little use of historical data which only suggests a poor sense of history among psychologists. However, for a proper appreciation of the adjustment problems of Pakistan society, it is important to know the historical basis of the social changes and the subsequent maladjustments. All developing nations have their human and social problems, but the problems of a new nation based on an ideology are special.

Studies of Sociocultural Factors and Mental Disorders

Psychologists and social psychiatrists generally have emphasized the role of sociocultural factors in causing of mental disorders: in recent years there has been a definite increase in their concern. One of the many hypotheses concerning the relation between sociocultural change and mental disorder brings out the effects of the acculturation process on social disintegration, subcultural conflicts, and a general state of frustration in society. I shall review some relevant studies concerning the cultural conflict hypothesis in order to show their significance for Pakistan.

In a general survey of studies concerning the effects of sociocultural factors causing mental disorders, Hunt (1959) classified them as demographic, ecological, cross-cultural, social stratification, and social mobility studies. He found that the demographic incidence of schizophrenia roughly equals all other mental disorders taken together. He also noted that institutionalized patients came predominantly from densely populated, low-income, high-delinquency areas. Cross-cultural studies which he surveyed indicated that the stress of acculturation may be one source of illness, and the other studies showed that the total incidence of psychosis was greater among the lower classes than others and that patient groups tended to be more socially mobile upward than was the population generally. Hunt also pointed out the vulnerability of the developing societies to mental diseases, tending to discount the common-sense notion that the incidence of mental diseases is greater in industrialized and affluent societies.

Leighton's (1945) observations on the social dislocation of Japanese Americans during World War II are highly pertinent to the recent history of Pakistan. These dislocations, Leighton pointed out, were detrimental to Japanese family structure and the feelings and values that go with it. Such social stress situations resulted in activities of a disorganizing sort and often in great changes in the organization of society. Other conclusions by Leighton *et al.* (1963) that in socially and culturally disintegrated communities far more people were found to have psychiatric symptoms than in integrated communities and that symptoms involving apathy, anxiety, and aggression were notably prominent may soon be true of Pakistan society which from all available evidence presently is more disintegrated than integrated.

Another relevant study is that of Hertz (1963) on the effects of urbanization in Liberia. He found that when groups and individuals moved into culturally, even though not geographically, foreign areas psychopathological conditions increased considerably. For the group of his patients with acute psychiatric disturbances, the experience of a strange, unfriendly, and hostile environment had become the source of anxiety-producing forces.

Another group of patients, whose problems were more difficult to handle because of increased intolerance demonstrated toward them, were the chronically ill who were no longer cared for by the basic family, which was undergoing radical changes.

De Macedo (1955), reporting on the effects of migration on mental health, observed that the process of intercultural contact gives rise in the individual to conflict taking the form of a struggle between the system of values of the immigrant and the values of the new social medium, conflict which is increased by forced mass immigration. He noted that the consequences of immigration appear more severely in second-generation immigrants than in those of the first generation. The immigration creates cultural conflict, and the subsequent maladjustment is evidenced in chronic emotional and psychosomatic disturbances. Lin (1960) pointed out that large-scale migration and resettlement, intensified communication, and universal yearning for education have created aspirations far beyond the resources of many countries.

One of the immediate consequences of social and population dislocation is the emergence of a group of unemployed individuals who find their environment hostile. The loss of financial security and the acute sense of social and emotional isolation more often than not result in psychiatric disturbances. Menninger (1948) found that about 60 to 80 per cent of unemployed individuals manifested signs of mental ill-health. The great majority gave evidence of their economic insecurity in their thinking and in their relations with other people. They often lost a fundamental necessity for good mental health—self respect. Even the threat of unemployment could be of particular significance. Roach and Gursslin (1965) also emphasized the significance of economic deprivation in initiating behavioral disorganization. Thus it seems reasonable to assume that a constant sense of economic insecurity in most of the developing countries of Asia and Latin America would make the people susceptible to most forms of neuroses and psychoses. Social scientists have demonstrated that sociocultural changes in traditional agricultural societies result in acute stress and social instability. Recent studies have presented sufficiently documented evidence that such societies are in a state of transition. Among sources of stress when a traditional social structure is being transformed into a twentieth-century industrial social system are rapid cultural change, conflict between an ideal and a real value system, unobtainable or unrealistic cultural goals, and the conflict of group and personal values (Opler, 1961). Stress also can come from the conflict between the old leaders and educated youth and from the conflict between the religious and secular demands of social change. Such stresses create circumstances contributing to mental illness even if not its cause. In dealing with mental disorders in Southeast Asia, Murphy (1957) listed immigration, nativity, minority status, occupation, education, social class, religion, primary group structure, birth order, and urban distribution as possible sources of mental disease.

Family structure and primary group affiliations have been emphasized by many investigators as very significant for the mental health of the
individual. Since the traditional family structure is sure to suffer from the
socioeconomic changes in developing countries, it may be appropriate to
look into the type of personality traits and attitudes generated by the traditional family pattern. According to Diaz-Guerrero (1955), the development
of neurosis within the Mexican family structure is founded on two fundamental propositions: the absolute supremacy of the father and the absolute
self-sacrifice of the mother. Mexican parents also emphasize the desirability
of a male infant and submission and obedience in the child. As a result, the
main areas of stress for a growing child are (1) submission conflict and
rebellion with authority; (2) preoccupation with sexual potency; (3) difficulty in superseding the maternal stage; (4) conflict and ambivalence
regarding his double role; and (5) problems before and after marriage
concerning mother love and the love of another woman.

Hoch (1957) in a discussion of psychiatry in India stated the
feeling that the joint family in which Indian children grow up does not
further emotional differentiation of individuals and endows them with a
lasting need for security. Recent industrialization is undermining this security without providing as a substitute greater prosperity and better administration. Govindaswamy (1958) reported as a result of industrialization in
India the heads of the families in villages are losing their authority, and
the unity of the joint family is being broken by the sons' migration to cities.
Simple religious ideas and beliefs and intense family loyalties are changing
with cultural change and being replaced by the "tyranny of modern existence." Emancipation of women is stated to be another of the changes
responsible for a great deal of neurosis and restlessness in young men and
women of the community.

The family structure and the pattern of child rearing in Mexico and
India, as reported by these investigations, are very similar to those in
Pakistan. The father's authority and the mother's submissive role are the
hallmarks of Pakistan society as well. Aggression in women is disapproved,
and children have exclusive female company in their early years. The recent
socioeconomic changes, however, have brought about some changes in these
respects. Parental authority is frequently violated and women are being
emancipated. The consequences therefore probably will be the same as in
India and Mexico. The young men and women also show signs of restlessness
and frustration. An extract from one of the popular Pakistan newspapers
may be relevant. Under the heading "1964—Social Change Telling on Student Behavior," Ahmad (1965) observed:

> Brimming with discontentment for a variety of
> reasons the students went into a headlong clash with the
> authorities as the year 1964 drew to a close . . . the age-old
> fraternity between the teacher and the pupil has been

shattered because the outlook of our youth is undergoing a metamorphosis. The Muslim society in undivided India was based largely on the family system. To-day that basis is tottering. Most middle class and higher middle class families have been hypnotized by Western culture, while the women who used to look after their children at home, have now come out of seclusion in search of employment. . . . These socio-economic changes have directly affected our youth.

The relevance of these conclusions to the problems of Pakistan society lies in the fact that almost all the developing countries, where some of these studies were conducted, are facing similar problems of cultural conflict and social disorganization. The major emphasis of development in these countries is on socioeconomic transformation of their traditional agricultural and rural social orientation. As a result of this emphasis, these societies are in a state of transition fighting hard to maintain their traditional social bases. It is this fight which should be the main focus of social psychiatric research in developing countries.

Indexes of Social Change

Using the basic facts and statistics put out by the Pakistan Government (1961, 1964), I shall apply the criteria of social change formulated by Allen and Bentz (1965) who arrived at four major indexes of socio-cultural change after an exhaustive factor analytic survey. These are: rising cost of living, growth of population, increasing industrial-technological and urban development, and increase in education.

The common man in Pakistan has been complaining of the rising prices of consumer goods for the last 15 years, and newspapers support his contention. The cost of living index for industrial workers in Karachi, Lahore, and Narayanganj for the year 1949–50 was 97, 90, and 101, respectively, and it was 132, 127, and 130, respectively, for the year 1963–64. Another cost of living index for the government and commercial employees in Karachi was 90 in 1950, 98 in 1954, 116 in 1960, and 122 in 1964. Both these indexes clearly point out the marked increase in the cost of living from 1949 to 1964.

Turning now to the growth of population, the two census surveys of 1951 and 1961 recorded the population of Pakistan at 75,842,000 and 93,690,000, respectively, showing an increase of 24 per cent in ten years. In explanation of this tremendous increase, however, the influx of about six million immigrants from India must be recalled, although about 50 per cent of them were already in Pakistan at the time of the first census.

The third index relates to urbanization and industrialization. At the time of independence in 1947 the urban population was less than 10 per cent. Government figures show a marked trend toward migration to cities between

1951 and 1961. The urban population increased by 56.1 per cent. The urban population represented 13.1 per cent of the total population in 1961 and over 16 per cent in 1965. As to industrial growth, the government figures indicate remarkable progress in the manufacture of consumer goods. Exports have increased and the volume of imports has gradually lessened. In 1954 only 4.5 per cent of the total national income came from manufacturing; by 1964 its share had multiplied manifold. For example, with a base of 100 in 1954, production in mining and manufacturing in 1950 was 39.5; in 1961 it was 204.5; and in 1964, 207. The pace of industrialization is increasing; should the third Five-Year Plan beginning in July, 1965, meet its targets the very basis of the economy may be changed.

The fourth index is education. The increase in literacy has not been as great as is desirable for a country changing from an agricultural to an industrial economy; however, physical plants have improved, the number of schools at all levels has multiplied, and public expenditures for education have increased greatly since 1950. In 1954 the expenditure was three times that in 1950. Since then, a number of new colleges and eight more universities have been established. A comparison of the fund allocations in the first and second Five-Year Plans indicates a 250 per cent increase (from 580 to 1,323 million rupees) in estimated expenditures on education.

Areas of Value Conflict

I shall illustrate my discussion on the conflict of values and the symptoms of disorganization in the rural social structure of Pakistan with data gathered in two villages of East Pakistan (Zaidi, in press). In order to focus the main theme of this chapter, namely, the incongruity of the social changes with the society's value system, I shall begin with a brief physical description of the traditional village with its value system, family relations, and socialization processes.

A typical village in East Pakistan is relatively small in area. The size of the landholding per family is also small, although the average family numbers about six persons. Transportation to and from such villages is difficult and time-consuming. During the rainy season all the dirt paths are submerged in water and the only practical means of transport is a small country boat. Generally a market (*haat*) is held weekly or biweekly to serve about a dozen villages. These bazaars are also the means for intervillage social and political contacts. Most villages have some sort of a religious elementary school and one or two mosques. The villagers are mainly Muslims. The village teacher, the *Imam* (the man who leads the Muslim prayers) and the traditional and often hereditary village *sardar* (headman) are the most prominent villagers. The *sardar* still holds authority in the affairs of the village. In addition, every village also has an informal council of *maatbars* ("elders"), who exercised many functions of the judiciary in the past and who still prescribe social control in the village society.

Social relations in the village are primarily based on kinship ties. Child-rearing practices in the villages are quite simple. The child is the responsibility of the mother till the age of six or seven. The father spends little more than an hour a day with the child. Both male and female are brought up by the mother or the grandmother until they are able to go out to school or to work in the fields. When a child misbehaves, the mother does not herself punish him but usually threatens to report him to the father. In the same way, she may threaten to leave the child in a dark or lonely place where ghosts and witches are supposed to lie in wait for naughty children. Thus for a child the image of a stern father (mostly made out to be such by the mother) and images of ghosts and witches may be the sources of early fear and anxiety. Though often a mere threat of punishment suffices, the father may actually punish the child for disobedience and unruly conduct. Thus it may be assumed that among Pakistani villagers the father is the early social control authority and that the development of a child's personality is affected by his ambivalent feelings of fear and respect for the father and by a passive affection for the mother. This ambivalence toward the father later may be generalized to include other authority figures—the ruler and god. To prevent giving a false picture, let me add that the village father's aloofness may be misunderstood unless his devoted attention to the material needs of his wife and children is taken into account. Although he may not overtly exhibit his affection, he often may starve himself in order to feed his family.

Children up to the ages of five or six get the unconditional love of both parents. It is, however, expected of every male child that on growing up he will take care of his parents and also enhance the name and prestige of the family. Financial support in old age, however, is the parents' most important expectation from male children. Such expectations and respect for age are reinforced by religious injunctions and are socially sanctioned by the joint pattern of the family. The tie with the family is never broken, and the authority of parents lasts as long as they live. As in many other Asian countries, the eldest son in an East Pakistan village family holds a slightly more privileged position than his siblings. This privilege, however, increases his responsibility to look after aged parents, younger brothers and sisters, and the family property or business.

The growing child in the village society also internalizes some other values of peasant communities. According to Redfield (1956) these values are an intense attachment to native soil; a reverent disposition toward the home, the habitat, and ancestral ways; a restraint on individual self-seeking in favor of the family and community; and a certain suspiciousness mixed with appreciation of town life. The village social structure in the two villages of East Pakistan in which I gathered my data is characterized by the following basic values: (1) respect for parents, old persons in the community, and the men of god; (2) strong attachment to dependents and to family property; (3) respect for persons who are senior relatives and love and affection for younger relatives; (4) charity for the weak and poor and hospitality to guests and outsiders; (5) self-sacrifice for the family and the community and emphasis on public good as contrasted with individual enhancement; (6) abhorrence of adultery and of violation of the religious injunctions; and (7) dislike for unnecessary display of wealth and material success (implying appreciation of modesty and selflessness). Redfield (1956) considered the culture of peasant communities an aspect of a larger culture represented by the refinements of religion, literature, art, and other higher forms of culture found in society outside the village community. According to this view, these values represent the value orientation of the entire Pakistan society.

All these basic values present a contrast to the value orientation of a modern industrial society. For example, the emphasis in Western urbanized and industrialized society is on personal achievement. Landy (1958) described the value orientation of the American culture as characterized by achievement, work, prestige, money, and leisure. Such a value system may lead to isolation of the individual, to loss of social and personal identity, and to increased importance of the peer group control. The values of Pakistan village society are not appropriate or conducive to adjustment and change to an industrial-urban society. It seems almost inevitable therefore that a serious value conflict will result with consequences of mental disorder and social disorganization.

In the West industrialization and urbanization usually followed a gradual course of social development. When the change came, it was familiar, expected, and that for which people had worked. The change naturally led to the development of institutions appropriate to the process. In the East, on the other hand, people have been caught in the tide. They are so used to their traditional way of life with its fatalism and resignation that to them these social changes appear a heresy. They tend to look at modernization attempts as something unwholesome and therefore unwelcome. As Lerner (1958) put it, "whereas the traditional man tended to reject innovation by saying 'it has never been thus,' the contemporary Westerner is more likely to ask 'does it work?' and try the new way without further ado."

This contrast between the perception and attitudes of the Westerner and those of the traditional peoples puts into clear perspective the value conflict, social disorganization, and the resulting problems of mental health and adjustment. A few of the significant areas are outlined below.

The most significant value conflict may occur in the area of family relations. In traditional societies the family provides the emotional, social, and even financial security of its members. In the joint family the resources are pooled, and the members look upon the head of the family as responsible for meeting all their needs and those of their wives and children. No one questions the loyalty of members to the family name, prestige, and property. It is taken for granted that wherever one may go he ultimately will come back to the family fold. His home offers the member of a joint family the greatest solace, comfort, and security in times of need. The family member never feels insecure even when unemployed or friendless. The family house and its members are always the last hope. The family is the real anchor for rich and poor alike. In the developing countries, however, the joint family is in a state of transition, of breaking up into numerous nuclear units. The sense of insecurity and loneliness is strong when a person is left to his own resources surrounded by strange people in a strange environment. As I wrote in 1959 of the village worker in the city:

> He faces the initial difficulty of adjusting to a largely urban and industrial environment for which his rural background is entirely unsuited. The stereotypes, beliefs, and attitudes appropriate to a rural family pattern make the adjustment to an industrial family pattern very difficult for him. The joint pattern of our large rural families comes into clash with the responsibilities of a new pattern. The worker is naturally inclined to this new pattern, but the affiliations with other members of the family keep him undecided. He mostly wants and tries to retain these affiliations with other relatives in the village, as evidenced by the large number of absences due to "urgent" business at home. Thus, he is torn between two loyalties.

Another difficulty for the village working man living in an industrial setting relates to his loyalty to the land and habitat. In the village social prestige and one's place in the social hierarchy are measured by the size of one's landholdings. Many of the industrial workers cannot get over this notion of social prestige easily. As a matter of fact, most of them come to work in the factory or mill with the specific objective of earning enough to hold on to the family property or to buy more land. They save for this purpose, although usually such savings compete with the desire for a better standard of living. Such attempts to maintain two "homes" lead to economic difficulties and to social frustrations affecting their physical and mental health. Evidence shows that a majority of workers in the large industrial centers of Pakistan are from the villages. They come to work in the factory or the mills because farming has become hazardous and because of frequent natural disasters; the yield from the land is always uncertain at best. They leave behind their wives and children to whom they regularly send money saved from their meager earnings. A pattern that is clearly indicated in the migration of villagers to industrial centers is that once a person gets a job and settles down to work, he writes back home; then relatives and friends are lured by his success to follow him to the city. Often small groups of workers from the same village or community work in the same industrial establishment, and this arrangement may provide each of them a sense of security and cohesion in a strange environment.

In a survey of migration from villages to towns in India, Deshmukh (1956) described the migrant as a marginal man in whom the conflict of the rural and urban culture traits is very active and who is consequently the most obvious sufferer from cultural shock. The majority of the workers in his sample remained completely undecided whether to pick up the new ways of living and settle down or to go back to the security of the familiar village life. These workers, he observed, relegated themselves permanently to a marginal status which further intensified their sense of personal frustration and resulted in various symptoms of maladjustment. Workers in Pakistan industrial establishments do not differ from those in India.

Another area of value conflict for people in developing countries is in personal versus community orientation in achievement. In the traditional village society of Pakistan a socially and financially successful person makes the entire community proud of him. He belongs to the community. For example, when a village youth or his family settles in a town or city in connection with his business or profession, any member of the community visiting the town makes it almost obligatory on himself to visit and even stay with him. Unless during their stay they have been "infected" with the selfish ways of the city life, the city-dwelling youth and his family welcome such visitors. In a traditional society the fruits of success and achievement are shared with the community. There is the highest degree of honesty and fellowship in such a relation. In the changing society of the developing countries, however, such a role expectation would generate a variety of conflicts in a city-dwelling family, involved with its new status symbols, personal achievement motivations, and the stress of maintaining or advancing its new-found social status. Such conflicts may cause many embarrassing and frustrating situations and may easily not be solved for decades.

Furthermore, the homeostatic balance of the traditional social hierarchy is likely to be disturbed in an important way by a shift in the pattern of social mobility now resulting from technological and social changes. Traditionally, as I said earlier, the village society (a major sector of Pakistan society) has had a well-defined and fairly permanent system of social stratification in which such matters as the size of landholding and family descent always have played a major role. Persons born in a certain family have an ascribed status in the village which is not altered by any achieved status. The son of a "lower-class" family, even though he has attained some position of power, on return to his village home may be expected to behave in the same humble way as his poor father did in the presence of the village elders. This pattern of social relation is sure to suffer under the impact of modernization. The criteria of social position will no longer be family descent, age, or the size of one's landholding in the village, because these have no value or functional utility in an industrial-urban social milieu. Readjustment of the traditional social system may mean a breakdown of the social structure and result in the destruction of various sociocultural institutions, aside from causing other associated maladjustments and behavior deviations.

Changes in the patterns of authority and village leadership, immediate targets of modernization, represent a fourth area of value conflict. In the village family authority is vested in the head of the family who is the eldest member both in age and relationship. Authority in the village rests with an informal council of elders who have had this privilege either through inheritance or through the usual channels of social stratification. As I mentioned before, the authority figures in the East Pakistan villages include the village teacher and the *Imam* in the mosque. There is no challenge to their authority as long as the traditional cultural pattern prevails, but the new wave of social change will bring increase in education; young people may go off to college and a university and later take positions in government and industry. There will be an inevitable flouting of the traditional authority and struggle between the old and the young for leadership in the village and beyond it. Even now when the basic village culture is intact, there are signs of conflict with, and violations of, traditional authority. This situation is not only detrimental to the village leadership but it also cuts at the root of some of the basic value orientations of the villager. Husain (1956) reporting a survey of factory workers mostly drawn from East Pakistan villages described the situation thus: "Finding parental discipline too irksome, they were enjoying their newly found independence and having a good time in the company of their mates and were not anxious to visit home or share in the family responsibility." This may be the general attitude of the semi-literate factory workers toward village and family authority. The consequences of widespread social change can easily be predicted on the basis of this attitude being shown even when industrialization had just begun.

Another vulnerable area of village society is connected with the present position of women in predominantly Muslim Pakistan. Although Islam places men and women on equal footing with appropriate division of labor, in practice the women in the villages have not been given the status they deserve. They stay at home and toil all day long with only occasional gossiping or quarreling to break the monotony. The village male generally is not convinced of the value of education for women. In such a society hostile to female education, the impact of social changes leading to universal education and job opportunities for all could be quite shattering. It could affect family solidarity, the relationship of parent and child, village attitudes and prejudices, and above all, the security and emotional support which the child enjoys at home at present because of the mother. Women might become economically self-supporting and, as many suspect, such changes may also make women less home-oriented and even emotionally insecure in the face of competition for marriage. In the present village society girls are secure in the knowledge that their parents or older relatives will find husbands for them. They also enjoy the security of the parental home if divorce occurs or the husband dies. It probably is true that for women the present pattern of family life in Pakistan is less anxiety-producing than that of the modern family in the industrial social structure. Even in Pakistan increasing divorce rates, extramarital relations, and prostitution in large urban centers are evidence on that score.

This chapter has outlined the precipitating causes and certain symptoms of a society under stress. While no definite conclusions can be formulated with the meager information available, the following observations seem warranted: (1) The social changes occurring in the developing countries, including Pakistan, seem to create a cultural milieu which in the early phases is likely to affect the values and beliefs adversely; (2) sociocultural changes in developing societies lead to conflicts and frustrations threatening the mental health of the people; and (3) the greater in span and wider in scope the anticipated sociocultural changes, the more widespread will be the social disorganization and the more intense the impact on the mental health of the people.

REFERENCES

Ahmad, F. 1965. 1964—social changes telling on student behavior. Morning News (Karachi), Sunday, January 17. P. 7.

Allen, F. R., and W. K. Bentz. 1965. Towards the measurement of sociocultural change. Social Forces 43:522-32.

Deshmukh, M. B. 1956. A study of floating migration. *In* Implications of industrialization and urbanization. Calcutta, UNESCO Research Centre.

Diaz-Guerrero, R. 1955. Neurosis and the Mexican family structure. American Journal of Psychiatry 112:411-17.

Govindaswamy, M. V. 1958. Some problems of mental ailments in India. Journal of the All-India Institute of Mental Health 1(2):1-6.

Hertz, D. G. 1963. Problems of urbanization in Liberia as reflected in the mental health services. *In* Proceedings of the Joint Meeting of the Japanese Association of Psychiatry and Neurology and the American Psychiatric Association, Tokyo. H. Akimoto, ed. Supplement No. 7 of Folia Psychiatria et Neurologia Japonica. Tokyo, Japanese Society of Psychiatry and Neurology.

Hoch, E. M. 1957. Psychiatrie in Indien. Praxis 46:1145-50.

Hunt, R. G. 1959. Socio-cultural factors in mental disorders. Behavioral Science 4:96-106.

Husain, A. F. A. 1956. Human and social impact of technological change in Pakistan. Vol. 1. London, Oxford University Press.

Husain, A. F. A., and A. Farouk. 1961. Problems of social integration of industrial workers in Khulna with special reference to the problem of industrial unrest. East Pakistan, Socio-economic Research Board, Dacca University.

Landy, D. 1958. Cultural antecedents of mental illness in the U.S. Social Service Review 32:350-61.

Leighton, A. H. 1945. The governing of men. Princeton, Princeton University Press.

Leighton, A. H., T. A. Lambo, C. C. Hughes, D. C. Leighton, J. M. Murphy, and D. B. Macklin. 1963. Psychiatric disorder among the Yoruba. Ithaca, Cornell University Press.

Lerner, D. 1958. The passing of traditional society. New York, Free Press.

Lin, T. 1960. Social change and mental health. World Mental Health 12(2):65–73.

Macedo, G. de. 1955. Imigracao, conflito de cultura, doenca psicosomatica. Medicina Cirurgia, Farmacia No. 228. (Abstracted in Review and Newsletter of Transcultural Psychiatric Research No. 3:10, 1957.)

Menninger, W. C. 1948. Psychiatry in a troubled world. New York, Macmillan.

Murphy, H. M. B. 1957. Unpublished material. Review and Newsletter of Transcultural Psychiatric Research No. 3:10 (abstract).

Opler, M. K. 1961. Epidemiology of mental health. Review and Newsletter of Transcultural Psychiatric Research No. 10:16 (abstract).

Pakistan Government. 1961. Pakistan: basic facts. Karachi, Government of Pakistan Publications.

_____. 1964. Pakistan: basic facts. Karachi, Government of Pakistan Publications.

Redfield, R. 1956. Peasant society and culture. Chicago, University of Chicago Press.

Roach, J. L., and O. R. Gursslin. 1965. The lower class, status frustration, and social disorganization. Social Forces 43:501–10.

Zaidi, S. M. H. 1959. Problems of human relations in industry in Pakistan. Journal of Social Psychology 59:13–18.

_____. 1964. Pakistan: a society in transition. Psychologia 7:15–21.

_____. (In press.) The village culture in transition: a study of East Pakistan rural society. Honolulu, East-West Center Press.

CONCLUSION

27. Cultural Psychiatric Research in Asia

E. C. WITTKOWER, M.D.

Department of Psychiatry
McGill University
Montreal, Canada

with the assistance of

P. E. TERMANSEN, M.D.

Department of Psychiatry
University of British Columbia
Vancouver, Canada

THE LONG-RANGE HISTORY of cultural psychiatric research in Asia has been reviewed repeatedly, most recently by Lin (1963). A brief résumé therefore may suffice. As may be remembered, Kraepelin (1904) was one of the pioneers in this field. Early in this century, inspired by regional differences in the behavior of the mentally ill which he had discovered in Germany and other European countries, he left for Java with the explicit purpose of studying cultural influences in the frequency and symptomatology of mental disorders in that country. He noted among other observations that manic-depressive psychoses were uncommon and that depressive reactions, if they occurred, seldom contained elements of sinfulness. The lead given by him was taken up by other Western psychiatrists after World War I. In 1920 Van Loon (1920) noted an increase in the frequency of major mental disorders in areas of Sumatra recently defeated by the Dutch. An estimate of the number of the mentally ill in China was published by McCartney in 1926 (1926a, 1926b). Seligman (1929) reported on schizophrenic psychoses among the Papuan of New Guinea in 1929. In the same year Woods (1929) published his observations on mental disorders in the Chinese. Dhunjibhoy (1930) noted a higher incidence of schizophrenia in Indians with Western education. Van Wulfften-Palthe (1936) described some apparently culture-specific mental disorders in the Javanese. He also corroborated Kraepelin's (1904) earlier findings of a rarity of severe depressive episodes in Javanese manic-depressives. Only prior to World War II did Asiatic investigators enter this field of research in significant numbers. Their studies were largely epidemiological in nature. Reference can be made to the classical studies of Uchimura *et al.* (1940) regarding prevalence rates of schizophrenia and morbidity rates of mental illness in Japan. Other Japanese authors reporting statistical findings in those years were Tsuwaga *et al.* (1942), Akimoto (1942), Oyama (1943), Ohta (1943), and Hanashiro (1943), to mention just a few. Yap's (1951) clinical study of mental diseases peculiar to certain cultures was followed by a number of further epidemiological studies, notably those of Lin (1953) and Yoshimatsu (1953). Bowman (1959) in a much-quoted study of culture and mental disease concluded from his experiences in China, Indonesia, the Philippines, and Thailand that the incidence and symptomatology of mental disorders in Asia are much the same as in other parts of the world.

In pulling together scattered observations and separating the wheat from the chaff, I shall concentrate my efforts on materials presented in our journal, *Transcultural Psychiatric Research,* i.e., on materials which have come under the purview of its editors during the last seven years. In all, 108 books, book contributions, published articles, and personal communications form the basis of this survey. They include not only reports on research but also, of necessity, impressions obtained by observers.

Geographical Areas

Most information has been obtained from India, with Japan a near second. Next in frequency follow reports from Taiwan, Indonesia, Hong Kong, Sarawak, New Guinea, and South Korea on account of a small number of scientifically active research workers in these countries. The conclusion must be drawn that cultural psychiatric research has been confined to certain areas of Asia, that virtually no observations are available for vast geographical and cultural areas of Asia, and that for this reason alone generalizations regarding mental disease in Asia are not permissible.

Observers and Investigators

Eighty-eight of the 108 presentations surveyed have been contributed by psychiatrists, 13 by cultural anthropologists and other social scientists, and 7 by psychologists. Hence, as would be expected, the bulk of the studies concerning cultural and transcultural *psychiatry* in Asia, in contrast to cultural and transcultural *psychology,* have been carried out by psychiatrists. Joint authorship, i.e., research co-operation between representatives of at least two of the three disciplines named, as in the studies of Caudill and Doi (1963), has been rare.

Fifty-nine senior authors were Asiatic and 49 non-Asiatic, mostly

Americans. As I stated earlier, Indian and Japanese observers have been prominent among Asiatic observers and investigators. Remarkable is the high percentage of non-Asiatics, especially Americans, reporting on observations of cultural psychiatric interest in Asiatic countries. This high percentage may be due to the great and growing interest in cultural psychiatry in North America (not present to the same extent in indigenous Asiatic observers); to the fascinating and intriguing aspects of Far Eastern peoples during and after World War II; and, last but not least, to the availability to Americans of research grants for such studies. On the other hand, the relative infrequency of cultural psychiatric research by Asiatics can be attributed to the sparsity of psychiatrists in most Asiatic countries (except Japan) which forces those available to concentrate on routine services rather than on research. Despite these difficulties, however, there has been a significant change in recent years. The ratio of Asiatic to non-Asiatic scientific contributions to the field of cultural psychiatry was 14:10 during the years 1962 to 1963 and has gone up to 21:8 during the years 1964 to 1965. Of course, the possibility cannot be entirely excluded that the ability to obtain access to materials from the Far East has improved as the years passed.

Topics and Problems

Topics which have been studied in relation to a given cultural milieu and in comparisons of this milieu with others include: (1) frequency of mental disorders, (2) frequency of nosological entities, (3) frequency of symptoms, (4) symptomatology, (5) specific syndromes, (6) etiological concepts, (7) patient care, and (8) community attitudes toward the mentally ill.

Specifically the following problems have been raised in Asiatic countries: Does the Oriental way of life with its emphasis on social and emotional withdrawal, on meditation and contemplation, increase or reduce a tendency to develop mental disease? To what extent is mental morbidity affected by prevailing Eastern value orientations—such as the traditional family structure, role and status of women—compared with prevailing Western value orientations? In which ways do mental disorders, quantitatively and qualitatively, differ between aborigines, native populations settled for many generations, and recent immigrants? To what extent do political change and cultural change—the breakdown of family traditions and of other social institutions, industrialization and urbanization—adversely affect mental health? To what extent do differences in belief systems between East and West influence the symptomatology of mental disorders? Are there any mental disorders specific to Asiatic cultures? Why are some forms of treatment for the mentally ill more acceptable to peoples in the East than those accepted in the West? Do community attitudes toward the mentally ill differ in the East from those in the West, and, if so, why?

Major Approaches and Methodologies

The questions listed, to which, of course, many others could be added, show that the principles underlying transcultural psychiatric research are correlation between psychiatric and sociocultural variables and comparison of observations made in one culture with observations made in one or several others. Consequently, there are two major approaches to transcultural psychiatric problems; the psychiatric, and the social science point of view. That is, the observer either may ask himself why in sociocultural terms certain psychiatric variants occur, or, starting off with sociocultural features, he may ask himself what effect those have on mental health.

Approaches may be either quantitative or qualitative, statistical or clinical. Statistical studies may be epidemiological, in which case they may be carried out by, or in conjunction with, an epidemiologist, while clinical studies may be descriptive or dynamic. There is an undercurrent of controversy between workers in the field about the merits and demerits of each of these approaches. Some investigators seem to believe that the absence of statistics impairs the scientific value of a paper. The facts are that none of the three major disciplines engaged in transcultural psychiatric research—psychiatry, cultural anthropology, and epidemiology—can make a significant contribution to the field in isolation, that epidemiology and descriptive psychiatry can produce valuable data, and that only cultural anthropology and dynamic psychiatry can offer explanations and interpretations of the data.

Methodologies of transcultural psychiatric research in Asia quite as much as elsewhere consist of application of the same investigative techniques to persons and situations in contrasting cultures, either by the same observer or by different observers.

As regards the investigative tools, they comprise: (1) clinical interviews, (2) field observations, (3) hospital and other records, (4) psychological tests, and (5) questionnaires. Clinical interviews were used in 40 per cent, hospital and other records in 28 per cent, field observations in 25 per cent, and psychological tests or questionnaires in the remaining 7 per cent of the research projects surveyed. These figures mean that only in one-quarter of the projects surveyed has research been carried out in the field. Since the subject studied is mental illness and since the bulk of the investigators are psychiatrists, however, it is hardly surprising that they use the investigative instruments to which they are accustomed, namely, clinical interviews and hospital records.

The term "clinical interview" refers to information obtained from patients by physicians, usually in their offices. Examples of studies of this kind are those of Yap (1963) and Rin (1963) concerning *koro* and those concerning differences in the clinical picture of schizophrenia, depression, and hysteria in contrasting cultures (Bhaskaran, 1963; Chakraborty, 1964; Grewal, 1959; Schooler and Caudill, 1964; Sukthankar, 1964; Vahia, 1963).

Evidence accumulated by examination of representative samples of patients of the same diagnostic category lends itself to statistical cross-cultural comparison, as in the study of the contents of the schizophrenic delusions in Japan (Asai, 1964) and of depressive ideas in India (Hoch, 1961a).

The term "field observation" signifies that the investigator, who may be a psychiatrist or a social scientist, studies phenomena, social situations, and groups of individuals in their natural environment. Matters which have been subjected to such a study are spirit possession in India (Freed and Freed, 1964; Harper, 1963); trance states in Indonesia (Pfeiffer, 1965); exorcism in Ceylon (Senanayake, 1961); the effect of acculturation in Mauritius (Raman, 1961); and mental morbidity in selected areas of Taiwan (Lin, 1953; Rin and Lin, 1962), of Korea (Yoo, 1961), and of India (Surya *et al.*, 1964). The mental hospital as such may be the subject of a field study provided that institutional aspects, as in Caudill's (1963) study of three Japanese hospitals, rather than the personal aspects of the patients are the focus of investigation.

Hospital records concerning admissions as well as outpatients have been used in research in Asia for (1) appraisal of differences in the distribution of diagnostic categories between Eastern and Western patients and between different population groups living in the same geographical area; (2) comparison between mentally ill migrants and nonmigrants; and (3) studying the relation between sibling rank within the family and frequency and nature of mental disorders. Examples of studies of these kinds are Gaitonde's (1958) comparison of patients attending outpatient departments in Bombay and Topeka; Murphy's (1965) study of mental hospital admissions in Southeast Asia; Pfeiffer's (1963) and Schmidt's (1961, 1964) work in Java and Sarawak, respectively; and Caudill's (1963) investigations, since repeated by others (Rin, 1965; Yamaguchi *et al.*, 1964), regarding the differential occurrence of schizophrenia in various sibling rank positions in Japan. Other records have been used for the study of the sociocultural background of persons who commit suicide and homicide.

Psychological tests and questionnaires have been sparingly employed in cultural psychiatric research in Asia. As regards the former, reference is made to the use of Shirley Star's vignettes and the social distance scale in Terashima and Nareta's (1964) study of community attitudes toward mental illness in rural Japan, and, as regards the latter, to our own global surveys of schizophrenic and depressive symptomatology (Murphy, Wittkower, and Chance, 1964; Wittkower *et al.*, 1960).

Some Data Obtained

In a brief survey of this kind, it is clearly impossible to cover comprehensively all the data obtained concerning cultural psychiatric research in Asia. Two selected research areas, the frequency and the nature of mental illness, must suffice by way of illustration.

FREQUENCY OF MENTAL DISORDERS

Various observers have made the suggestion, chiefly based on their impressions, that the total frequency of mental disorders in the East is the same as, higher than, or lower than in the West. The fact is that nothing definite is known about differences in total incidence and that no method exists to give valid information on this point. As I mentioned before, attempts have been made to estimate differences in the *relative* frequency of mental disorders by means of hospital records and by means of census examination of selected population samples. In contrast to Stoller (1959), I seriously doubt whether the use of hospital records, even in areas of similar cultural evolution, is suitable for comparative purposes because of the composition of a mental hospital. The method of census examination is more suitable for this purpose, though with it cross-cultural comparison is exceedingly difficult because of differences in the population resistance to being surveyed, as Surya *et al.*, (1964) has shown, and differences in sampling, intensity of investigation, criteria of mental disorder, and methods of computing data used by different investigators. Census examinations, as evidenced by the study of Lin *et al.* presented in Chapter 5, lend themselves particularly well to comparison of total and relative frequency of mental disorders between different subcultural groups. Both methods have been used successfully for the study of the frequency and the nature of mental illness in relation to such social factors as age, sex, residence, education, social class, caste, and religion.

Bearing these methodological difficulties in mind, the following general conclusions can be drawn: (1) infectious psychoses play a greater part in the East than in the West (Dorzhadamba, 1965; Hoch, 1959, 1961b; Rin and Lin, 1962); (2) general paralysis of the insane—no longer a problem in the West—continues to be a problem in the East, though perhaps except in Thailand, Burma, and Indonesia it is on the decline (Dorzhadamba, 1965; Grewal, 1959; Pfeiffer, 1963; Ratanakorn, 1960; Yoo, 1961); (3) schizophrenia all over the world is the most common functional psychosis requiring hospitalization; (4) manic-depressive psychosis is less common—or at least reaches psychiatrists less often—in the East than in the West (Gaitonde, 1958; Pfeiffer, 1963); (5) post-partum psychoses have been reported as particularly frequent in some Asiatic countries (Dorzhadamba, 1965; Gaitonde, 1958); (6) conversion hysteria in its gross forms, which has almost vanished in the West, is common in some Asiatic countries (Burton-Bradley, 1962; Gaitonde, 1958; Maguigad, 1964; Vahia, 1963); (7) obsessive-compulsive neurosis has been reported as rare in Taiwan and Indonesia (Lin, 1953; Pfeiffer, 1965) but is by no means uncommon in the big cities of India and Japan; (8) psychophysiological reactions have been noted to be common in India (Gaitonde, 1958); (9) presenile and senile psychoses are seen less often by Eastern psychiatrists than by Western psychiatrists (Hankoff, 1958; Schmidt, 1961); (10) opium addiction, at one time prevalent among the Chinese, seems to be on the decline (Dorzhadamba, 1965); and (11) alcoholism has increased in Japan and other Far Eastern countries since World War II (Chafetz, 1964; Stoller, 1959; Yoo, 1961).

The explanation of some of these phenomena is obvious; in others exploration is required; still others defy explanation in the light of our present knowledge. For instance, it is obvious that in countries in which the risk of infection is abundant and in which medical services are inadequate infectious psychoses are prevalent while the frequency of general paralysis of the insane depends on availability of early treatment for syphilis. Schizophrenia, it is true, is ubiquitous, but nobody knows whether there are numerical differences between East and West. It is conceivable that, for culturally inherent reasons, in non-Western countries different population groups are prone to be affected. The alleged rarity of depressive states in Asia may be an artifact; there is good reason to believe that quiet retarded depressives are retained in and looked after by the family. Conversely, if the rarity is genuine, as it well may be in some Asiatic countries, the fact may be accounted for by the protective effect of the extended family against mourning over object loss; the effectiveness of funeral rites in working through object loss; the effectiveness of projective mechanisms as a defense against depression; and a predominance of a collective superego in primitive societies versus a predominance of an individual superego in Western and Western-type societies.

The high frequency of puerperal psychosis in some Asiatic countries has been attributed to the great importance of fecundity among women, the numerous taboos related to pregnancy and parturition, the reality of the dangers of delivery, and high infantile mortality.

The frequency of gross forms of conversion hysteria among the uneducated in the East, as in illiterates elsewhere, has been attributed to deficient repression, and their recession in the West, to the emancipation of women and an increasing sophistication of the population. The infrequency of obsessive-compulsive neurosis in rural Asia may be due, as it is generally, to the disinclination of obsessive-compulsives to seek psychiatric help, leniency in toilet training in some Asiatic countries; externalization of a threatening superego in the form of popular beliefs and superstitions; and to absorption of obsessional defenses in culture-dictated rituals. Knowledge about the occurrence of psychophysiological reactions in at least some Asiatic countries is so inadequate that generalizations regarding their frequency should be treated with caution. As far as primitive sections of the population are concerned, however, it appears likely that they are apt to somatize emotional tension and conflict. Reference is made to Rin's careful study in Taiwan (Chapter 7). Religious and legal prohibition account for the low rate of alcoholism in Asia (Chafetz, 1964); its recent increase is one of the doubtful privileges bestowed by Westernization. Differential prevalance rates of mental illness were observed by Rin and Lin

(1962) in a study of four Formosan aboriginal tribes at different levels of acculturation. Finally, once again mention should be made of Caudill's (1963) sibling rank study. He attributed the seemingly higher incidence of schizophrenia in first-born males and in last-born females among hospitalized patients to their special positions in traditional Japanese families.

NATURE OF MENTAL DISEASE

Information about differences in the symptomology of mental disorders in Asia has been derived predominantly from clinical interviews with patients in mental hospitals and to a lesser extent with patients attending outpatient departments. Patients seen in private practice and hospital records also have been used for this purpose.

Most researchers and observers agree that in comparing East and West, similarities in the symptomatology of the major functional psychoses are far greater than dissimilarities. Some differences, however, in the clinical manifestations of schizophrenia and of manic-depressive psychoses in Asiatic patients have been noted.

For instance, it has been reported that more often than in Europe schizophrenia in India is restricted to the primary symptom or colored by hysterical manifestations; that in Indian schizophrenics apathy is often the main presenting symptom; that catatonic rigidity, negativism, and stereotypy are fairly common; that there is less "method in the madness" of Indian patients (Hoch, 1959, 1961a); and that they are more emotionally and socially withdrawn than their Euro-American counterparts (Wittkower *et al.,* 1960). Contradictory statements have been made regarding assaultive behavior of Asiatic schizophrenic patients; according to some observers (Schooler and Caudill, 1964) Asiatic patients are more assaultive and according to others (Hankoff, 1958; Stoller, 1959), less assaultive than Euro-Americans. It goes without saying that the content of delusions and hallucinations is influenced by the sociocultural environment of the patient. Persecutory ideas center around in-laws, other members of the joint family, the stars and the spirits of the dead in tradition-rooted uneducated Indian patients (Hoch, 1959). According to Asai (1964) and Hasuzawa (1963) paranoid schizophrenia has increased in Japan since World War II. Since then, in replacement of delusions regarding the Emperor, paranoid delusions have concerned themselves increasingly with the United States, the Communist Party, radio, and television. Concurrently, there has been an increase in delusions of possession by powerful deities, sacred animals, or figures of primitive mythology. Equally, political elements related to current political events in Taiwan (Rin *et al.,* 1962) and in Indonesia (Pfeiffer, 1963) are noticeable in delusional schizophrenic patients in these countries.

As regards manic-depressive psychoses, the manic phase comes more often to the observation of psychiatrists in some Asiatic countries than does the depressive phase (Rin and Lin, 1962). In the clinical picture of the latter, the classical features of depressive mood, insomnia with early morning wakening, and loss of interest in the social environment have all been encountered in Asia. However, some distinctive features have been described. For instance, diurnal mood changes, anorexia, and constipation have been reported as uncommon among Indian patients, and religious preoccupations, loss of sexual interest, and theatrical grief as infrequent among Japanese depressives (Murphy, Wittkower, and Chance, 1964). Guilt feelings were rarely a part of the depressive syndrome in Java (Pfeiffer, 1963) and the Philippines (Maguigad, 1964). Hoch (1961a) carried out a study of the contents of depressive ideas in Indian patients and found that a simple preoccupation with the body, the mind, and the family predominated over other ideas. She demonstrated differences in content according to caste and religion and according to degree of education and Westernization. Much research has been devoted to the frequency and motivation for suicide in Japan, India, and Hong Kong. Reference is made in this connection to the studies of Yap (1958), Satyavati and Rao (1961), Sakamoto and Kasahara (1963), Ohara (1963), and DeVos (1966).

As for psychoneuroses, the frequency of gross forms of conversion hysteria and the rarity of obsessional neuroses in Asiatic rural populations have been mentioned. In view of their tendency to somatize, it is hardly surprising that neurotic patients, if they present themselves at all, hardly ever connect their bodily symptoms to emotional conflicts (Maguigad, 1964).

Finally, there is a special group of unusual symptom patterns which constitute so-called culture-bound disorders, also described as folk illness, such as possession states, *latah, koro, mata gelap,* and *amok.* These disorders have been described and discussed in Yap's presentation in Chapter 3.

What do all these findings mean? In trying to explain the reported differences between East and West, one should bear in mind (1) that in some parts of Asia mental disorders are precipitated, aggravated, and influenced by such biological factors as infection and vitamin deficiency to an extent and in a manner not fully explored; (2) that most of the patients from whom conclusions were drawn were examined in mental hospitals and, owing to the tendency to admit only grossly disturbing and disturbed patients, retaining the others at home, constitute therefore a highly selected sample; and (3) that cultural differences in thought, feeling, and behavior —and even in value orientation—between educated Westerners and educated highly Westernized Asiatics become somewhat blurred, but that uneducated people all over the world, whether mentally healthy or sick, have in common certain characteristics, such as weakness of ego control, unconscious preference for denial versus repression, and ample use of projective mechanisms as ego defenses. Hence, if a large proportion of the population consists of illiterates, as in many parts of rural Asia, one would expect to and actually find that mental phenomena universally common in the uneducated frequently occur. On these grounds, the occurrence of short-term, violent episodes of psychoses in unacculturated tribes, the frequency of gross forms of conversion hysteria, the rarity of obsessional neurosis, and the paucity of delusional content may be plausibly explained.

Nevertheless, enough differential features remain which lend themselves to cultural interpretation. For instance, the high frequency of social and emotional withdrawal in Indian schizophrenics, also observed in other Asiatic schizophrenics, may be related to the teachings both of Hinduism and Buddhism that withdrawal is an acceptable mode of reacting to difficulties; and the frequency of catatonic rigidity, negativism, and stereotypy in Indian schizophrenics (a view not shared by Stoller), to a traditional passive-aggressive response to a threatening world. As regards hallucinations and delusions, obviously their contents everywhere are determined by elements in the cultural environment of the sufferers. Interesting is the change in the contents of hallucinations and delusions of schizophrenics in post-World War II Japan, with a concurrent increase in perceptual disturbances concerning technological advances and mythological figures. It appears conceivable that the widely felt disquieting effect of a change in political structure is reflected in a regressive revival in psychotic patients of the old and the accustomed. Of so-called culture-specific diseases only *koro* will be discussed here. In many respects *koro* resembles castration anxiety so common in the West, but it differs in the way in which the threat to the genitals is experienced by the Chinese—as a fear of the penis retracting into the abdomen—and in the manner in which the irrational fear is dealt with by the patient and members of his family—by fixing the penis to a box and making efforts to pull it out. Psychodynamically the presenting symptom presumably both in the East and West is based on an unresolved Oedipal conflict, but, as Rin (1963) has pointed out, it also is rooted deeply in fundamental Chinese concepts of sexuality. Moreover, it has been suggested that the susceptibility of the Chinese to symbolic castration threats may be related to their oral orientation and to fear of oral deprivation.

Summary and Conclusions

An outline of cultural psychiatric research in Asia has been given, dealing with the geographical areas in which research has been carried out, the identities of the investigators, the topics investigated, the problems raised, the major research approaches, and the methodologies employed. Frequency and nature of illness were chosen as examples of data obtained.

What general conclusions can be drawn from the materials presented? Some of the questions posed are unanswerable. Asia is such an enormous continent with such a conglomeration of different cultures and subcultures that the question of whether there are more or fewer mental disorders in Asia than in Europe or in America is meaningless.

The methods used for cultural psychiatric research are often ill-suited to answer the questions posed. For instance, for reasons given analysis of hospital records can supply only limited information about the epidemiology of mental disease. Methodologically, too, disregard of such social variables as education has made compared samples incomparable and has given rise to erroneous cultural interpretations.

Those foremost in the field probably would be the first to admit the limitations of the epidemiological approach to mental disease. For example, even though much can be learned through the correct application of statistical methods in research, such methods cannot lead to the heart of human behavior and its motivations.

As regards clinical observations, integration of psychiatric and social theories is far from complete. It is hoped that, to a much greater extent than hitherto, psychiatrists, cultural anthropologists, and psychologists will combine their efforts in cultural psychiatric research. Very few research workers in our field live up to the "principle of intense marginality."

Team co-operation between indigenous researchers and foreign researchers, whether in cultural psychology or psychiatry, seems to be desirable because the indigenous investigator knows his culture but is often not sufficiently detached from it to be perceptive and unbiased, while the foreign investigator does not know the culture but is perhaps more perceptive and objective because of his detachment.

As regards clinical studies, I believe that the descriptive approach and even a refinement in phenomenology will not lead much further. At the present state of knowledge, whether in the understanding of differences in psychotic symptomatology or of such syndromes as *koro*, more can be gained from a dynamic approach. Asiatic psychiatrists are at a disadvantage in this respect because of the descriptive orientation in psychiatric training at their universities.

In particular it appears to me that: (1) because of the numerous variables inherent in cross-national psychiatric research, the comparative study of members of subcultures different in tradition within the *same* nation is preferable and more profitable; (2) in cross-national and cross-cultural psychiatric research, safeguards should be taken to make the data obtained comparable; (3) whenever and wherever possible, the statistical approach should be combined with a clinical approach; and (4) the problems chosen for research should be of manageable proportions.

REFERENCES

Akimoto, H. 1942. Demographische und Psychiatrische Untersuchung der abgegrenzten Kleinstadtbevolkerung. Psychiatria et Neurologia Japonica 47: 351–74.

Asai, T. 1964. The contents of delusions of schizophrenic patients in Japan: comparison between periods 1941–1961. Transcultural Psychiatric Research 1:27–28.

Bhaskaran, K. 1963. A psychiatric study of paranoid schizophrenics in a mental hospital in India. Psychiatric Quarterly 37:734–51.

Bowman, K. M. 1959. Culture and mental disease, with special reference to Thailand. Archives of General Psychiatry 1:593–99.

Burton-Bradley, B. G. 1962. Psychiatric observations in Papua, New Guinea. Review and Newsletter of Transcultural Psychiatric Research No. 12: 35–38.

Caudill, W. 1963. Social background and sibling rank among Japanese psychiatric patients. Review and Newsletter of Transcultural Psychiatric Research No. 15: 20–22. (Paper presented at the Second Conference on the Modernization of Japan, 1963.)

Caudill, W., and L. T. Doi. 1963. Interrelations of psychiatry, culture and emotion in Japan. *In* Man's image in medicine and anthropology. I. Galdston, ed. New York, International Universities Press.

Chafetz, M. E. 1964. Consumption of alcohol in the Far and Middle East. New England Journal of Medicine 271:297–301.

Chakraborty, A. 1964. An analysis of paranoid symptomatology. Transcultural Psychiatric Research 1:103–106.

DeVos, G. 1966. Role narcissism and the etiology of Japanese suicide. Transcultural Psychiatric Research 3:13–17 (abstract).

Dhunjibhoy, J. E. 1930. A brief résumé of the types of insanity met with in India, with a full description of Indian hemp insanity peculiar to the country. Journal of Mental Science 76:254–64.

Dorzhadamba, S. H. 1965. The epidemiology of mental illness in the Mongolian People's Republic. Transcultural Psychiatric Research 2:19–22.

Freed, S. A., and R. S. Freed. 1964. Spirit possession as illness in a north Indian village. Ethnology 3:152–71.

Gaitonde, M. R. 1958. Cross-cultural study of the psychiatric syndromes in outpatient clinics in Bombay, India and Topeka, Kansas. International Journal of Social Psychiatry 2:98–104.

Grewal, R. S. 1959. Mental disorders in Burma. Review and Newsletter of Transcultural Psychiatric Research No. 6:20–21.

Hanashiro, S. 1943. Zur Belastungsstatistik der Durchschnittsbevolkerung in Japan: Geschwister und Eltern von 342 Patienten der inneron Abteilungen. Psychiatria et Neurologia Japonica 47:282–307.

Hankoff, L. D. 1958. Letter. Review and Newsletter of Transcultural Psychiatric Research No. 4:19–20.

Harper, E. B. 1963. Spirit possession and social structure. *In* Anthropology on the march: recent studies of Indian beliefs, attitudes and social institutions. Bala Ratnam, R. K., ed. Madras: The Book Centre.

Hasuzawa, T. 1963. Chronological observations of delusions in schizophrenics. *In* Proceedings of the Joint Meeting of the Japanese Society of Psychiatry and Neurology and the American Psychiatric Association, Tokyo. H. Akimoto, ed. Supplement No. 7 of Folia Psychiatria et Neurologia Japonica. Tokyo, Japanese Society of Psychiatry and Neurology.

Hoch, E. 1959. Psychiatrische Beobachtungen und Erfahrungen an indischen patienten. Praxis 48:1051–57.

_____. 1961a. Contents of depressive ideas in Indian patients. Indian Journal of Psychiatry 3:28–36; 3:120–29.

————. 1961b. Letter. Review and Newsletter of Transcultural Psychiatric Research No. 11:65–71.

Kraepelin, E. 1904. Vergleichende Psychiatrie. Zentralblatt fur Nervenheilkunde und Psychiatrie 27:433–37.

Lin, T. 1953. A study of the incidence of mental disorder in Chinese and other cultures. Psychiatry 16:313–36.

————. 1963. Historical survey of psychiatric epidemiology in Asia. Mental Hygiene 47:351–59.

Loon, F. H. Van. 1920. The problem of lunacy in Acheen. Mededellingen van den Burgerlijken Geneeskundigen dienst in Nederlansche-Indie 10:2–49.

McCartney, J. L. 1926a. Neuropsychiatry in China: a preliminary observation. China Medical Journal 40:617–26.

————. 1926b. Neuropsychiatry in China: a report of diagnosis. China Medical Journal 40:831–42.

Maguigad, L. C. 1964. Psychiatry in the Philippines. American Journal of Psychiatry 121:21–25.

Murphy, H. B. M. 1965. The epidemiological approach to transcultural psychiatric research. *In* Transcultural psychiatry. A. V. S. de Reuck and R. Porter, eds. London, Churchill.

Murphy, H. B. M., E. D. Wittkower, and N. A. Chance. 1964. Cross-cultural inquiry into the symptomatology of depression. Transcultural Psychiatric Research 1:5–18.

Ohara, K. 1963. Characteristics of suicides in Japan—especially of parent-child double suicide. American Journal of Psychiatry 120:383–85.

Ohta, K. 1943. Uber die psychiatrische Belastungsstatistik durch Stichprobe in der Provinz, Akita. Psychiatria et Neurologia Japonica 47:319–28.

Oyama, K. 1943. Uber die Statistische Untersuchung Psychischer Belastung in der Otarugegend. Psychiatria et Neurologia Japonica 47:308–18.

Pfeiffer, W. M. 1963. Vergleichende psychiatrische Untersuchungen bei verschiedenen Bevolkerungstruppen in West Java. Review and Newsletter of Transcultural Psychiatric Research No. 15:32–36.

————. 1965. Versenkungs und Transcezustande bei Indonesischen Volksstammen. Transcultural Psychiatric Research 2:106–10.

Raman, A. C. 1961. The effect of acculturation on mental health. Review and Newsletter of Transcultural Psychiatric Research No. 10:29–35.

Ratanakorn, P. 1960. Studies of mental illness in Thailand. Review and Newsletter of Transcultural Psychiatric Research No. 7:27–28.

Rin, H. 1963. Koro: a consideration on Chinese concepts of illness and case illustrations. Review and Newsletter of Transcultural Psychiatric Research No. 15:21–23. '

————. 1965. Family study of Chinese schizophrenic patients: loss of parents, sibling rank, parental attitude and short-term prognosis. Transcultural Psychiatric Research 2:24–26.

Rin, H., *et al.* 1962. A study of the content of delusions and hallucinations manifested by the Chinese paranoid psychotics. Journal of the Formosan Medical Association 61:47–57.

Rin, H., and T. Lin. 1962. Mental illness among Formosan aborigines as compared with the Chinese in Taiwan. Journal of Mental Science 108:134–46.

Sakamoto, K., and Y. Kasahara. 1963. Family dynamics and attempted suicide of depression in Japan. *In* Proceedings of the Joint Meeting of the Japanese Society of Psychiatry and Neurology and the American Psychiatric Association, Tokyo. H. Akimoto, ed. Supplement No. 7 of Folia Psychiatria et Neurologia Japonica. Tokyo, Japanese Society of Psychiatry and Neurology.

Satyavati, K., and M. Rayo. 1961. A study of suicide in Bangalore. Transactions of the All India Institute of Mental Health 2:1–19.

Schmidt, K. E. 1961. The racial distribution of mental hospital admissions in Sarawak. Review and Newsletter of Transcultural Psychiatric Research No. 11:17–18 (abstract). (Annual Report of the Sarawak Mental Hospital 1959.)

_____. 1964. Folk psychiatry in Sarawak. *In* Magic, faith and healing. A. Kiev, ed. Glencoe, Free Press.

Schooler, C., and W. Caudill. 1964. Symptomatology in Japanese and American schizophrenics. Ethnology 3:172–78.

Seligman, C. G. 1929. Temperament, conflicts and psychosis in a stone-age population. British Journal of Medical Psychology 2:187–202.

Senanayake, I. A. 1961. Exorcism, the art of curing in Ceylon. Paper presented at the Third World Congress of Psychiatry, Montreal.

Stoller, A. 1959. Assignment report on mental health situation in Thailand. WHO Project: Thailand 17. Mimeographed document No. 7.

Sukthankar, H. K., and N. S. Vahia. 1964. Influence of social and cultural factors in schizophrenia and hysteria in Bombay (India). Presented at the First International Congress of Social Psychiatry, London.

Surya, N. C., *et al.* 1964. Mental morbidity in Pondicherry. Transactions of All India Institute of Mental Health 5:50–61.

Terashima, S., and T. Nareta. 1964. A rural community's opinion and knowledge about mental illness in Japan. Presented at the Annual Convention of the American Psychiatric Association, Los Angeles.

Tsuwaga, T., *et al.* 1942. Uber die psychiatrische Zensusuntersuchung in einem Stadtbezirk von Tokyo. Psychiatria et Neurologia Japonica 46:204–18.

Uchimura, Y., *et al.* 1940. Uber die vergleichend-psychiatrische und erbpathologische Untersuchung auf einer Japanischen Insel. Psychiatria et Neurologia Japonica 44:745–82.

Vahia, N. S. 1963. Cultural differences in the clinical picture of schizophrenia and hysteria in India and the United States. Review and Newsletter of Transcultural Psychiatric Research No. 14:16–18 (abstract). (Paper presented at the Postgraduate Centre for Psychotherapy, New York City, 1962.)

Wittkower, E. C., H. B. Murphy, J. Fried, and H. Ellenberger. 1960. A cross-cultural inquiry into the symptomatology of schizophrenia. Annals of the New York Academy of Sciences 84:854–63.

Woods, A. H. 1929. The nervous diseases of the Chinese. Archives of Neurology and Psychiatry 21:542–70.

Wulfften-Palthe, P. M. Van. 1936. Psychiatry and neurology in the tropics. *In* A clinical textbook of tropical medicine. C. D. de Laugen and A. Lichtenstein, eds. Batavia, Kloff.

Yamaguchi, T., H. Makihara, H. Nagai, N. Hagiwara, T. Ishikawa, U. Anazawa,

S. Yano, and T. Kobayashi. 1964. Sibling rank in schizophrenia and neurosis. Seishinigaku 6:578–86. [in Japanese.]

Yap, P. M. 1951. Mental diseases peculiar to certain cultures. Journal of Mental Science 407:313–27.

—————. 1958. Suicide in Hong Kong with special reference to attempted suicide. Hong Kong, Hong Kong University Press.

—————. 1963. Koro or Suk-Yeong—an atypical culture-bound psychogenic disorder found in Southern Chinese. *In* Proceedings of the Joint Meeting of the Japanese Society of Neurology and Psychiatry and the American Psychiatric Association, Tokyo. H. Akimoto, ed. Supplement No. 7 of Folia Psychiatria et Neurologia. Tokyo, Japanese Society of Psychiatry and Neurology.

Yoo, P. S. 1961. Mental disorders in the Korean rural communities. Paper presented at the Third World Congress of Psychiatry, Montreal.

Yoshimatsu, S. 1953. Zur Frage einer Belastungsstatisik der Durchschnittsbevolkerung, Geschwisterschaften von 100 Paralytikerchegatten. Psychiatria et Neurologia Japonica 47:274–81.

28. Cultural Relativity and the Identification of Psychiatric Disorders

ALEXANDER H. LEIGHTON, M.D.
Department of Behavioral Sciences
Harvard School of Public Health
Boston, Massachusetts

ONE OF THE FRUITS evident in the conference which produced this volume was the spreading of skepticism about cultural stereotypes. As one or another participant leaned on a stereotype about Asiatics, Americans, the Japanese, or somebody, others quickly pointed out the range and diversity that can occur within a particular culture. Our ability to be realistic and avoid oversimplification thus was greatly strengthened, while at the same time we continued to realize the importance of culture.

Another fruitful outcome was conceptual development, beautifully exemplified in Chapter 14 by Sasaki on the shaman. Progressive, shared clarification is not common in meetings, especially when one has to move back and forth between such widely different concepts as individual psychology, culture, social process, population studies, and the measurement of demographic features.

Fig. 1 is a device for keeping in mind some of the relations between these various orientations and approaches. For example, most work in psychiatric epidemiology (such as that in Chapter 1 by Stoller, Chapter 4 by Jayasundera, Chapter 5 by Lin et al., and Chapter 6 by Kato) occupies a position somewhere between the interests of clinical psychiatry and those of a census. Weidman's chapter on "Cultural Values, Concept of Self, and Projection: The Burmese Case" lies toward the top of the diagram, though not at the very top.

A question raised a number of times during the conference on Mental Health Research in Asia and the Pacific was: What should be the focus of future meetings? I should like to list five proposals that have to do with experimental programs aimed at improving mental health.

1) *Services*: It would be useful to have a conference to review the various strategies that have been developed in recent years as alternatives to the big state hospital and classical outpatient service. These alternatives generally attempt to bring treatment closer to the patient in his community and home and also closer in time to the beginning of his disorder. By and large, they rely heavily on ancillary personnel, such as nurses and assistants. In some instances, notably in Nigeria, native healers have been trained and employed to work with psychiatric units. While it is obvious that many things can be said for and against these attempts, a conference which discussed only the pros and cons would have limited value. A discussion is needed of how such ideas can be put to some kind of experimental testing in order to see if they are feasible and whether they yield worthwhile results. It is becoming more and more obvious in many countries that the number of people needing psychiatric attention far outruns the services available or ever likely to be available. This situation calls for bold experimentation, and such experimentation can yield better results if it is done comparatively with co-ordination between different teams trying out different approaches.

2) *Identification of factors influential in the success of mental health programs*: What are the procedural, situational, social, and cultural factors that are of key importance in the acceptance of a psychiatric service aimed at treatment and prevention? There are grounds for supposing that the successful establishment of a mental health service is not a matter of executing a predetermined blueprint, but rather a procedure involving successive stages, with each stage calling for different sets of policies and actions. The kind of thing I have in mind is reflected in Chapter 11 by Hsu and Lin on the development of counseling in schools. It also is dealt with in a report written some years ago (Leighton and Longaker, 1957) on the "phases" that occurred during the establishment of a psychiatric outpatient clinic in a rural area where the people were somewhat hostile to the plan—a situation not unlike that described by Terashima in Chapter 12. Much might be gained if we could become acquainted with and discuss some of the main findings that have been reported in the fairly large body of anthropological and sociological literature on problems of establishing new institutions in an existing sociocultural system.

3) *Effectiveness of various native healing techniques*: An important question is whether native healers are effective. If they are, is there anything we can learn from them? The suggestion has some rashness about it, since research that adequately evaluates the effectiveness of treatment is problematical even in centers where psychiatry has been long established. If we cannot deal satisfactorily with the question of effectiveness in formal psychiatric clinics, can we do better with regard to the native healer? I do not

Figure 1: Relations between Various Psychiatric Orientations and Approaches

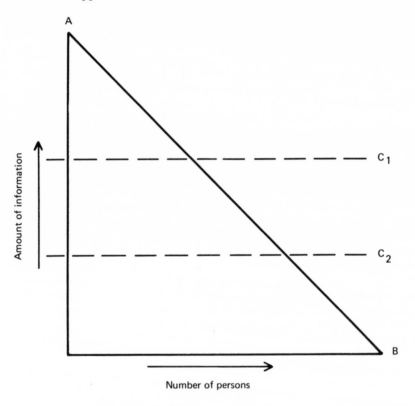

A   = A personality study with maximal information about one individual as in clinical psychiatry.

B   = A census; minimal individual information but about large numbers of people.

C_1 = A sample survey of a small number with a large amount of information on each individual.

C_2 = A sample survey of a large number, but with less information on each individual.

think that the difficulty is reason enough for delay. The problems of establishing a critical test of therapy are not necessarily more difficult in situations involving native healers than in those involving psychiatrists, and in some instances they might even be easier. The need is to attack the problem on several fronts comparatively, and such an approach could well lead to better techniques for evaluating psychiatric therapeutic results.

4) *Development of preventive psychiatry*: The model I have in mind is one in which experiments are conducted to reduce the frequency of psychiatric disorders in selected populations of limited size with clearly marked boundaries. When I say "psychiatric disorders," I refer not only to the major mental diseases, such as schizophrenia, but also to the host of disabling psychoneurotic and personality disorders and to some of the socio-pathic conditions, such as alcoholism, use of drugs, and juvenile delinquency. I am, in short, including the whole range of disturbances generally found in textbooks on psychiatry. Preventive efforts require action not only by the people engaged in preventive psychiatry as such—that is, social psychiatrists —but also by those concerned with other aspects of health, and especially those concerned with economic development and education. The research focus that most involves psychiatry, however, is the measurement of any change in disorder frequency that comes about as the result of the efforts. A conference which focuses on this kind of issue would inevitably question the relation of psychiatry to preventive medicine and also to economic, educational, and social development. It is common for the latter programs to operate independently, not only of psychiatry, but of each other as well. It might be that a conference with a psychiatric orientation would point up the necessity for co-ordination and begin to elucidate some means to achieve it.

5) *Techniques for measuring social and cultural factors*: If psychiatric disorder is looked upon as a dependent variable and social and cultural influences as independent variables, means need to be devised for measuring the independent variables. So far, the great bulk of effort in psychiatric epidemiology has concentrated on the measuring of prevalence or incidence of psychiatric disorders in populations. The independent variable has been treated in terms of traditional categories developed in sociology and anthropology, such as culture and socioeconomic class. Are these in fact the best ways to categorize social processes in order to reveal etiological relations?

The Categorization of Psychiatric Phenomena

In turning now to my topic—"Cultural Relativity and the Identification of Psychiatric Disorders"—I should like to take note of Chapter 2 by Phillips and Draguns and Chapter 9 by Katz, Gudeman, and Sanborn and accuse them of disturbing the peace. What they are saying is that the diagnostic categories commonly employed in clinical psychiatry cannot be researched. Theorists in psychodynamics and psychotherapists long have felt dissatisfied with the way psychiatric phenomena are classified, and now these authors term them an obstacle to scientific investigation. The condemnation apparently is sweeping, applying no less to the system advocated by the World Health Organization than to the one presented in the American Psychiatric Association's *Manual* (1952). There is implication that the typologies used do not refer to real recurrent phenomena in nature. These authors probably would not insist that every traditional category is useless, but they do seem to be saying that many do not constitute a packaging of natural phenomena in a way which enables one to make progress toward understanding natural processes. In short, someone needs to do for psychiatry what Linnaeus did for botany.

Having made this accusation, I must now associate myself with it. In 1952 my colleagues and I undertook the assessment of mental health and mental illness in the population of a small town and rural area in the northeastern part of North America. This assessment involved collecting data on a sample of individuals and rating each one of them with regard to his psychiatric status. The data consisted of the results of a questionnaire interview, observations made during the interview, and collateral information gathered from a variety of sources about each individual. It was an attempt to devise a rating system which forced us to abandon the traditional patterns of diagnosis, partly because of the difficulty in achieving agreement between psychiatrists making independent ratings and partly because of the fact that most diagnostic categories contain built-in etiological assumptions which bias the assessment of the causal role of social and cultural factors.

After experimenting with a variety of alternatives, we found that if we limited ourselves to considering symptom patterns—such behaviors as depressive states, anxiety, gastrointestinal disturbances, asthma, alcoholism, mental deficiency, hallucinations—we could develop a codified system with explicit definitions and rules for decisions. We utilized the labels presented in the American Psychiatric Association's *Manual* (1952), but revised the definitions to exclude as far as possible all considerations of etiology.

It is interesting to note that we began at an edge of the mental health field opposite to that of Katz, Gudeman, and Sanborn (Chapter 9) and Phillips and Draguns (Chapter 2). Our approach was to examine and sift a population in its natural setting, rather than patients in a hospital. We therefore emphasized the milder rather than the more severe kinds of disorders. Despite this difference, we have apparently come to very similar methodological conclusions.

Although habituated to the use of the words "symptom patterns" we have gradually come to realize that they have meaning which contradicts our intent. "Symptom" implies a medical frame of reference in which symptoms are indicators of an underlying disease. They are the surface manifestations of a phenomenon that has to be identified by penetrating study. Thus, pain in the abdomen in the right lower quadrant is a symptom of appendicitis, and an Argyll-Robertson pupil is a symptom of tabes dorsalis. While it has been natural for psychiatry as a branch of medicine to attempt to follow this sort of conceptualization, it is often misleading because psychiatrists generally lack the etiological evidence which characterizes diagnostic entities such as appendicitis and tabes. What psychiatrists have been calling symptom patterns are not so much indicators as manifestations of the disorder itself. The question of causal factors (underlying or otherwise) is left open, because this is what the research is concerned with. It is more accurate, therefore, to say that psychiatrists deal in *behaviors of psychiatric interest*. It appears that what psychiatrists have done is to select out of the total range of human behavioral patterns a rather heterogeneous collection to which attention is attracted because in the branch of medicine known as psychiatry they turn up over and over again in those people who, for a variety of reasons, are designated patients.

In speaking thus it must be understood, however, that "behaviors" include not only movement and appearance but also the individual's verbal reports of his subjective state. Thus, the "depressive pattern" includes slowed movement, dejected appearance, and statements about being in a blue mood.

The qualifier "psychiatric" in *behaviors of psychiatric interest* means that this particular collection of behaviors has its origin in centuries of clinical observation and experience. This heritage is the justification for grouping together such a miscellaneous assemblage of phenomena. One must be prepared, however, as his research goes along, to modify, to eliminate, and to enlarge as a result of the findings.

Having made these comments about the *behaviors of psychiatric interest* and taken note of the unwanted implications in the word "symptom," I shall continue with "symptom patterns" for the sake of continuity with previous writings.

A Method for Identifying Psychiatric Disorders in Populations

In order to approach the problem of identifying psychiatric disorders cross-culturally, let me first describe a little more fully than I did above the method which employs symptom patterns as the basic unit. Visualize a psychiatrist sitting down to examine a protocol of data that contains the result of a questionnaire which reviewed medical history and the systems of the body and asked a number of questions about emotional states. The protocol also contains observations made by the interviewers and data derived from other sources, such as general practitioners and various kinds of hospital records. The psychiatric evaluator's first task is to make 39 dichotomous choices pertaining to symptom patterns. (The precise number of symptom pattern categories has varied somewhat from survey to survey according to purpose and stage of development of the method.) The evaluator has to look at the data in the protocol to decide whether any of the behaviors described fit any of the 39 symptom patterns. He has to decide "yes" or "no" for each pattern category. For each of the

Figure 2: Evaluation Scheme*

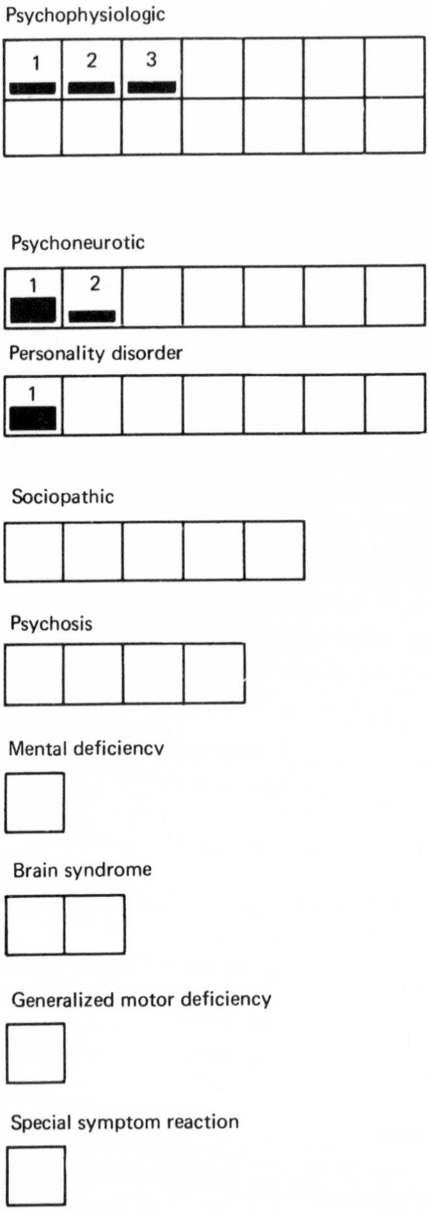

Psychophysiologic

1	2	3				

1. Gastrointestinal
   Impairment:
   Minimal
   Time: Current
   Duration:
   2 + years

2. Cardiovascular
   Impairment:
   Minimal
   Time: Current
   Duration:
   Uncertain

3. Headaches
   Impairment:
   Minimal
   Time: Current
   Duration: 1 year

Psychoneurotic

1	2					

1. Anxiety
   Impairment:
   Moderate
   Time: Current
   Duration: 1 year

2. Other
   Impairment:
   Minimal
   Time: Current
   Duration:
   Uncertain

Personality disorder

1						

1. Emotionally
   Unstable
   Impairment:
   Moderate
   Time: Current
   Duration:
   2 + years

Sociopathic

Psychosis

Mental deficiency

Brain syndrome

Generalized motor deficiency

Special symptom reaction

_____

Rating as a Case: A
Total Impairment: Moderate

* This figure previously appeared in Leighton, Leighton, and Danley (1966). It is reprinted with permission of the Canadian Psychiatric Association Journal. The height of the black bar denotes the degree of impairment in a specific symptom pattern.

symptom patterns for which he has said, "Yes, this exists in the protocol data," he makes four additional ratings, each of which has a scale: the time of the occurrence of the symptom pattern; its duration; the degree of impairment; and, finally, the degree of confidence the psychiatric evaluator has in his categorization of the particular symptom pattern.

Having made the symptom pattern ratings, he next makes two overall judgments drawing on his clinical training and experience. The first of these requires deciding whether the individual is a psychiatric case within the ordinary clinical meaning of the word. To express this decision, the evaluator rates the subject on a four-point scale of A, B, C, and D. A means undoubtedly a psychiatric case—that is to say, he is clearly a psychoneurotic or psychotic or a person who is senile, mentally deficient, or exhibiting sociopathic behavior. D is at the other end of the scale and means that the evaluator has a high degree of certainty that this person is not a case. B represents a degree of conviction that is fairly strong, but less strong than A; the evaluator feels that there is about a 75 per cent chance that this person has some kind of psychiatric disorder. C is the doubtful category; here are classified the people about whom the evaluator feels uncertain. The final judgment is an overall rating of the degree of impairment the individual shows as a result of all his symptoms.

I have grossly oversimplified in this summary account of the evaluation procedure, my aim being to furnish only a general idea. A detailed account of the procedure is to be found elsewhere. (A. H. Leighton *et al.*, 1963; D. C. Leighton *et al.*, 1963). Fig. 2 presents the evaluation steps of a particular case in schematic form.

It is important to note that in this system a person can exhibit symptom patterns without being impaired or being considered an instance of psychiatric disorder. Further, he can exhibit symptoms and be regarded as a case and still not be very much impaired. These distinctions are of value in trying to explore relations with social, cultural, and situational factors and also in following changes of disorder status that occur with time. As one might expect, symptoms, impairment, and identification as a psychiatric case do not necessarily vary in a closely co-ordinated manner. For example, an individual can be rated as having depressive behavior and yet not be regarded as a case. Thus a man recently bereaved undoubtedly would get a check in the depressive category if he showed sadness and inability to eat and appeared slowed up, but he would not get a rating of A, B, or C because under his circumstances he would not be considered a psychiatric case on these symptoms alone; or, if a man clearly had anxiety symptoms, the impairment from which fluctuated considerably from time to time, he could well get an A rating but no mark for current impairment.

These conceptual separations which are mandatory during the rating process are often exceedingly difficult for a clinician to learn. Yet it is by avoiding interpretive judgments regarding the effect of environmental factors during evaluation that the opportunity for discovering relations and meaning is achieved when it comes to the quantitative analysis.

Psychoneurotic depression illustrates this point of view. Depressive symptoms are apt to get this classification in the ordinary clinical context if they are not sweeping enough to be psychotic and so long as there is no readily visible, common-sense or plausible cause. Once, however, such a cause is recognized, clinical judgment runs toward considering the individual normal and removing him from further psychiatric attention. The point I wish to make is that this assignment of boundary is a highly arbitrary and subjective matter, which I do not think one can afford in research. As yet not enough is known about the meaning of "visible," "common sense," "plausible," or of "normal" as opposed to "abnormal" patterns of depression. They are all behaviors of psychiatric interest, and the research focus needs to be on a comparative analysis of their form, content, and changing context and on a determination of the conditions which make them impairing and on the conditions which render them not impairing. Levy's (Chapter 22) "On Getting Angry in the Society Islands" is an example of the kind of thing I have in mind when stressing the importance of following these behaviors of psychiatric interest through their various contexts without trying to decide a priori whether they constitute neurosis, psychosis, and so on. The data promise to be much more powerful for discovery purposes than when they are gathered according to diagnostic categories.

The independent evaluation of symptom patterns not only helps us to see their relations to sociocultural factors but also helps to reveal something about their relations to each other. It would appear that many of them can occur in virtually every conceivable combination, as Phillips and Draguns point out in Chapter 2. The matter deserves much study, but it is obscured in most systems of diagnosis. For instance, schizophrenia is readily classified as showing or not showing paranoid manifestations, but it seems highly probable that paranoid thinking actually occurs in many other associations, such as with depression, senile brain disorders, personality disorders, and sociopathic disturbances. Because of the way the diagnostic labels are commonly used, these other combinations are apt to get buried.

Despite its advantages, this manner of categorizing psychiatric phenomena as symptom patterns raises a number of immediate questions, which I should like to note briefly. The first is whether it is possible to build a bridge into the more usual forms of diagnosis. I believe that it is. If one wants to convert an individual's rating in terms of sympton patterns, and A, B, C, and D and impairment into a rough approximation of one of the standard diagnostic categories, he can look first to see if the A, B, C, or D rating suggests that the person is a case. If so, an inspection of the symptom patterns that have the highest rating for impairment gives a clue to the diagnosis that would most likely be applied.

A second major question is about the reliabiity of the method. Do two clinicians independently confronted with the protocol data tend to agree in their ratings? This question has been tested with numbers of psychiatrists, and the results are generally adequate. For example, two psychiatrists compared with regard to their A, B, C, or D ratings in some 900 protocols had a correlation of .793. (Owing to the nature of the ratings, the assessment of agreement is a complicated matter and difficult to summarize accurately. The reader is referred to: D. C. Leighton *et al.*, 1963.)

A third question is of validity. How do these ratings based on survey data compare with what a clinician would make if he conducted an actual face-to-face examination? In considering this question, one must be aware, of course, that a clinical psychiatrist does not constitute a standardized instrument. As is well known, psychiatrists often differ considerably in appraisals made of individual patients. In comparing psychiatric examinations with the results of a survey, two instruments are being compared, both of which can be in error. With this reservation in mind, my colleagues and I have made one study in which 123 people were rated by the survey technique and then re-rated independently by means of a psychiatric interview. Here, again, it is possible to report that the results were reasonably satisfactory (Leighton, Leighton, and Danley, 1966).

The panel of 123 are being followed over a five-year period and revisited annually by a psychiatrist. This method is in line with the thought expressed by Yap in Chapter 3 that real diagnosis is achieved only when the patient is followed through time. We hope that at the end of five years a reasonable basis will have been established for assessing these individuals and comparing them both with the original survey rating and with the clinical psychiatric independent rating.

Work continues on improving this method of classifying and rating psychiatric phenomena. The definitions are under revision, and attempts are being made to clarify the rules of procedure to make the instrument more reliable and valid. During the last two years we have been giving particular attention to the possibility of using a computer to replace the human evaluator; since more progress has been made than we at first thought likely, it is possible that we shall convert to this technique (Smith, Taintor, and Kaplan, 1967).

Cultural Relativity

Having summarized a method for estimating the prevalence of psychiatric disorders in populations, let me now report on its employment in an effort to reach across a cultural line. This research was done in collaboration with Dr. T. A. Lambo at the Aro Hospital near Abeokuta in Nigeria (A. H. Leighton *et al.*, 1963).

In the interest of brevity, much of the detail involved in the preparation for this research must be omitted, such as studying the language of the Yoruba tribe, who were the subjects of the research, and investigating existing anthropological literature pertinent to the region. The team that conducted the research was interdisciplinary, composed of anthropologists and psychiatrists. Among the psychiatrists, Lambo and Asuni, were themselves Yoruba and played a major role in the translation of the questionnaire and in adjusting the rating criteria. After development to a certain point, the questionnaire and rating techniques were tried out on a known population of patients in the Aro Hospital and again in a village which was not included in the later study. Extensive work was done in selecting the villages, mapping them, and drawing a probability sample of the people to be interviewed.

The aspect of the work that I wish to place in the foreground here is a study of Yoruba ideas regarding mental health and mental illness. This aspect was conducted primarily by Murphy, an anthropologist, with some help from myself and with the co-operation of several native healers and other Yorubas knowledgeable about their culture.

Having discovered early and easily that in the traditional Yoruba view there is a conception of mental illness, our next question was what kinds of disorder they distinguish. When asked to give examples of mental illness, the informants said such things as, "There is a kind of dwindling or sapping of a person's inner self that is caused by someone making an image of him and putting it on a fire," or, "If the god of smallpox is about to trouble a man and he does not have the usual skin eruptions to show he has smallpox, often the god will run into his brain and make him insane." Numerous long conversations resulted in many pages of such descriptions, and at first it was difficult to make very much out of them. On stepping back, as it were, and getting perspective, it seemed apparent that certain formulations could be made. For example, it was evident that there were four criteria involved in deciding whether or not a person had a psychiatric disorder. These were: type of symptoms, degree of impairment, fit with theories of causation, and response to treatment. This conclusion suggested that we could divide our analysis in terms of each of these four Yoruba categories and examine them separately.

Following this line of thought, Murphy invited the Yoruba informants to describe all the different kinds of symptoms they recognized as possibly involved in psychiatric disorder. She also asked two native healers to report on particular cases, giving all the information they could on each individual. Then four of the psychiatrists in the team interviewed 12 patients while one of the Yoruba psychiatrists talked to the relevant healers about these same patients.

These several efforts led to a compilation of symptoms, but when we asked outselves if these conformed to all the main patterns with which psychiatry is concerned, it was apparent that they did not. The collection was composed of symptoms primarily associated with mental deficiency, schizophrenia, epilepsy, paresis, and other brain disorders. For the most part, symptoms characteristic of psychophysiologic, neurotic, personality, and sociopathic disorders were not mentioned. We were particularly struck by the fact that brain syndromes, especially the senile type, were not included.

Tactics shifted at this point and we began describing to our informants the missing symptom patterns and asking if they had ever heard of such conditions. The response was, on the whole, affirmative. For example, as soon as we described senile behavior, they said it was well known that older people become childish, do not answer questions properly, cannot remember things, "beat around the bush," and generally lose their capacities, but from the Yoruba viewpoint this kind of behavior is not "illness"; it is a normal part of life. Just as a child cannot do many things, so an older person cannot do many things; one does not take people to native healers for this kind of behavior because there is no treatment for it.

It was apparent, then, that although the description of senile behavior was not volunteered under the category of mental illness it nevertheless was well known to our informants. Most psychoneurotic symtoms, certain manifestations of depression, and a good many kinds of personality disorders also were known but were not regarded as illness; rather, they were considered to be uncomfortable, undesirable, impairing, and in some instances unusual.

To sum up, the Yoruba in the area we studied apparently recognized on a symptomatic basis the major types of mental illness. They also recognized the minor types of psychiatric disorder but did not classify them as illness. It should be noted in passing that while the latter is quite different from the psychiatric frame of reference, it is a very common point of view among nonpsychiatrists (including physicians) in Europe and America. The only patterns apparently unknown among people of Yoruba culture were phobic and obsessive-compulsive symptoms.

When we turned to impairment, no difficulty was encountered. The Yoruba regarded it as undesirable and based their estimates of degree on work and ability to perform roles in the family and in the community. Similarly, the criteria of whether a condition responded to treatment appeared as clear as our own.

It was when we came to the topic of etiology that we found utter divergence from the ideas of the Yoruba informants. Their conceptions of cause were altogether different from the psychiatric. Highest on their list were magical and supernatural malignant influences. Then came, more or less in order, drugs and poisons, heredity, contagion, and having committed an act that violated one's destiny. While physical and even psychological traumata were included, they were considered rather rare and unimportant. It thus became apparent that if one were to think in terms of diagnostic categories little ground for comparison and discussion could be found between the Yoruba healers' viewpoint and that of psychiatry. The outlook on the nature of cause differs radically. The Yoruba bring together symptoms and causal ideas in ways that have no counterparts in psychiatry.

On the other hand, if attention is limited to the comparison of symptom patterns rather than diagnostic categories, a great part of the cross-cultural obstacle disappears. What is left points to the need to ask about particular symptoms under headings other than illness and to realize that there are special problems regarding the symptom patterns represented by the psychiatric words "phobic" and "obsessive-compulsive."

It is clear that our study has been limited to one ethnic group, the Yoruba, and to mostly a rural subsample of it. Nevertheless, the experience suggests ways of conceptualizing psychiatric phenomena and approaching cross-cultural comparisons that may have wider use. In other words, the concept of *behaviors of psychiatric interest,* or symptom patterns, which was developed in order to study prevalence in one cultural group does appear adaptable to the study of psychiatric disorder in another. It provides a framework for making and comparing observations with sufficient objectivity to permit replication and validity checks by independent observers. The separation of phenomena from notions of etiology strengthens the possibility of discovering rather than assuming causal relations. Further, the approach avoids becoming paralyzed by considerations of cultural relativity which are apt to prevail when one tries to employ the traditional categories of diagnosis. By our method, one can pose the question of cultural difference, and, beginning with a common ground of mutually recognized symptom patterns, discover wherein culture does and does not invoke serious problems for cross-cultural comparison.

The survey of the Yoruba villages and the small segment of the town of Abeokuta involved a sample of 326 adults. In evaluating the data we had, of course, the benefit of the Yoruba psychiatrists. We also were able to consult with a variety of other people who had been reared in this culture. The team thus was sensitized to the problem of cultural differences and its implications for meaning; at the same time the team had considerable resources for discussing and resolving such questions. It turned out in practice that in only 2.5 per cent of the interviews did questions of cultural meaning intrude themselves in any significant way. For example, one of the doubtful cases was a religious leader who went into states in which he apparently talked to the deity. We were uncertain whether this should be regarded as hallucination or as a religious pattern. While it was easy to find out from our Yoruba informants that this man did not display a common or well-recognized cultural pattern, it was still possible that he was performing according to the procedures of a small sect, rather than as a person showing psychiatric disorder. A follow-up of this particular individual and the gathering of additional biographic data made it seem more likely that he was, in fact, an instance of mental disturbance, but the question never was settled completely.

In reflecting on this case, one has to recognize that problems of cultural and social interpretation also occur in European and American samples. In one of the North American surveys we had a good deal of similar debate about an individual who was a preacher in a fundamentalist sect in which hearing voices and being possessed was not uncommon. This particular man resolved the problem for us eventually by becoming a patient in a psychiatric clinic, but for a time we wondered whether to regard him as one who was expressing the cultural pattern of a small group or as one who was manifesting psychiatric disorder.

It seems probable that any population studied will present problems of cultural and subcultural interpretation. In Nigeria we had all the usual difficulties that are inherent in making a survey, and a few additional ones specific to this particular culture, but not in a proportion to give us reason to feel that they seriously affected the main outline of the results (*see* A. H. Leighton *et al.*, 1963, Chapter 8).

One of the caveats that commonly is put forward to those approaching a cross-cultural study of psychiatric disorder is to be aware that what you consider illness will be considered by your subjects the result of bewitchment and magic; for example, hallucinations and delusions cannot be considered illness. In other words, you are going to find people who believe things which to you seem impossible or untrue but which in their culture are considered all right. The work with the Yoruba showed that the fact that it is acceptable in Yoruba culture to hear voices and to believe that witches put spells on people does not make it impossible to identify psychiatric disorders, because the Yoruba consider witchcraft and magic explanations of cause, but they do not think that such explanation removes the person from mental illness. On the contrary, it accounts for why he is ill. This point was brought home to me vividly on one occasion when a native healer was describing one of his patients. The healer said that the patient was normal now but six months ago had been suffering "from hallucinations and delusions." When I asked what he meant by this statement, the healer said that the man was standing close to where we were standing now, looking up at the top of a palm tree in which he saw his uncle, who was talking to him. He also thought that instead of being at the healer's village, he was in a town about 50 miles away. Said my informant, "I don't know what you think about that in America, but we consider it crazy here."

In concluding I should like to return to the question of future meetings to suggest in this cross-cultural context that it might be worthwhile to have a workshop type of session. Hopefully, it might be in Hawaii and demonstrate the use of various survey techniques, such as those of Phillips and Draguns, Katz, Gudeman, and Sanborn, and ourselves.

ACKNOWLEDGMENT
This work has been conducted as part of the Cornell Program in Social Psychiatry and has been supported through funds provided by the Milbank Memorial Fund, the Carnegie Corporation of New York, the Ford Foundation, the National Institute of Mental Health, and the Dominion Provincial Mental Health Grants of Canada.

REFERENCES

American Psychiatric Association. 1952. Diagnostic and statistical manual: mental disorders. Washington, American Psychiatric Association.

Leighton, A. H., T. A. Lambo, C. C. Hughes, D. C. Leighton, J. M. Murphy, and D. B. Macklin. 1963. Psychiatric disorder among the Yoruba. Ithaca, Cornell University Press.

Leighton, A. H., D. C. Leighton, and R. A. Danley. 1966. Validity in mental health surveys. Canadian Psychiatric Association Journal 11:167–78.

Leighton, A. H., and A. Longaker. 1957. The psychiatric clinic as a community innovation. *In* Explorations in social psychiatry. A. Leighton, J. Clausen, and R. Wilson, eds. New York, Basic Books.

Leighton, D. C., J. S. Harding, D. B. Macklin, A. M. Macmillan, and A. H. Leighton. 1963. The character of danger: psychiatric symptoms in selected communities. Vol. III. The Stirling County study of psychiatric disorder and sociocultural environment. New York, Basic Books.

Smith, W. G., Z. C. Taintor, and E. Kaplan. 1967. Computer evaluations in psychiatric epidemiology. Social Psychiatry 1:174–81.

29. The Family as a Strategic Focus in Cross-cultural
Psychiatric Studies

LYMAN C. WYNNE, M.D., Ph.D.
Adult Psychiatry Branch
National Institute of Mental Health
Bethesda, Maryland

TWO INTERTWINED major concerns of this conference which produced this volume were: What questions are meaningful to ask concerning mental health research in Asia and the Pacific? For which of these questions are practicable research methods available? I suggest that a focus upon the family constitutes an especially strategic orientation for developing research that is both meaningful and methodologically feasible. I shall cite examples supporting this view both from my own work and from other chapters in this volume.

First, however, I wish to review briefly the theoretical basis for stressing the family in cross-cultural mental health research. My primary assumption is a commonplace: that a given population and a given set of concrete phenomena can be observed from a number of distinct vantage points (frames of reference, or "systems" of observation and conceptualization). Each of these systems can provide a valid basis, within its own context, for selecting, abstracting, classifying, and conceptualizing phenomena which are seen differently, less well, or not at all from the vantage point of another system or frame of reference. In mental health research four systems for observation and conceptualization have evolved and generally have been acknowledged to have characteristics which are not directly reducible to the terms of any of the others—biology, psychology, social structure, and culture. Each of these four systems involves phenomena that for many purposes can be studied usefully in their own right given a degree of control over intrusions from the other systems. For example, neuroendocrine studies have shown the positive and negative feedback connections betwen the hypothalamus, the pituitary, and the adrenal cortex. To the extent that these neuroendocrine functions tend to be self-equilibrating, we can speak of a neuroendocrine physiologic system. This system, however, like all living systems, is not closed but is open to trans-actional exchange with other systems. For example, muscular activity, depressive psychological states, and intense interpersonal relations all have been shown to affect the neuroendocrine system.

Another example: A mother and a small child or a psychoanalyst and patient, as dyads, may for substantial periods develop complementary relations on many overt and covert levels, in which the dyadic relation for a time tends to be a self-equilibrating system with boundaries. Even when the participants try to maintain such relations as though they were enduring closed systems, however, they are susceptible to the impact of other linked systems sooner or later. Disruptions may arise because of changes in the psychological or physiological systems of one or the other participants or because an external event or person—such as another family member—challenges the primacy and affects the functioning of the mother-child or patient-therapist pair.

Mental health research necessarily is concerned deeply both with understanding such open systems in their own terms and with clarifying the links between systems (von Bertalanffy, 1950; Kroeber and Parsons, 1958; Caudill, 1958)—how the connections of one system with another may help a given system maintain a steady state or may contribute to change, sometimes to disturbed disruption and sometimes to developmental growth. Because cross-cultural mental health and psychiatric studies in-volve variables of such great diversity, ranging from individual biology and genetics to cultural value orientations, it is quite easy to neglect alto-gether certain classes of variables and to overlook important but researchable connections between diverse kinds of data and concepts. My central proposi-tion is that the family is an especially strategic focus for cross-cultural psychiatric research because in the family it is both feasible and "natural" to study *directly* variables from all four of the primary conceptual systems (biology, personality, social structure, and culture) with which mental health issues are concerned. Family studies therefore lend themselves particularly well to the investigation of links between these systems. Let me be more explicit:

1) *Families and social structure*: The family can be regarded as being a small but ordinarily distinct unit of social structure. As a subsystem of society (Parsons and Bales, 1955), nuclear families are open to inter-change with larger units of the broad social structure, such as lineages and community social networks. Indeed, I have suggested (Wynne *et al.*, 1958)

that the lack of such openness is a feature of certain disturbed families in which "the family members try to act as if the family could be a truly self-sufficient social system with a completely encircling boundary." Such efforts eventually turn out, apparently, to contribute to psychologically disastrous failure (including reactive schizophrenia) of the individual family members to develop skills which are adaptive in later life outside the family in the broad society. Such observations make especially striking the links between the personality systems of individual family members, the family as a small social system in its own right, and the broad social structure of which the family is only a component.

2) *Families and culture*: Families tend to have rules of behavior, norms, and values which are to some extent idiosyncratic for each family and to some extent shared with other families having the same cultural traditions. Families, through the socialization of children, are primary transmitters of cultural patterns from one generation to the next and at the same time contribute significantly to cultural divergency and change. Thus families provide a fruitful locus for empirical investigation of the details of cultural phenomena.

3) *Families and personality*: The family constitutes the largest naturally occurring social unit in which there is ordinarily some practicable prospect of obtaining direct research data from all or a significant portion of the members, seen both individually and interacting together. Social units such as lineages and community networks are usually too large for systematic personality studies. Empirical studies of the links between aspects of personality functioning (including psychiatric breakdown) and aspects of directly observable social organization and social relations therefore are at present most feasible in family studies. Certain peer-group studies sometimes offer similar opportunities, but peer groups are much more variable cross-culturally in their occurrence and functions.

4) *Families and biology*: Because of the relatively small size of families, biologic, including genetic, studies can be carried out readily within the family context and in turn linked to other variables within the family context. As an example, in family studies at the National Institute of Mental Health (NIMH), the genetic biology of family members, as observed in twins who are identical genetically but discordant for schizophrenia, is being linked systematically both to the personality functioning of the individual members and to the interpersonal relations and subculture of the family as a whole (Pollin, Stabenau, and Tupin, 1965).

Thus the family is a unit of social structure which regularly occurs and usually can be identified in diverse cultures, in all social classes, in both rural and urban settings, industrialized or not, and, with relatively infrequent and temporary exceptions, at all stages of the life cycle. Because certain family functions, such as parenthood and the socialization of children, the regulation of preferential sexual practices, and the establishment of primary interpersonal ties, are nearly universal, the family provides a context for comparative cross-cultural studies of numerous critical mental health issues. From the standpoint of the etiology and pathogenesis of psychiatric disorders, as well as their treatment and prevention, the family commonly is regarded as a primary setting in which both normal processes and psychological disorders arise—a viewpoint which is relevant whether these disorders are regarded as stemming from biologic inheritance or from learning and identification processes. A deliberate focus on the family can help avoid the pitfall of seeing individuals as isolated from the social context in which they are embedded. Both intrafamilial relations, such as husband-wife, parent-child, and relations of the family with the broad community and culture can provide a context to help make meaningful and understandable the behavior and experience of individual persons.

As I see it, a number of serious conceptual and methodologic pitfalls can be reduced by deliberately focusing upon the family in mental health research. This is not to say by any means, of course, that there are not also many pitfalls in family studies as well as new difficulties which are especially vexatious with this approach. I believe, however, and will try to illustrate that at the present stage of thinking and methodology the family serves as a strategically useful social unit for attention—intermediate in size between isolated individual persons and unwieldly larger social units; bringing together crucial emotions, learning experiences, and maturational processes; and available to currently practicable research methods.

I now wish to turn to a series of examples from my own work and from the chapters in this volume to illustrate some of the above rather abstract propositions.

Internal Family Social Structure

There have been, of course, many studies of intrafamilial relations in which a family member, usually an offspring, is schizophrenic, delinquent, or has a behavioral disorder such as school underachievement. Most of these studies have not, at the same time, also examined or controlled for cultural variables. Conversely, studies which have emphasized cultural factors in personality functioning and psychiatric disorder usually have not examined family role relations in much detail. Weidman, however, in Chapter 16, reviews her Burmese observations in which she explicitly describes the three-way connections between the age-graded status hierarchy within Burmese families, cultural emphasis on the evil and dangers that can be expected from persons who are at a psychological or social distance, and a tendency in Burmese personality functioning and self-development to make extensive use of projective mechanisms.

Phon Sangsingkeo reports in Chapter 17 a triangulated connection also between in this case Thai family role relations, Buddhist cultural values, and the apparent tendency of Thai children to be happy, merry, polite, obedient, submissive, and to suffer from psychosomatic manifestations. As he noted, his impressions are tentative at the present time and systematic research is needed for which he provides interesting leads.

Sechrest (Chapter 19) believes that the Philippine culture apparently is not one strongly conducive to the development of anxiety, perhaps to the degree that the individual is protected from stresses by the support available in both a nuclear and extended family. Although Filipinos are said to kill family members less often than do Americans but to kill strangers more often, it is not clear whether there is any connection between Filipino family relations and the apparent high degree of extrafamilial interpersonal stress and symptomatic difficulties in the expression of hostility.

Turning to a different part of the intrafamilial role structure, Rin in Chapter 7 reports on a three-way relation between sibling rank, type of mental disorder, and culture. This study provides a preliminary basis for comparing Taiwanese patients with those previously studied in Japan and in the United States by Caudill (1963) and Schooler (1961). Caudill's data emphasized an overrepresentation of schizophrenics in particular sibling ranks, depending upon the cultural group. Rin's present study in Taiwan suggests also a significantly high rate of psychophysiological reactions in youngest-born females. Such work provides especially valuable and illuminating evidence concerning connections between distinct conceptual frames of reference and does so on a basis that allows for definite statistical comparisons. Caudill has made a further breakdown between two subcultural Japanese styles of family life—traditional small-business families versus families in which the principal earner is a salaryman in a large organization (Caudill, 1963). Thus it appears that intrafamilial social structure can be linked to individual psychiatric difficulties but that this connection is affected by cultural factors which can be regarded as moderator variables, that is, moderating the extent to which the family-individual link actually is manifest. Such studies promise to help make possible the separation of variables which ordinarily are jumbled together, sometimes so that potentially positive findings are obscured.

The sibling rank studies nearly all point to sex differences as well as birth-order differences in intrafamilial structure. Usually these differences have appeared sensible in the light of what is known about points of special stress in families of a given cultural group—for example, the stress of the eldest son in traditional small-business Japanese families, particularly this son's problems in establishing autonomy in his relation with his mother. Although generalizations of this kind have been supported by case illustrations, more detailed, direct study of the relations within the families on a statistically significant sample eventually will be necessary to confirm the interpretation of these findings. In any event, it is clear that a variety of interesting and important investigations are suggested by specifying and controlling for intrafamilial role structure. This methodology provides leverage for systematic studies of family relations which too often have been left at the level of general clinical and anthropological impressions.

Problems of sex differences in relation to family roles and the cultural values associated with these roles provide an especially easy, but too often neglected, starting point for comparative studies. In American studies of families of schizophrenics being carried out at Yale, NIMH, and elsewhere, consistent evidence is accumulating that it is of the utmost importance to separate out female and male patients, both because their symptomatic manifestations may be quite different and because their family relations may be markedly different, indeed, inverse in some respects. If these data from still relatively small samples are confirmed, it will be quite clear why what would otherwise look like contradictory findings, or at least highly variable findings, start to make sense when subgroups are specified by sex. The data Caudill and Schooler report in Chapter 8 on symptom patterns among Japanese psychiatric patients are replete with evidence about the importance of distinguishing male and female patients. The biologic fact of sex thus combines in many interesting ways with the social and familial variables.

In Asian countries opportunities are especially rich to study sex role differences. In my own work I have been impressed by the importance of these differences in a country, Lebanon, at the other end of the Asian continent from the Pacific. In a relatively traditional and relatively isolated Muslim village, Williams (1968) has made a detailed study of adolescents and their life directions, which to Williams (and also to me in more limited observations in the same village), appeared to be almost inverse in girls compared to boys. Girls in this village have a life direction which has a very definite upward sweep. The birth of the girl, which is often a grievous disappointment to the family, marks the low point of her life curve. She is taught soon and effectively that she is overtly regarded as of less worth than her brothers, and various privileges and freedom of opportunities are withheld from her, but even quite early in childhood she is simultaneously provided with consistent evidence of her usefulness within the particular household sphere when she starts to care for younger children of the extended family. The household that extends to her so little verbalized esteem nevertheless becomes dependent upon her contributions for its effective functioning. She also gradually learns that the esteem that has been initially withheld will accrue to her in her middle and old age after she has competently filled an active work role. In contrast, the boy's life does not have nearly the upward sweep of the girl's. One could almost say that the boy's life curve reaches its apex with his birth as a male. The high esteem in which he is held carries with it few specific expectations, attributes, or behaviors. Although in the past his qualifications for manhood may have been measured in terms of working skill, this expectation no longer appears to be much the case, especially since farming methods have changed. Although his masculinity is still highly extolled, what he can do with it depends very much on his family or lineage, which, among other things, affects the likelihood of his having educational and financial resources. He ordinarily has considerable latitude to define his own role and behavior in contrast to the demeaned, but sharply delineated and circumscribed role and behavior of the female. These greater role opportunities for the males than for the females seem to be associated with greater opportunities for ambivalence, anxiety, hypochondriacal preoccupations, and a tendency to a kind of indolent, directionlessness, and purposelessness. These male-female differences seem apparent both from interviews and from psychological tests currently being reviewed with these and related questions in mind.

External Family Social Structure

So far, I have been discussing the problems of the *internal* structure of nuclear families, that is, families of two generations, consisting of one set of parents and their immediate children. Especially in Asian countries, many rich opportunities exist for studies of the *external* relations of nuclear families, involving both the *boundary* between the nuclear family and the broad social structure and *interchange* between the nuclear family and other social units. Especially important are the links of the nuclear family to larger kinship units (extended families, lineages, clans) and to community social networks (Bott, 1957).

As Surya (Chapter 23) and others point out in this volume, in some cultures, as in the traditional Hindu pattern, the joint family and extended family may be much more prominently in view than is the nuclear family. The transition from the nuclear family of orientation (or origin) to the nuclear family of procreation (or marriage) may be demarcated much less sharply than it is in America and Europe, for example. Because social relations may be spread over a considerable number of kin outside the immediate nuclear family, the intensity of emotional ties within the nuclear family may be reduced. Responsibilities for socialization of children are shared more fully by parents with others, a pattern also found in the Israeli kibbutzim. Although theoretically one would expect the intensity of the emotional ties with particular persons to be reduced and somewhat diffused under these conditions, the actual degree to which this situation is the case has not yet been sufficiently studied empirically. A number of observers in the Israeli kibbutzim have noted that even though the parents spend only a couple of hours a day with their children and do not take part in many of the functions ordinarily conceived as parental in Europe and America, for example, nevertheless, the emotional involvement of children with the parents is actually quite intense and certainly stated to be more emotionally significant than is that with any of the surrogate parents who may spend more chronological time with the children (Nagler, 1963). Thus the problem of evaluating psychological and emotional relations of nuclear family units is not necessarily the same as formal living arrangements and responsibilities might suggest.

Boundary problems of psychiatrically disturbed families are especially complicated. Certain disturbed families appear to have special difficulties in maintaining culturally appropriate interchange with other relatives and with the community. Some of these families appear to shut themselves off from interchange, whereas other nuclear families appear quite chaotic in the way in which relatives, doctors, and agencies are induced to take over and share in the intrafamilial life and problems. Cross-cultural observations are needed especially to interpret adequately such variations. My own working hypothesis is that it is not so much the degree of openness or intrusiveness that creates problems, but rather the extent to which a particular family operates with norms which are idiosyncratic in relation to the rest of the culture or, in some cases, behaves with a seeming normlessness. This hypothesis could be examined cross-culturally regardless of the specific kind of family boundaries and kinship units found in a given society.

Chapter 21 by DeVos and Wagatsuma on the outcastes of Japan provides an excellent illustration of the way in which the primary, nuclear family may have an impact upon the behavior of individual family members because of difficulties of interchange between a disadvantaged minority group and the broad society. DeVos and Wagatsuma described the way in which many persons in severely disadvantaged groups tend to react with apathy and lack of involvement in educational and other achievement aspects of the broad culture, retreating into protective identifications with the submerged group and the primary family. This material suggests that in such circumstances the primary family can serve as the vehicle for negotiating the problems between individual members and the broad culture.

Such matters can be vividly illustrated in the case of members of disadvantaged minority groups, in which apathy and delinquency, as defined by the large culture, appear to be especially frequent outcomes. The same principles presumably apply in families of other groups, however, including families which are self-defined as different from the broad community. In my clinical work with disturbed families, I have been impressed by the regularity with which these families carry a picture of themselves as a kind of one-family minority group—different or special, inferior or superior, compared to the rest of the human race. Often, it is implied that one or more of the offspring manifests apathy or grandiosity which is vividly understandable in the light of the special beliefs of the family about itself in comparison to the surrounding community and culture.

Let me now cite a further example of the ways of families which are marginal in the community of which they are a part, with indications of possible consequences for the personality functioning of individuals within these families. In the Muslim village in Lebanon, to which I referred above, Williams and Williams (1965) made a detailed census of the village and its structure of lineages, extended families, and nuclear households. In this village of 875 persons, there were some 24 lineages. Ten lineages consisted of a number of households, the largest having 27 nuclear family units with 156 members, another with 16 nuclear family units, another with 11. The smallest lineage included 38 persons. On the other hand, 14 smaller kin groups of isolated nuclear families or small groups of related nuclear families ranged in size from 4 to 23 persons. In Williams' study (1968) of the adolescents of this village, a very striking finding emerged when she looked at their position in lineages versus marginal families. It turned out that a total of six adolescents in the village in the age range of 15 to 18 were delinquents. All six were in small, detached, isolated nuclear families, despite the fact that they represented about half of all the adolescents in this age range from these families. In striking contrast, no delinquency was either observed or reported in the adolescents of the same age in the large, well-integrated lineages. Because the observers lived in the village prolongedly and had a well-developed network of informants, it is unlikely that there were examples of significant delinquency which were unreported or unknown. Such data suggest the merit of looking at the overall social structure of family units in relation to individual behavioral disorders—a provocative idea that, so far as I am aware, has not been considered elsewhere.

Family Communication Patterns

During the last decade a number of investigators in the United States and in the United Kingdom have directed their attention to the detailed direct examination of communication patterns of family members, particularly in relation to psychopathological disorders of one or more individual family members. In this work communication patterns can be regarded as an aspect of the family subculture. Indeed, other aspects of the family subculture can be deduced from the empirical study of the interaction and communication of family members, for example, the norms and rules governing family interaction and restraints or encouragement given to interchange of family members with persons outside the family.

These communication studies, in general, have been of two kinds. First, individual family members have been studied in communication with a tester or interviewer, with the data about the family as a whole assembled from the various family members. A series of such studies has been carried out by Singer and myself (Wynne and Singer, 1962a, 1962b, 1965a, 1965b) over the past decade. We have worked with some 350 American families varying considerably in age, social class, education, and psychiatric disturbance. So far, the emphasis has been on use of the Rorschach, the Thematic Apperception Test, and the Object Sorting Test. Using test protocols as samples of communication, we have developed methods for evaluating and scoring the protocols which emphasize formal, structural, or stylistic aspects of communication. The clarity with which thoughts are organized, the extent to which closure on an idea is achieved, the extent to which a focus of attention is shared with the other person, and the structure of the language used are examples of the kinds of features scored (Singer and Wynne, 1966). This scoring contrasts with the usual methods of scoring the Rorschach which emphasize the content of the so-called projections. We have not found content to be a very useful feature of test material in our family studies and particularly feel that content does not lend itself to cross-cultural studies, in which consistencies across cultures associated with variety of psychopathology are sought. It is clear that delusions as well as normal thought content vary widely from one cultural group to another as well as from one social class and educational group to another, whereas structural or stylistic features appear to have more constancy despite social variations (Wynne, 1963).

We have shown statistically significant differentiations between the parents of adolescent and young adult schizophrenics and the parents of matched neurotics and normals (Wynne and Singer, 1962a, 1962b, 1965a, 1965b). The scoring procedures recently have been simplified so that they can be used reliably by relatively untrained raters and still maintain a highly significant differentiation between groups of parents (Singer and Wynne, 1966). We also have shown that criteria for differentiating the parents of childhood schizophrenics from the parents of children with nonpsychotic and medical disorders are not the same as those for differentiating the parents of late adolescent and young adult schizophrenics. This difference makes sense on theoretical grounds and has held up empirically (Singer and Wynne, 1963).

These findings on family communication patterns have been tentatively shown to be useful cross-culturally. M. T. Singer and M. I. Caudill (in an as yet unpublished work) have scored a number of protocols from the families of Japanese schizophrenics, finding that essentially the same scoring procedures are possible with the Japanese protocols and that they appear to differentiate along lines also found in the American samples. We also have a smaller sample from Lebanon in which a similar finding is emerging. In addition, another sample from Japan of the parents of childhood schizophrenic patients indicates that this differentiation is possible among Japanese as well as Americans. The sample size in these cross-cultural studies is not yet sufficient to make a definitive statistical evaluation, but it is quite definite that the methods themselves are usable cross-culturally.

In a second type of communication study, family members are stimulated to communicate and interact directly with one another, with or without a tester or interviewer in the room, with the communication and interaction data recorded on tape recorders or other electronic devices. This group of procedures has now been structured into a variety of interaction experiments in which standard situations of problem solving (Mishler and Waxler, 1966; Reiss, 1967) and projective test card interpretation (Loveland, Wynne, and Singer, 1963) are presented to the family as a conjoint matter for them to discuss. Thus the investigators obtain data having a comparable starting point which can be judged and scored with a variety of techniques that are currently evolving rapidly. So far as I am aware, family interaction experiments have not yet been reported on a cross-cultural basis, although Loveland recently has demonstrated in unpublished studies that her procedure of the Family Rorschach (Loveland, Wynne, and Singer, 1963) can be used successfully in a variety of European countries with families having no psychiatric disturbance or neurotic or schizophrenic family members. Although certain methodologic problems, mainly of scoring, require further work, these experimental interaction procedures are sufficiently well developed that they will soon lend themselves to potentially fruitful means of cross-cultural comparisons.

Family Subculture:
Problems of Social Change

Lindemann (Chapter 30) and others discuss problems of social change from a number of interesting vantage points in this volume. I would like to add here a few comments about aspects of social change which are particularly relevant to family relations. Parsons (1952), among others, has hypothesized that characteristics of social systems and culture are internalized into the personality structure of individuals. I have emphasized specifically the idea that the patterns within the family are internalized in such a way as to shape character structure—not so much as a simple identification with only one parent but rather a broad, complex internalization of the relations of the family members with one another (Wynne *et al.*, 1958).

These general ideas have been applied specifically to the defective ego functioning of schizophrenics whose characteristics are illuminated by family patterns. DeVos and Wagatsuma in Chapter 21 apply a similar line of thinking to the outcaste group in Japan in which they note that the fragile and deviant family patterns in this minority group appear to be internalized into the individual members of the group. They suggest this hypothesis to help account for resistance to social change. Clearly, if a pattern of behavior has become ingrained or built into an individual's character structure, mere external change in the social environment will not readily bring about a change in the individual's behavior. Rather, changes early in life or changes having effects which are cumulative across several generations, may be necessary to bring about a character change.

Considerable suggestive evidence along these lines has been proposed in the United States in the last year or two in connection with the problems of bringing about change in disadvantaged groups, in which it is apparent that external changes which may start to affect individuals at school age or later may be too late to affect some basic features of learning ability and personality functioning. Also, critical aspects of the family structure remain unchanged—for example, the ways in which the father fails to assume leadership and function as a model for identification for his sons because of deficiencies in his development of self-esteem and learning of skills. Such observations are rather sobering with respect to possibilities of producing intended social change and also provide a caution in interpreting the effects of unintended rapid social change in relation to the appearance of personality disorders and other psychiatric problems.

These theoretical ideas about change are relevant to a "three-generation hypothesis" for the emergence of schizophrenic illness, originally proposed by Hill (1955). His idea was that schizophrenic disorders involve profound defects in the very fabric of personality structure which are not likely to be influenced in a schizophrenic direction in adults because of external changes, however drastic, unless the person already is predisposed to schizophrenic difficulties. It is possible that such vulnerability (sometimes called "schizotypy") can emerge on biological and genetic grounds or alternatively arise from the build-up of difficulties on an experiential or learned basis across generations. The "three-generation hypothesis" suggested that in the first generation, the "fit" between the pair was such as to lead to rather serious character disorders or neurotic problems in the next generation, which were maximized in the third generation.

This "three-generation hypothesis" may be of a special interest in relation to the data Lin *et al.* (Chapter 5) report in their follow-up epidemiologic study in Taiwan in which they found that after 15 years there was relatively little shift, associated with migration and related rapid social change, in the prevalence of schizophrenic disorders, but a marked increase in the prevalence of nonpsychotic disorders, notably mental deficiency, psychoneurosis, and psychopathic personality. All the recent work with families of schizophrenics unequivocally leads to the hypothesis that the kind of social change associated with migration would not be likely to affect schizophrenic illness in the migrating generation, either on a genetic or an experiential basis, but that symptoms such as anxiety and regression, and probably also psychophysiologic disorders and delinquency, would be likely to be evoked under such conditions of social change.

It is worthwhile to keep in mind Vogel's interesting report (Chapter 24) on family life in urban Communist China with respect to possible evidence of long-term changes in the patterning of psychiatric disorders. Unfortunately, the problems of interpretable statistical data are especially great in Communist China at present, but there may be opportunities in other countries undergoing rapid social change for obtaining base lines of data, both about family patterns and about the individuals within these families, in order to see what both the short-term and the long-term multigenerational effects of social change may be.

The Muslim village which I studied in Lebanon has begun to be the focus of considerable change in the last few years with the introduction of water supply, roads, and educational facilities. The same village had been studied 15 years previously by Williams and Williams before any of these changes began. It proved especially interesting to evaluate processes of change in relation to the family structure of the village. Data were obtained on whether individuals who showed evidences of special change, such as having achieved more education than usual, being more geographically mobile, introducing improved farming methods, buying land rather than serving as tenant farmers, were members of the large lineages or of the isolated nuclear families. In this particular village, it appeared very definite that the large extended families and lineages actually facilitated social change and made change possible by providing economic and interpersonal resources to the individuals who then served as representatives of the family. The extended family, even when it became widely scattered in residence remained functionally intact and integrated. Indeed, as Williams and Williams (1965) wrote:

> this high level of integration of the extended family seemed
> to be a prime factor in making change possible. In turn,
> change has enhanced extended family cohesion, reinforced
> and preserved the lineage structure, at times at the expense of
> nuclear units. Ties which have always had social, political,
> and ethical function have been given a more immediate,
> pragmatic base and a new economic one.

These observations obviously are very much in contrast to the usual notion that breakdown of extended family ties occurs with social change and economic development, which heighten emphasis on nuclear family units which usually are thought to facilitate mobility and change. My point is to indicate that by looking at the family in some detail variations in processes of cultural change may be more fully understandable. In this Lebanese village it may be that the present situation is transitional, with the lineage and extended family system serving functions which will no longer be needed after the economic and related changes have been consolidated for a generation or two.

Another factor appears to be the question of whether changes have been brought about through the initiative of the persons themselves or have been imposed by external forces. For example, when slum dwellers are moved out without consultation about their resettlement, the effect may be much more psychologically and socially disorganizing than change that they initiate and bring about themselves. In another part of the Middle East, the effects of enforced change brought about by war conditions were studied in a Palestinian village. There the processes of family distintegration and disruption seemed to have been accelerated especially in the large family units, so that the reverse of the situation in the Lebanese village occurred.

In conclusion, I wish to underline my view that a research focus upon the family as a social and cultural unit can be a useful part of a considerable variety of studies and may help clarify the connecting links between diverse variables. At the same time the advantages of family studies cannot be maximized unless investigators are prepared to conceptualize and study data from more than one vantage point, as illustrated by studies contained in this volume.

REFERENCES

Bertalanffy, L. von. 1950. The theory of open systems in physics and biology. Science 3:23–29.

Bott, E. 1957. Family and social network. London, Tavistock Publications.

Caudill, W. 1958. Effects of social and cultural systems in reactions to stress. Social Science Research Council Pamphlet No. 14.

————. 1963. Sibling rank and style of life among Japanese psychiatric patients. *In* Proceedings of the Joint Meeting of the Japanese Society of Psychiatry and Neurology and the American Psychiatric Association, Tokyo. H. Akimoto, ed. Supplement No. 7 of Folia Psychiatria et Neurologia Japonica. Tokyo, Japanese Society of Psychiatry and Neurology.

Hill, L. B. 1955. Psychotherapeutic intervention in schizophrenia. Chicago, University of Chicago Press.

Kroeber, A. L., and T. Parsons. 1958. The concepts of culture and of social system. American Sociological Review 23:582–83.

Loveland, N., L. C. Wynne, and M. T. Singer. 1963. The family Rorschach: a new method for studying family interaction. Family Process 2:187–215.

Mishler, E. G., and N. E. Waxler. 1966. Family interaction and schizophrenia: an approach to the experimental study of family interaction and schizophrenia. Archives of General Psychiatry 15:64–74.

Nagler, S. 1963. Clinical observations on kibbutz children. Israel Annals of Psychiatry and Related Disciplines 1:201–16.

Parsons, T. 1952. The superego and the theory of social systems. Psychiatry 15:15–25.

Parsons, T., and R. F. Bales. 1955. Family, socialization and interaction process. Glencoe, Free Press.

Pollin, W., J. Stabenau, and J. Tupin. 1965. Family studies with identical twins discordant for schizophrenia. Psychiatry 28:60–78.

Reiss, D. 1967. Individual thinking and family interaction. Archives of General Psychiatry 16:80–93.

Schooler, C. 1961. Birth order and schizophrenia. Archives of General Psychiatry 4:91–97.

Singer, M. T., and L. C. Wynne. 1963. Differentiating characteristics of parents of childhood schizophrenics, childhood neurotics, and young adult schizophrenics. American Journal of Psychiatry 120:234–43.

————. 1966. Principles for scoring communication defects and deviances in parents of schizophrenics: Rorschach and TAT scoring manuals. Psychiatry 29:260–88.

Williams, H. H., and J. R. Williams. 1965. The extended family as a vehicle of culture change. Human Organization 24:59–64.

Williams, J. R. 1968. The youth of Haouch el Harimi: a Lebanese village. Cambridge, Massachusetts, Harvard Middle Eastern Monograph Series No. 20.

Wynne, L. C. 1963. The transcultural study of schizophrenics and their families. *In* Proceedings of the Joint Meeting of the Japanese Society of Psychiatry and Neurology and the American Psychiatric Association, Tokyo. H. Akimoto, ed. Supplement No. 7 of Folia Psychiatria et Neurologia Japonica. Tokyo, Japanese Society of Psychiatry and Neurology.

Wynne, L., I. Ryckoff, J. Day, and S. Hirsch. 1958. Pseudo-mutuality in the family relations of schizophrenics. Psychiatry 21:205–20.

Wynne, L. C., and M. T. Singer. 1962a. Thought disorder and family relations of schizophrenics. I. A research strategy. Archives of General Psychiatry 9:191–98.

_____. 1962b. Thought disorder and family relations of schizophrenics. II. A classification of forms of thinking. Archives of General Psychiatry 9: 199–206.

_____. 1965a. Thought disorder and family relations of schizophrenics. III. Methodology using projective techniques. Archives of General Psychiatry 12:187–200.

_____. 1965b. Thought disorder and family relations of schizophrenics. IV. Results and implications. Archives of General Psychiatry 12:201–12.

30. Mental Health Aspects of Rapid Social Change

ERICH LINDEMANN, M.D.

Department of Psychiatry
Stanford University Medical Center
Palo Alto, California

THE DISCUSSION of mental health issues both in practice and research would be incomplete without a consideration of the social matrix in which disordered behavior occurs. In counting the number of psychiatric conditions in any given population, one is inclined to think of the social structure as relatively static with little change over time. Over the last two decades, however, we have learned to think of social systems, whether at the community, family, or group level, as dynamic organizations subject to continual change, faster in some segments of the structure and slower in others. Casualties are expected only when rapid changes occur in individual opportunities and role expectations and in collective arrangements for the maintenance of the social order. The psychiatric profession is interested in certain types of casualties, among them the psychoses, which are discussed at length in this volume.

The scope of mental health considerations must be broadened to include casualties involving not only the psychoses, psychoneuroses, and psychosomatic disorders but also persons who fail to function effectively as useful members of society. It is this range of casualty which must be considered in planning for urban change, patterns of industrialization, manpower procurement, and providing facilities for newcomers at the time of rapid population shifts.

The sociology of knowledge has taught us to distinguish different types of professional organization. Among psychiatrists there are at least two forms of interest and professional behavior. One group, working in mental hospitals where persons with disturbed behavior have been segregated for the protection of others and to some degree of themselves, has been concerned with methods of case finding, prediction of case loads in order to make adequate provision of hospital facilities, and determination of rates of return of persons able to re-enter the community. These psychiatrists are interested particularly in severe cases requiring maximum effort for their care and treatment. The interests characterizing the psychiatrists of the second group started from the study of the psychogenic forms of somatic disorders. Their initial interest was in hypnosis and psychotherapy, but extended to a dynamic interpretation of the social and motivational factors leading to disordered behavior. Recently, their concern with the social processes influencing motivation and disturbed emotional equilibrium has developed into a study of events of social change. These interests also have led to the study of the effect of early psychological experience on personality growth and development in primates in addition to humans in the hope of finding clues to preventive measures in infant care, family organization, and social planning.

The conference from which this volume evolved constituted in itself an event which could accelerate social change by altering the mental health arrangements in Eastern or Western countries as a consequence of sharing the findings and methods in this wide field. While in the Western industrialized countries social change has been equated automatically with improvement and success, many Eastern countries are concerned with controls against too rapid and ill-advised arrangements for change which would destroy significant values of the past and undermine existing communal safeguards for emotional well-being and assistance in times of life crises. The recurrent theme of dependency in interpersonal relations and the value of a supportive network in kinship and community in Eastern approaches in contrast to the Western idea of the independent, autonomous individual who can adapt to a great variety of circumstances serves as a warning not to oversimplify notions about social change, as though psychiatry and mental health in the East were expected to take over without drastic revision the conceptual orientation and the methods of behavioral scientists of the West. Among Easterners, there seems to be a wish to underline the existence of value patterns with respect to social relations and individual support, a point which should be carefully considered by Westerners.

I propose to review briefly some of the essentials of the organization of caretaking and maintenance functions in social systems which provide for the survival of the community and the majority of its members, even if at the cost of differential access to opportunities and differential exposure to social stress. Then I will consider certain forms of drastic

Figure 1: Diagram Showing the Different Types of Community
Concern Which Appear as Institutions and as Professional
Prerogatives*

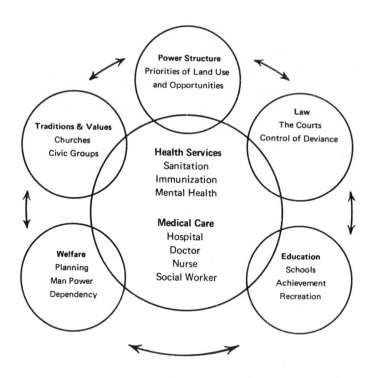

*The overlapping areas represent an expanding field of joint concern with opportunities
for co-operation but also for controversy.

social change which, no matter where they occur, challenge the adaptive potential of group members. Such change may lead to casualties but also to forms of social learning, as can be well demonstrated in the study of bereavement reactions. It can be illustrated by two forms of planned social change as seen in arrangements for the reception of newcomers in a middle-class suburb in contrast to the arrangements for the displacement of a slum population at the time of urban renewal. In both instances it appears that the fate of the individuals and the likelihood of their developing unfortunate behavior reactions, including mental disease, depends on the way in which the various professions in the community collaborate and that health services often become involved only after many other things have gone wrong and the individual's breakdown is in a late stage.

It may be of interest to consider for a moment how the medical profession relates to other caretaking professions in a society. Medical and health services and professional activities can be thought of as constituting certain prerogatives of access to a segment of the population which becomes eligible for such services by exhibiting a certain kind of behavior which Parsons (1958) has described in some detail as the "sick role." Much effort has been spent on circumscribing behavior which fits into disease categories, thereby establishing without question the right as well as the obligation of the health services to segregate this population as "their cases." The boundary between these services and other community agencies and professions, however, is fluid, and this boundary determines much of the uncertainty about the nature and care of disturbing, undesirable, and suffering individuals, particularly at times of rapid social change (Fig. 1).

The medical profession likes to be the gatekeeper to all those who can be defined as sick. They vie in this prerogative with at least four other professional or quasi-professional groups in the community, each of which has an important separate function. In Western countries at the present time there is much discussion about whether alcoholism and drug addiction constitute diseases to be treated by medical methods or are forms of criminal behavior to be handled by punishment and deterrent methods. Many forms of intense preoccupation with phantasy life in Eastern countries can be considered withdrawal into a religious world of traditional imagery but also may constitute an illness incapacitating the person for effective collaboration in the social order. Priests and shamans both have long traditions about permissible and objectionable forms of withdrawal from social participation, and their methods of treatment or restoration to acceptable conduct vie with approaches of scientific medicine. In different societies an equilibrium develops between different professional groups which is liable to displacement in the process of social change. The chapters on shamanism in this volume are fine examples of this fact.

There are, furthermore, the ubiquitous societal arrangements for child rearing and education of new members of society and for assistance to members who are unsuccessful in self-support or in helping their families. These areas of education and welfare again have their own definitions of permissible and nonpermissible deviance. The underachiever in school may be considered lazy and in need of punishment or sick and in need of medical care. The chronically unemployed person may be considered a legitimate beggar, a punishable pauper, or a person to be counseled and in whose favor opportunities should be rearranged. Again, the point at which a pattern of conduct becomes a legitimate concern of the medical profession is uncertain and shifts from society to society. Furthermore, as described in this volume, for instance, in chapters on Burma and Pakistan, a style of dealing with emotions, particularly aggression, is developed and enforced through tradition and child-rearing methods.

One of the most significant developments in mental health research both in the West and in the East seems to be the gradual acceptance of social science concepts and procedures for the description and interpretation of potentially comparable patterns of child rearing, educational arrangements for individual welfare, control of deviance, and distribution of opportunities for growth and satisfaction in various societies. It now is possible to forget about rivalries and mutual derogation between different professional groups and to recognize the common concerns and the many occasions for co-operation in the recognition and care of emotional disturbances.

Events of drastic social change have been of particular interest precisely because the relative contributions to effective problem solving by various professional groups could be appraised and bridges for understanding could be found. Social changes caused by bereavement, i.e., the loss of an emotionally significant member of an intimate social network, have been the object of a number of studies (Lindemann, 1944; Engel, 1961; Schmale, 1958). It has been possible to circumscribe the processes of mourning and grief and to delineate the adaptive and maladaptive consequences both for the individuals and for social groups. Diagnosis under such circumstances refers not so much to a disease picture as to categories of disturbed behavior in relating to the time and sequence of psychological events expected after such crises. A variety of disease pictures; psychosomatic, psychoneurotic, and criminal behavior; and identifiable psychoses then can be referred to as adaptive patterns in the mastery of a particular crisis of rapid social change. It was Adolf Meyer who pointed out that it is indispensable in assessment and diagnosis of any sort of disordered behavior to study the adaptive crisis at hand, the equipment and resources of the individual and his group to deal with it, and the role of the psychiatrist as a participating caretaker, who has to mesh his efforts with those of other professional and nonprofessional persons with other responsibilities for the disturbed person's life. A comprehensive diagnosis obviously demands much more investment of time and effort than is possible in the frame of population surveys.

John Gordon used to point out that contemporary psychiatry counts behavior patterns in much the way that decades ago forms of hives might have been counted as symptoms of infectious disease. A bold statement could be made that patterns of disordered behavior involve not individuals, but clusters of individuals related to one another in meaningful ways; that much of the disturbance results from feelings, expectations, and responses of others to the individual under consideration; and that for mental health work the development of sociopathology is a necessary correlate to that of individual pathology. Studies of particular social constellations possibly preceding the development of psychosomatic disease, such as ulcerative colitis, following bereavement led to the recognition of pathogenic social settings. In cases of ulcerative colitis excessive dependence on a special type of mother may be found, or in schizophrenia defective patterns of communication may exist in the family structure.

The intervention of the psychiatrist becomes then an effort at dealing with forms of social pathology which are precursors to more severe forms of disturbed behavior. Categorizing the pathology of social systems, including families, and the periods of disorganization which can be expected at times of rapid social change is just beginning.

It is useful to look carefully at the provisions made by communities to deal with the necessary events of social change. I will not review here the large number of studies which have been made concerning the rate of mental disorder after migration and change of habitat. Excellent overviews have been provided recently by Murphy (1961) and Fried (1964). Murphy showed dramatically the great diversity of findings which at present are not susceptible to systematic interpretation because of the diversity of methods of counting of casualties and the lack of adequate description of the social processes involved.

Studies on bereavement and separation reactions, as well as the analysis of acculturation problems under a variety of conditions, have shed some light on the complexities of the coping mechanisms involved in role transition and crisis behavior. The work of Engel (1960), Schmale (1958), and Coelho, Hamburg, and Murphy (1963), dealing primarily with individuals in crisis and small groups, encouraged further work concerned with the responses of large population groups. My own concern has been with the details of community arrangements to assist persons in transition, rather than with counting the cases of illness among migrant and nonmigrant members of the population. The first study dealt with community arrangements to facilitate the entry of newcomers to a middle-class suburb and their problems in integrating with the existing population and finding opportunities for productive participation.

A survey of newly arrived families during the years 1959 and 1960 (Thoma and Lindemann, 1961) showed that real estate agents functioned as agents to select those who were deemed acceptable to the town and could be expected to be integrated readily. Certain middle-class persons, preferably of white Anglo-Saxon background, had appropriate education and jobs and acceptable manners. Persons of different ethnic origin were discouraged from seeking homes or were shown undesirable dwellings. After this selection process, there followed a series of efforts on the part of commercial interests, schools, and churches to facilitate acquaintance and integration. Social contacts were provided by a large variety of hierarchical clubs, providing membership at first at lower levels, with gradual rises in prestige and in influential participation in community affairs. Emotional distress was found more often in children than in adults, since little thought had been given to the crisis of transition which they faced at their respective age levels.

Quite different were the adaptive problems studied in a sample of 400 families of a 10,000-person slum population who were involved in a forced relocation as a result of a slum clearance project (Fried and Lindemann, 1961). Instead of the small, middle-class family unit, which was assisted by impersonal, professional, and commercial agencies in the suburb, we found a population with a closely knit, extended kinship system. Emotional and material support was largely guaranteed by the complex bonds of large family and quasi-family groups. The fragmentation of these social networks caused by the relocation of individual households brought about a great many grief-like reactions and a variety of pathological responses, which are still under detailed study. Arrangements to facilitate the transition were quite inadequate, consisting mostly of some social work and financial help. Until very shortly before the destruction of the existing houses began, the attitude of the population, as well as of the neighborhood agencies, was one of disbelief. The life-span of these persons had been restricted to their particular neighborhood. One of the investigators described them aptly as a group of "urban villagers" who had maintained within the metropolitan area a peasant style of neighborliness. Transplantation into other metropolitan situations demanded a profound alteration of their way of thinking and feeling and a reorganization of their daily role behaviors and routines. Paranoid and depressive reactions, which were common, are illustrated by the following sequence: An Italian couple in their mid-thirties were transplanted to a suburban neighborhood. The wife, who had been the food-gatherer at corner grocery stores, an occasion for much interchange with other women and for acquiring informal knowledge about the neighborhood, in the new suburban setting had to rely on her husband to bring home the groceries from the supermarket because she did not drive. She also found it impossible to make social contacts with socially superior neighbors. She had very little to do, became depressed, and then severely suspicious of her husband, without any insight into the psychological determinants of her state of distress.

The research team found that under the stress of relocation this type of population is quite unable to make use of the separate services of different agencies and professions which might be available to them. In consequence of these findings, it is planned in future crises of transition arising as a result of forced relocation to provide multiservice centers organized around suitably trained social workers, in which medical, legal, educational, and job problems can be handled within one building, with a regular program for sharing information and collating the respective contributions of the different professional agents.

The team also was impressed with the great difficulty of the psychiatric approach to case finding in the traditional sense. The population in the slum area harbored a number of psychotic persons who were tolerated and accepted in the neighborhood and not defined as being medical problems. In the process of transplantation, it was impossible to accommodate them and psychiatric help appeared appropriate.

In dealing with crises of transition, the psychiatrist, co-operating with other professions, will be called upon much less to diagnose mental disorders than to give advice about the best preparation and supportive measures for the most vulnerable segment of the population in crisis. Together with social scientists, he will try to assess the mental health consequences of social processes, such as changes in roles and hierarchy, opportunities for communication, and shifts in prevailing values. The rapid processes of urbanization and industrialization throughout the developing countries in Asia require from the mental health worker a fresh appraisal, not only of individual defenses against breakdown, but also of collective attitudes and traditional procedures, such as ceremonials to be safeguarded.

Several chapters in this volume show the serious preoccupation of investigators with cultural phenomena which protect the population to some degree against emotional breakdown, but represent at the same time a form of social pathology which victimizes certain members of the community, as is well exemplified by the studies of witchcraft. There should be careful evaluation of the levels of tolerance for various ways in which certain individuals are made scapegoats in order to satisfy collective paranoid tendencies.

There is also the problem of tolerance for deviant or abnormal behavior. The apparent increase in the number of persons with mental abnormalities of old age, who constitute a very large percentage of those admitted to mental hospitals in the West, appears, according to Gruenberg, to be related to the decreased tolerance of the industrialized society for the presence of the elderly, even when they are only mildly disturbed.

It is clear from all I have been saying that I advocate a change in role and value orientation for the psychiatrist who engages in mental health work. He still will have to be a fully established clinical diagnostician. but he also will have to have knowledge of the possible precursors of disease (as exemplified by grief reactions) and, together with social scientists, will have to address himself to social systems, whether family, kinship circle, small group, work team, institutional, or whole community. Problems of transition and crises of adaptation are challenges for the right kind of mental health services, and they are also opportunities for investigation. The study presented in by Bulatao Chapter 18 of the multiple facets of gradual acculturation and Westernization in the Philippines illustrates the value of this kind of inquiry.

My experience in a large metropolitan hospital in Boston has shown that such a role change by the psychiatrist is important even for consultation with the other medical departments. Here, also, the social processes involved in the arrival and departure of the patient, the social structure of individual wards, and the opportunities for social reintegration of the patient upon return to the community have become significant factors in appraising the nature and probable outcome of a given medical condition.

While each contributor to this volume has presented with pride the accomplishments in his particular sphere of operations, he also has had to come to terms with very great differences in research technology and organization skills. The more advanced the level of technology, the better the opportunities appear for comparative studies. Epidemiological surveys with respect to clear-cut clinical entities are obviously the most promising. The less quantitative, rather exploratory studies, however, which combine social science and psychodynamic and clinical observations, do much to develop a high level of motivation and involvement, creating a community of issues which must precede the evolution of methods of collaboration.

Finally, carrying out the plans for further work in mental health research at the East-West Center will provide an auspicious opportunity for the development of methods to approach the solutions of many of the problems I have only been able to touch upon in this chapter. Having effectively joined forces at the Conference on Mental Health Research in Asia and the Pacific, from which this volume derived, we now must continue to move forward together.

REFERENCES

Coelho, G. V., D. Hamburg, and E. B. Murphy. 1963. Coping strategies in a new learning environment: a study of American college freshmen. Archives of General Psychiatry 9:433–43.

Engel, G. L. 1960. A unified concept of health and disease. Perspectives in Biology and Medicine 3:459–85.

————. 1961. Is grief a disease? Psychosomatic Medicine 23:18–22.

Fried, M. 1964. Effects of social change on mental health. American Journal of Orthopsychiatry 34:3–28.

Fried, M., and E. Lindemann. 1961. Sociocultural factors in mental health and illness. American Journal of Orthopsychiatry 31:87–101.

Lindemann, E. 1944. Symptomatology and management of acute grief. American Journal of Psychiatry 101:141–48.

Murphy, H. B. M. 1961. Social change and mental health. Milbank Memorial Fund Quarterly 39(3):385–445.

Parsons, T. 1958. Some trends of change in American society: their bearing on medical education. Journal of the American Medical Association 167: 31–36.

Schmale, A. H. 1958. Relationship of separation and depression to disease. 1. A report on a hospitalized medical population. Psychosomatic Medicine 20:259–77.

Thoma, L., and E. Lindemann. 1961. Newcomers' problems in a suburban community. Journal of American Institute of Planners Vol. 27, No. 3.